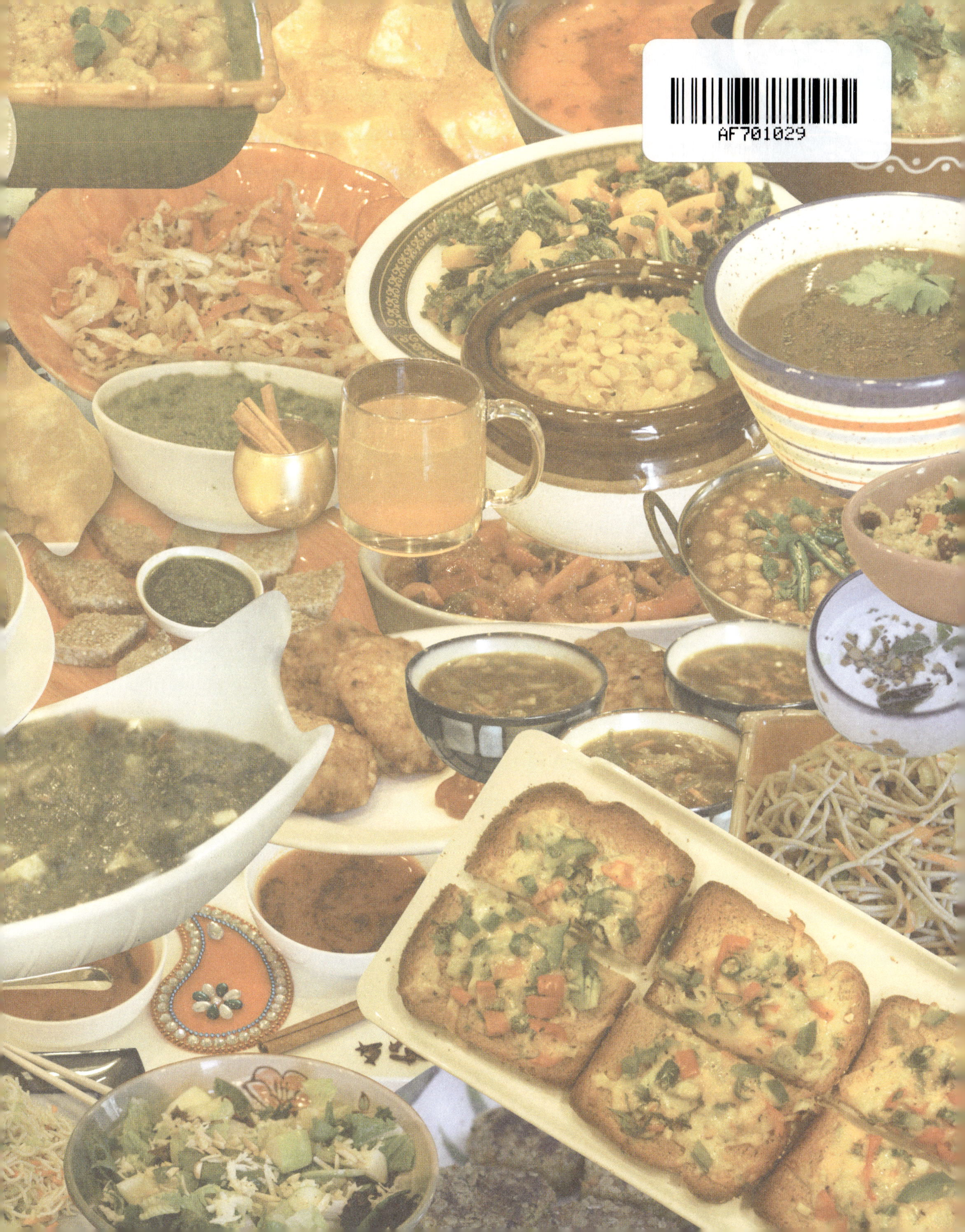

The JKYog COOKBOOK

Delicious Vegetarian Recipes

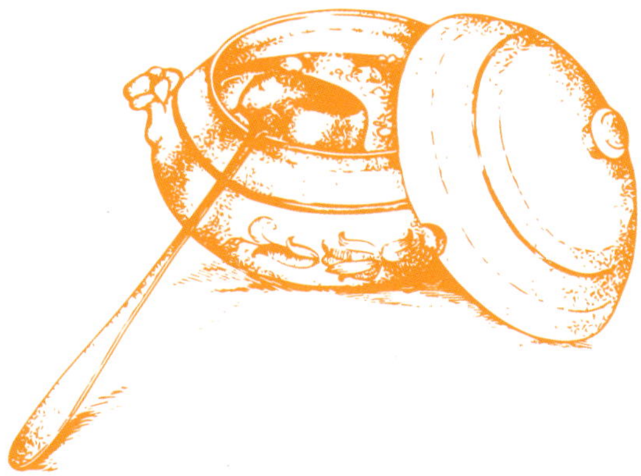

Published by:
Jagadguru Kripaluji Yog
7405 Stoney Point Dr
Plano, TX 75025

www.jkyog.org
www.natural-cure.org

ISBN: 978-0-9968693-5-5

Printed in the USA
Signature Book Printing, www.sbpbooks.com

Disclaimer:
The ideas and suggestions in this book may be practiced at the reader's own discretion. The author and publishers cannot take responsibility for any consequences from their practice. All liability arising from the implementation of the information and suggestions in this book is expressly disclaimed.

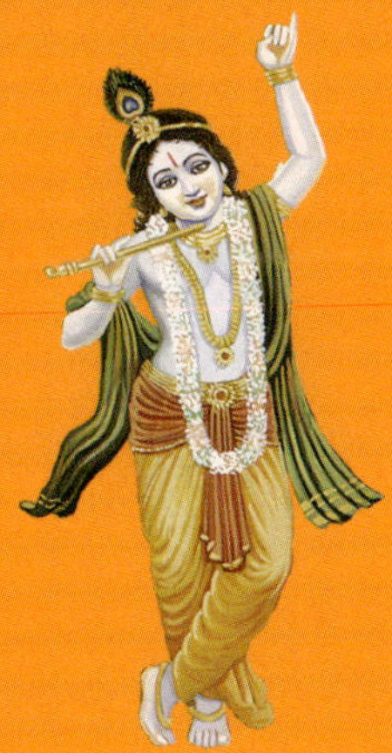

DEDICATION

This book is dedicated to Jagadguru Shree Kripaluji Maharaj, the embodiment of divine love and grace, who compassionately revealed sublime knowledge for the welfare of humankind. He taught the importance of enriching our life by blending both spiritual and material sciences. He emphasized that we must not separate devotion from our daily life. He taught us to pour the love of our heart into every act we perform; to see even the kitchen as a sacred space where cooking is an act of worship.

From him, we learnt the value of culinary science in devotion to Lord Krishna. He revealed the beautiful sentiments with which the gopis prepare gastronomic delights for their Beloved Radha Krishna in Divine Vrindavan. He trained us to see cooking as a fun activity to indulge in, as an art to master, and as a way of expressing our devotion to the Lord of the Universe.

I sincerely hope that with his blessings, readers will be benefitted with happiness, health, fulfillment, and bliss by the recipes and knowledge presented in this book.

Swami Mukundananda

PREFACE

The food choices we make in life deeply influence every aspect of our personality. The nutriment we eat and drink creates the cells that compose our body. Even more significantly, it impacts the thoughts our mind generates. "By eating pure food, the mind becomes pure," states the Chhāndogya Upaniṣhad (7.26.2). Thus, the wise partake of foods that are conducive to good health and have a peaceable impact upon the mind.

Such foods are juicy, naturally tasteful, mild, and beneficial. They bestow good health, virtue, happiness, and satisfaction. In the book, "Science of a Healthy Diet," we have discussed this in detail. However, the secret to good food does not lie only in the ingredients that compose it, but also in the bhav (love) with which we cook it. The Bhagavad Gita states:

patraṁ puṣhpaṁ phalaṁ toyaṁ yo me bhaktyā prayachchhati
tadahaṁ bhaktyupahṛitam aśhnāmi prayatātmanaḥ,

"If one offers to me with devotion a leaf, a flower, a fruit, or even water, I delightfully partake of that article offered with love by my devotee in pure consciousness." This is the wonderfully merciful nature of God. He is not concerned with the material value of our offering, as he is with the love with which we make it.

When Lord Krishna went to Hastinapur, Duryodhana invited Him to a lavish feast of fifty-six items. But, the Lord preferred, instead, to have his meal in the humble abode of Vidur. Vidurani was so overwhelmed with love that she fed Shree Krishna with her own hands. But in her devotional trance, she did not realize that she was dropping the banana fruit and putting the peels in His mouth. Shree Krishna not only ate the peels with relish, but he also exclaimed that he had never eaten anything so delicious.

When food is prepared with loving devotion, and offered to God and Guru, it is elevated to a whole different level. After the offering, devotees partake it as prasad (grace), and every morsel that is eaten is akin to divine nectar. Food cooked with this bhav (divine sentiment) as a key ingredient does not just provide nourishment to the body, but transmits a bliss to those who partake it with devotional hearts.

In this way, the culinary science is holistically connected to the wellbeing of our body, mind, and soul. It also provides an excellent medium for expressing our devotion to the Lord and engaging in His loving service. In recent years, as the JKYog system of yoga, consisting of the five sciences—yogasan, pranayam, meditation, subtle body relaxation, and the science of healthy diet—has grown in popularity, devotees have become interested in learning the art of devotional and healthy cooking.

Consequently, there were growing requests to JKYog for publishing a cookbook. We found the perfect team for it, led by Parag and Sonali Birla, and Hina Patel. By virtue of their sanskars, they have a natural love for the culinary science, and a passion for pleasing devotees with the most mouth-watering recipes and innovations. They were ably assisted by JKYog devotees around the country who repeatedly cooked, tasted, and honed these recipes to delectable perfection.

The JKYog Cookbook, true to its name, was put together by a large and dedicated team of devotees. I would like to thank all of them for their contributions.

The recipes were devotedly tried and tested multiple times until they were truly mouthwatering. They also went through a rigorous selection and elimination process. The devotees who contributed recipes and tested them were: Hina Patel, Sonali Birla, Sangeeta Sadachar, Archana Gupta, Mrs. T. Ragi Rao, Parag Birla, Rashmi Halker, Renu Bagri, Shashi Birla, Somi Nangalia, Suma Addagadde, Anoopama Dhar, Babita Savitsky, Bharathi Pothan, Deval Bhatt, Harita Patel, Jayesh Patel, Neela T. Moorjani, Neeta and Umesh Chokshi, Rashmi Mohunta, Seema Kabra, Shashi Bannuru, Shobha Sarayia, Sunita Upadhyay and T.V. Avinash Chandra.

I wish to thank Neela T. Moorjani for photographing and editing this Cookbook. I am grateful to Sangeeta Sadachar for her suggestions in the recipe selection process. I also wish to acknowledge the help of Arati Nemani, Vijoya Tanty and Manisha Shreshta in cooking and testing recipes; Harish Sukhwani for additional support with photography and Stacey Sprenz for some of her recipe photographs included in this book. I would like to thank Anand Rao for facilitating the publication and printing processes; Rajiv Kumar for the design, layout and formatting of the book; and, Shreya Bhat for providing the team guidance and support at various stages of the project.

Finally, the team is ready to share these recipes with you and the world. We hope they will bring joy, sublime bliss, and fulfillment to your dear ones and you, and enable you to serve your Lord in many more tasteful ways!

Swami Mukundananda

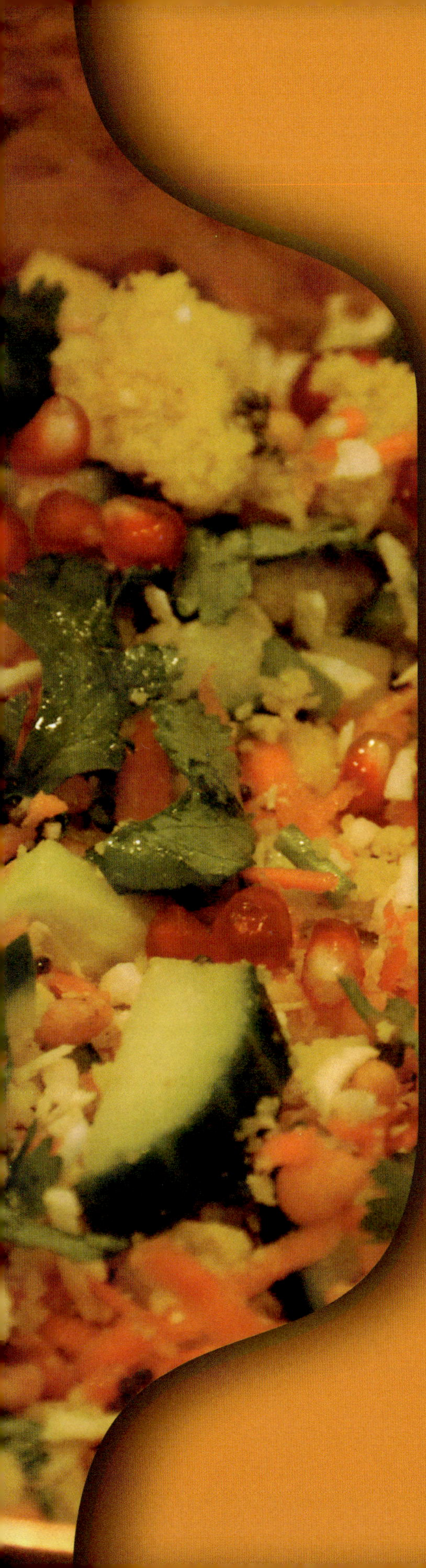

CONTENTS

DRINKS

1. Panchamrit
2. Mango Lassi
3. Aam ka Panna
4. Apple Cider
5. Herbal Tea

SOUPS AND SALADS

1. Clear Vegetable Soup
2. Tomato Soup
3. Rasam Thai Soup
4. Minestrone Soup
5. Black Bean Soup
6. Mixed Bean Soup
7. Hot and Sour Soup
8. Dhokla Salad
9. Couscous Salad
10. Quinoa Salad
11. Spicy Taco Salad
12. Toasted Almond Apple Salad

SNACKS – APPETIZERS

1. Lentil Dhokla
2. Buckwheat Dhokla
3. Masala Rava Idli
4. Masala Oats Idli
5. Oats Healthy Tikki
6. Vegetable Bean Cutlet
7. Kale Pakoras
8. Chana Dal Vada
9. Sabudana Vada
10. Samosa
11. Paneer Chilli
12. Albeli Chaat

SNACKS – MINI MEALS

1. Avocado Sandwich
2. Cream Cheese Sandwich
3. Chili Cheese Toast
4. Sooji Toast
5. Buckwheat Chilla
6. Uttapam
7. Mixed Lentil Masala Dosa
8. Healthy Cereal Chivda
9. Pizza
10. Pasta
11. Hakka Noodles

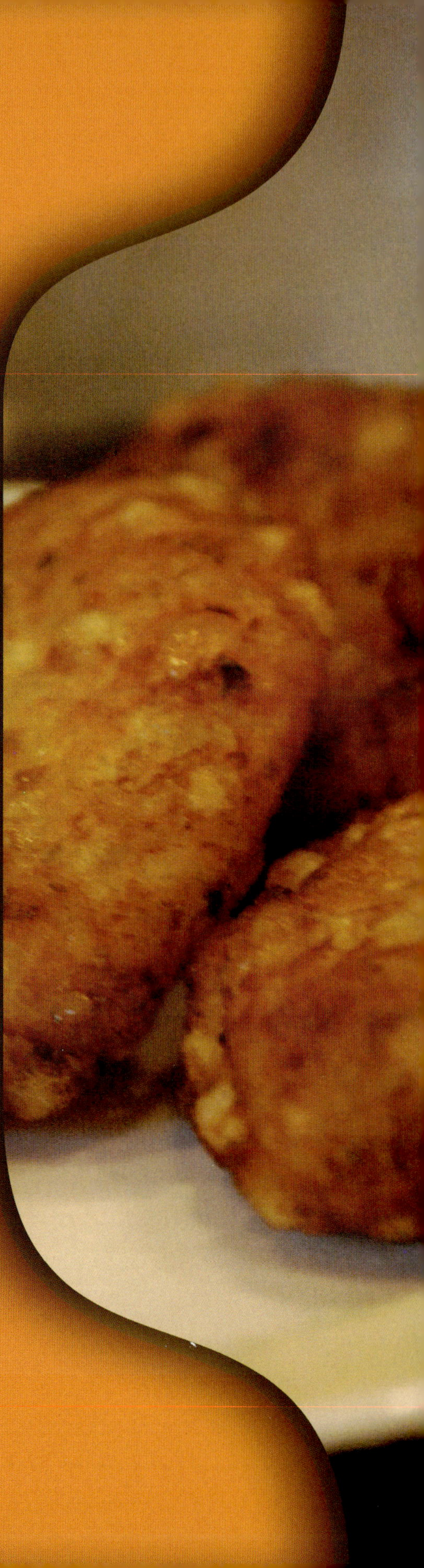

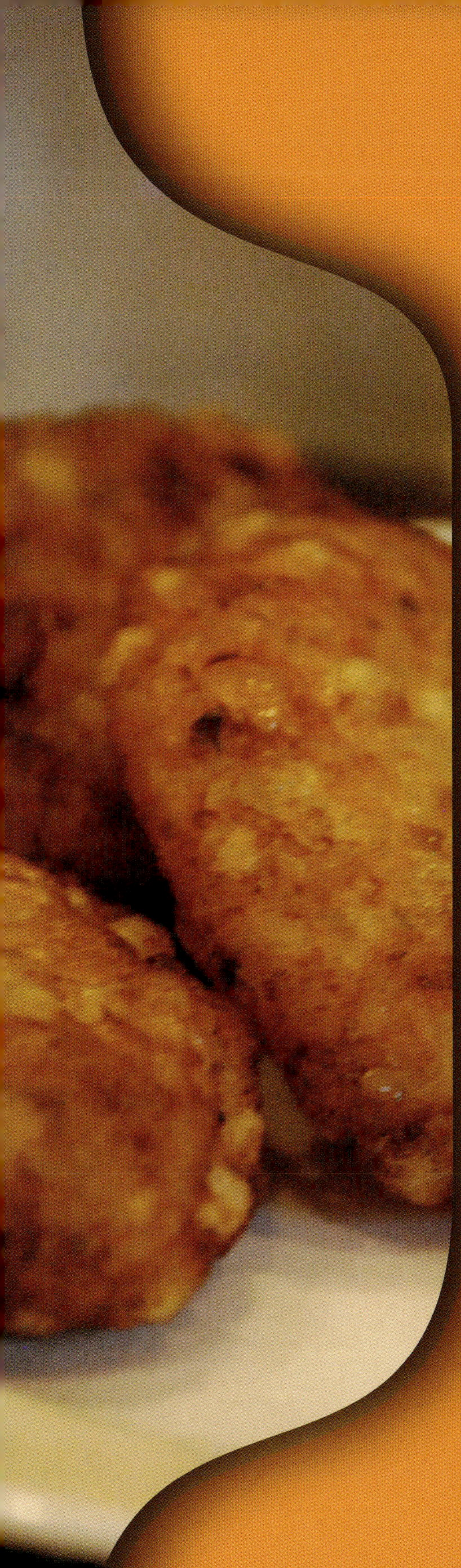

CHUTNEYS, PICKLES AND CONDIMENTS

1. Apple Cilantro Mint Chutney
2. Tamarind Date Chutney
3. Apple Butter Chutney
4. Almond Chutney
5. Coconut Chutney
6. Tomato Chutney
7. Hummus
8. Mango Salsa
9. Instant Lemon Pickle
10. Carrot and Green Chilli Pickle
11. Mango Pickle
12. Vegetable Raita

SABZIS, DALS AND CURRIES

1. Almond Sagu
2. Palak Paneer
3. Paneer Makhani
4. Cabbage and Red Pepper Flax Seeds Vegetable
5. Bharwaan Baingan with Aloo
6. Baingan Bharta
7. Kurkuri Bhindi
8. Gatte ki Sabzi
9. Kale and Peppers Sabzi
10. Aloo Gobi Masala
11. Kashmiri Mini Dum Aloo

12. Lauki Chana Dal
13. Pineapple Dal
14. Karela Dal
15. Gujarati Dal
16. Dal Makhani
17. Cabbage and Chana Dal Curry
18. Mixed Vegetable Curry
19. Punjabi Kadhi
20. Chole
21. Sambar

ROTIS, BREADS AND RICE

1. Thepla
2. Paneer Parantha
3. Kale and Cheese Parantha
4. Muli Aloo Parantha
5. Jowar Methi Parantha
6. Mixed Grain Roti
7. Cranberry Walnut Bread
8. Oatmeal Whole Wheat Bread
9. Focaccia Bread
10. Carrot Lemon Rice
11. Spinach and Corn Rice
12. Tamarind Rice
13. Bisi Bele Bath
14. Himachali Pulao

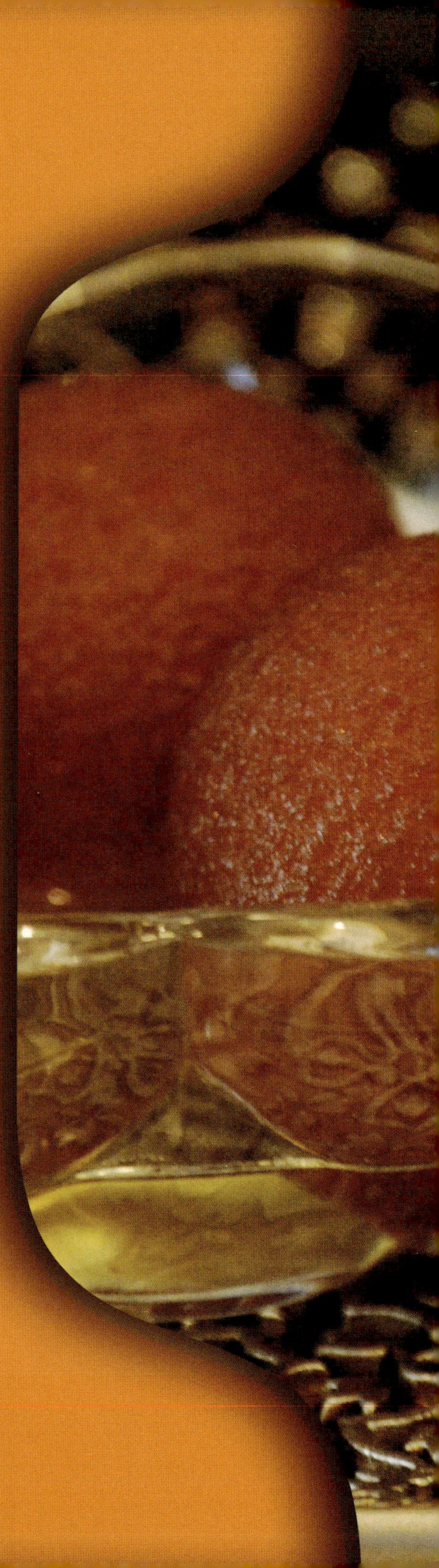

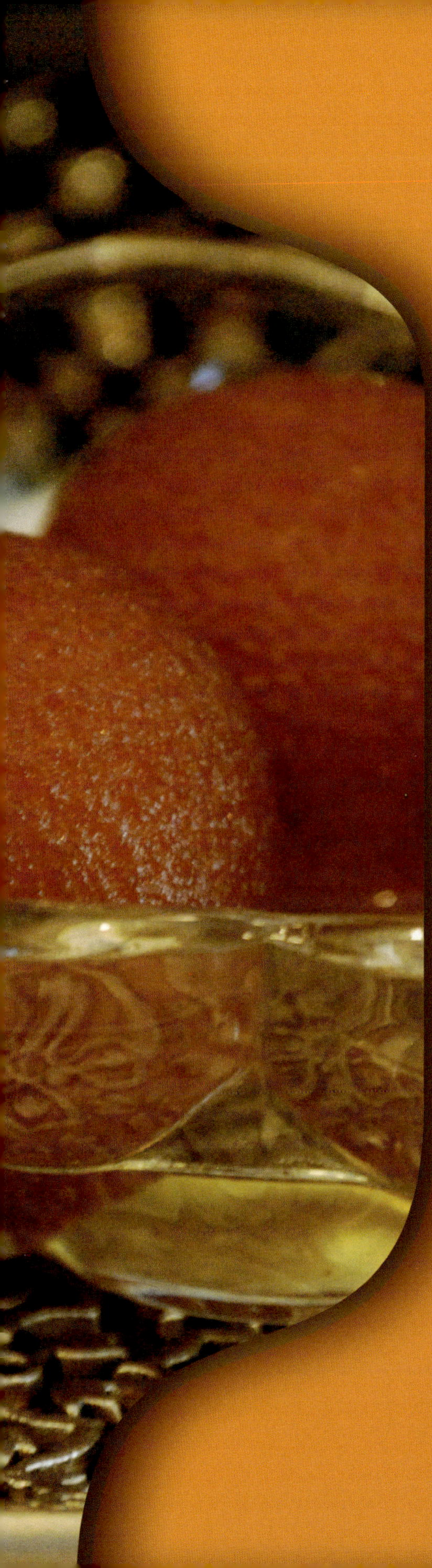

MITHAI

1. Double ka Meetha
2. Gulab Jamun
3. Besan Burfi
4. Walnut Burfi
5. Peda
6. Kopra Pak
7. Date Nut Roll
8. Gud Papdi
9. Sesame Peanut Flax Chikki
10. Almond and Cashew Cookies
11. Rasagulla
12. Mango Shrikandh
13. Kulfi

CAKES AND PUDDINGS

1. Banana Nut Cake
2. Date Nut Cake
3. Chia Orange Cake
4. Whole Wheat Mango Cake
5. Sooji Cake
6. Chia Berry Bowl
7. Mango Coconut Delight
8. Kheer

INTRODUCTION

Food is central to our very existence and is a necessity of life. It is believed that the thoughts of the chef infuse the food with subtle properties and energy. Thus, food cooked with divine sentiment or bhav as a key ingredient does not just provide nourishment to the body, but is also a delight for the senses, and a joy to the soul. This JKYog cookbook is a collection of 108 such vegetarian recipes compiled lovingly by devotees for the pleasure of the Lord.

According to the Shreemad Bhagavatam, culinary skills was one of the sixty-four traditional arts. The cowherd maidens (gopis) of Braj, displayed the perfect blend of the culinary science combined with the sentiments of divine love. It was with this combination that they selflessly served Shree Krishna. Their offerings of butter, buttermilk (chaach), etc. left Him longing for more, so much so that He would repeatedly steal these items from their houses!

In the Vaishnava tradition, the Bhagavad Purana tells us about chappan bhog. Chappan in Hindi translates to fifty-six, while bhog is a meal offered to God. Legend has it that when Shree Krishna lifted the Goverdhan Hill on his little finger, sheltering the residents of Braj (brajwasis), from the wrath of Indra, he did not eat. The rain ended after seven days once Indra realized his folly and pleaded forgiveness from Shree Krishna. At that time, people offered the Lord chappan bhog to show their profound appreciation, gratitude, and love. The number fifty-six was calculated based on the logic that Shree Krishna used to eat eight meals a day.

Indian cooking is widely accepted as a complex, creative art, since it requires not only a deep understanding of food and nutrition but also of the fruits, vegetables, nuts, and spices, and their overall impact on the human body. Keeping this in mind, the recipes shared in this book have been through a rigorous quality control check, and tweaked and refined in multiple ways and multiple times by a dedicated team. As the ingredients changed again and again, the dishes were tested each time to ensure that the spices used do not clash with each other or leave an unfavorable after-taste. The end result is a collection of delectable items that further the Indian culinary tradition.

These recipes were primarily collected from devotees and their circle of family and friends. Several guidelines were followed for the selection process. Each dish should be servable as bhog and at the same time be included in everyday meals too. While care was taken that they constitute healthy, wholesome, and nutritious meals, taste was always the primary criteria.

The taste and flavors of the dishes are enhanced using herbs and spices that not only make them nutritious but are also a delight for the taste buds. Recipes presented here do not require any special skillset as some can even be prepared by young children and amateur cooks. Then, there are others that will tease the hobbyists' palate and grow their repertoire.

One unique characteristic of Indian cooking is that ingredients are used by estimation (andaaz). Ingredients are skillfully added simply by eyeballing and using hands, palms, and flicks of fingers, unlike western cooking which is very specific and measure dependent. While, on the one hand, this makes it difficult to pen down a recipe, on the other hand, it provides the reader an opportunity to tweak them to suit their tastes and needs. In some recipes, variations are suggested that make them more nutritious or suitable for more festive occasions. Additionally, while we list onion and garlic in various recipes, their use is optional. While those preferring more sattvic preparations, or preparing bhog dishes can omit them, others may use them for health benefits or to enhance the taste. According to Ayurveda, ghee or clarified butter prepared from cows' milk, is considered an elixir of health. We leave the choice of using ghee or alternative fats to the readers.

The recipes in this book are organized in nine sections: drinks; soups and salads; snacks – appetizers; snacks – mini meals; chutneys, pickles and condiments; vegetables and entrées (sabzis, dals and curries); rotis and rice dishes (rotis, breads and rice); desserts (mithai); cakes and puddings. The recipes from each section may be used as a stand-alone meal, or paired with others to make a whole meal. A typical Indian meal is a balanced mix of whole grains such as roti or rice, vegetables, dal, and some elements of dairy, such as cottage cheese (paneer) and yogurt (raita). In addition, one may serve condiments such as chutneys or pickles, and if desired, the meal can be completed with a dessert too. Together these form an elegant combination of proteins, carbohydrates, fats, dairy, sugar, and fiber that constitute a nourishing and balanced meal.

This cookbook offers a variety of dishes representative of various Indian cultures and cuisines – from dhoklas and theplas of Gujarat in the west to rasagullas of Bengal in the east; from dum aloo of Kashmir in the north to south Indian delights like idlis and dosa. International recipes such as pizza, pasta, and many fusion recipes round out this compilation. In addition, we also expanded the choice of ingredients used, to go beyond the traditional and include some of

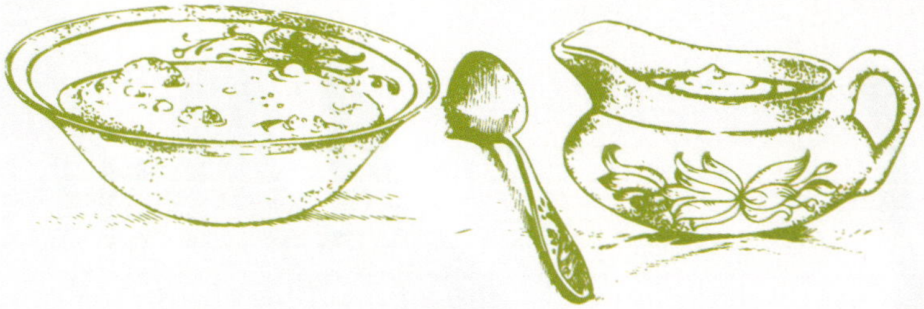

the more recent "superfoods" such as quinoa, sorghum (jowar/white millet), coconut oil, avocados, walnuts, chia seeds, and kale to provide a wide variety of choices for everyone.

The Prasadam Mantra of the Bhagavad Gita guides us to view God in everything.

brahmārpaṇaṁ brahma havir brahmāgnau brahmaṇā hutam
brahmaiva tena gantavyaṁ brahma-karma-samādhinā (4.24)

"For those who are completely absorbed in God-consciousness, the oblation is Brahman, the ladle with which it is offered is Brahman, the act of offering is Brahman, and the sacrificial fire is also Brahman. Such persons, who view everything as God, easily attain Him." Additionally, in verse 9.27 of the Bhagavad Gita, Shree Krishna states:

yat karoṣhi yad aśhnāsi yaj juhoṣhi dadāsi yat
yat tapasyasi kaunteya tat kuruṣhva mad-arpaṇam

"Whatever you do, whatever you eat, whatever you offer as oblation to the sacred fire, whatever you bestow as a gift, and whatever austerities you perform, O son of Kunti, do them as an offering to me."

Keeping this in mind, with gratitude and loving devotion, we offer this garland of 108 culinary beads (manakas) to our beloved Gurudev. We hope you enjoy cooking these dishes as much as we enjoyed putting them together.

Drinks

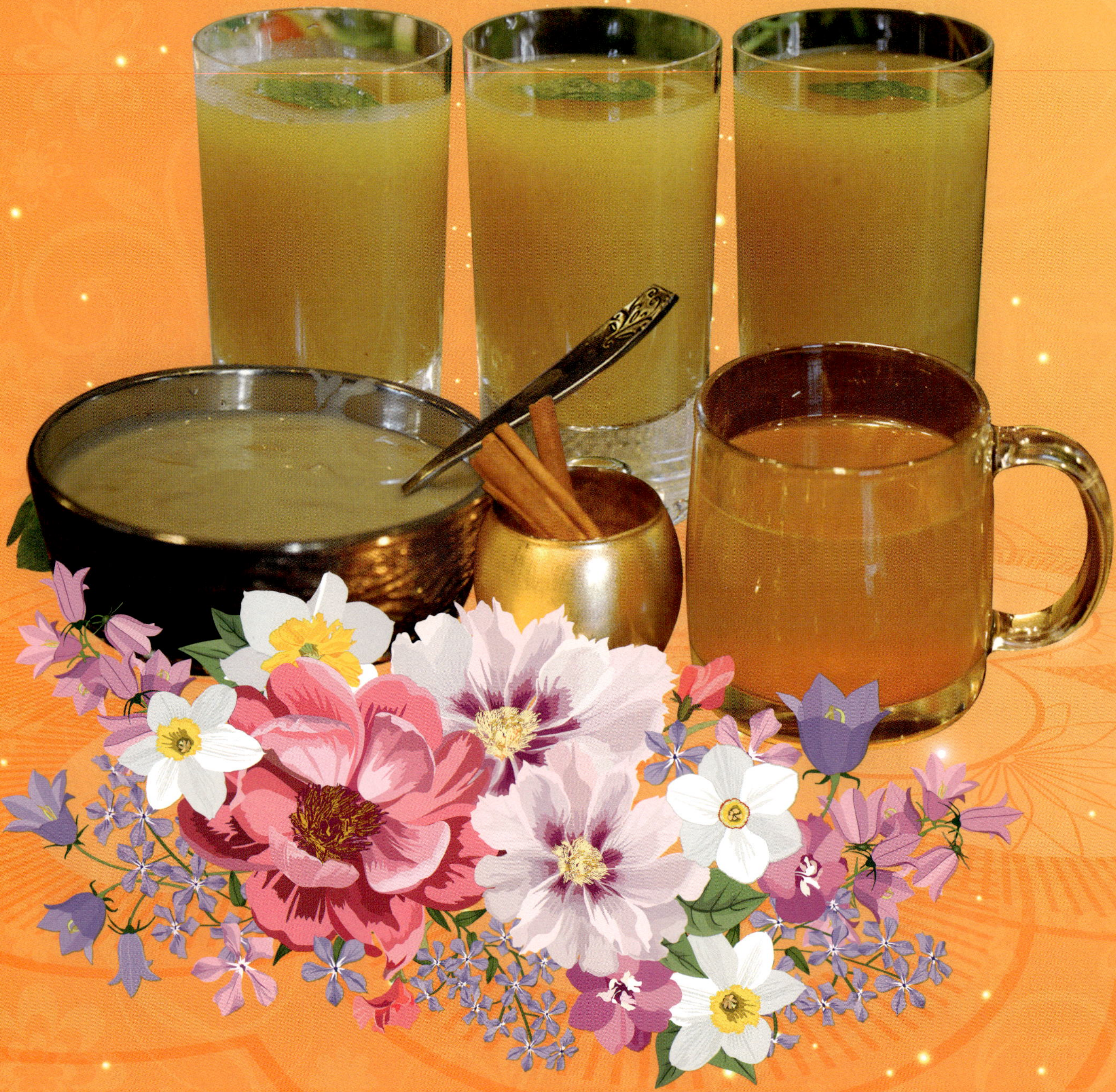

We begin this first section by offering our very first bhog recipe in this cookbook - *Panchamrit* – "the nectar of Gods" to our revered Gurudev and God alone with whose blessings this project was undertaken. Served as a bhog to the Lord in temples, and distributed as prasad to the devotees, there could not be a better choice to begin this cookbook.

Other beverages may be served as meal starters or as simple refreshments. All of them have different fruity and spicy flavors. *Mango lassi* and *aam ka panna* are cooling and refreshing choices best enjoyed during hot summer months whereas, *apple cider* and *herbal drink* simmered in warm spices provide soothing comfort in cold weather.

1. Panchamrit
2. Mango Lassi
3. Aam ka Panna
4. Apple Cider
5. Herbal Tea

Panchamrit

"Nectar of the gods"–traditionally made from five ingredients–yogurt, milk, sugar, honey and ghee

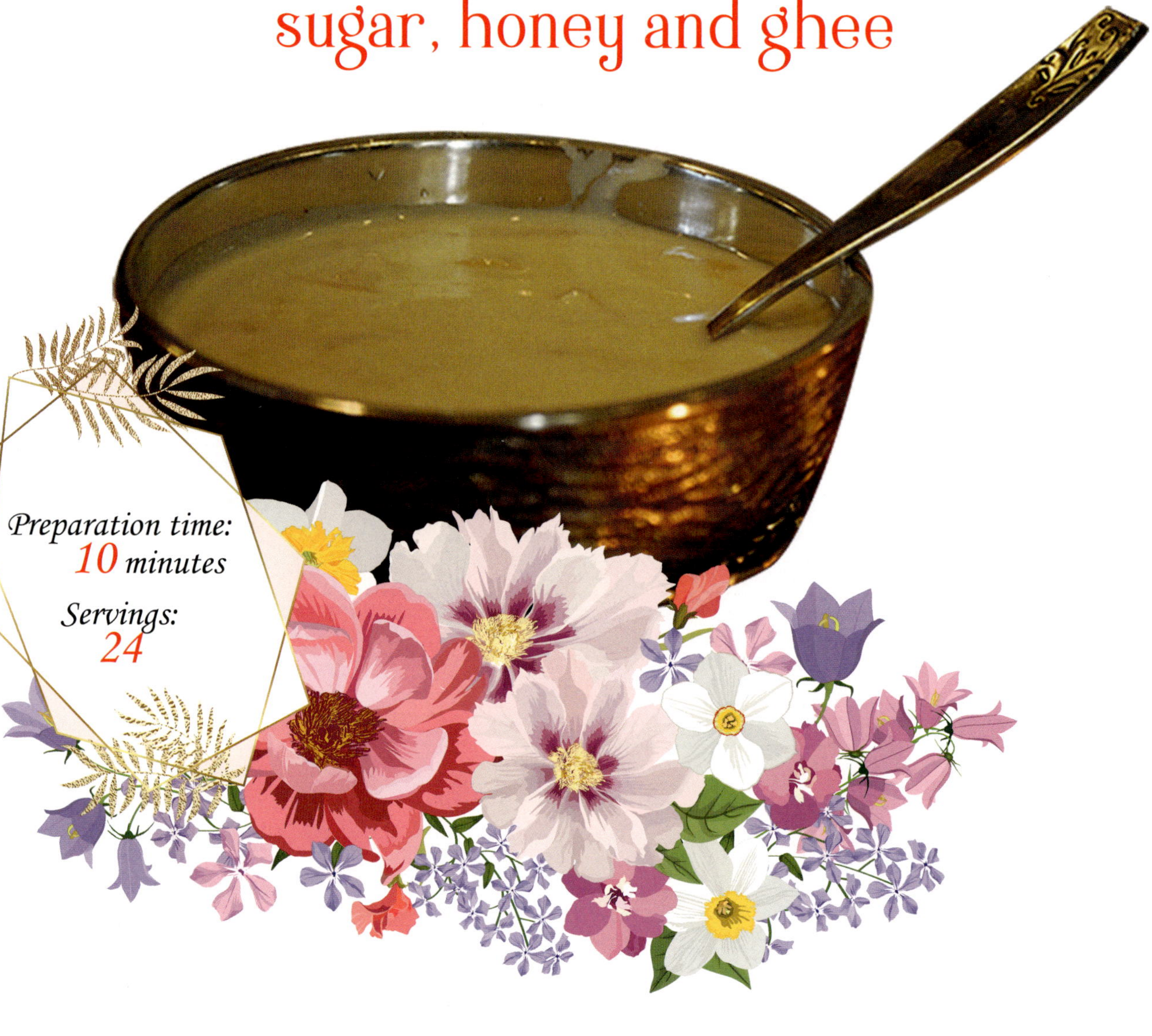

Preparation time: 10 *minutes*

Servings: 24

Ingredients

- 16 oz. yogurt
- ¼ cup milk
- ½ cup sugar
- 1 tablespoon honey
- 1 teaspoon ghee
- ½ cup mixed dry fruits chopped fine (almond, cashew, makhana, coconut, golden raisins) (optional)

Process

1. Mix all ingredients together. If it is too thick then add some more milk.
2. Refrigerate for at least 30 minutes before using.
3. Offer as bhog and serve as prasad to devotees.

Photo note: The panchamrit depicted in the photo does not have all the dry fruits listed in ingredients.

Alternate option: Saffron and tulsi leaves may also be added if desired.

Mango Lassi

A popular traditional yogurt-based summer drink

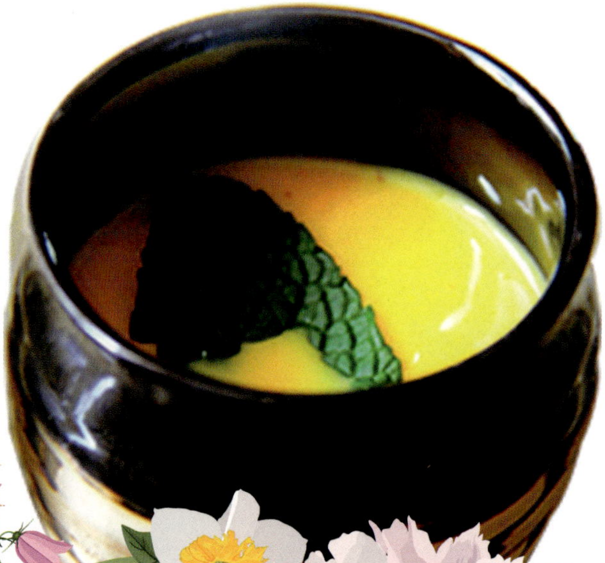

Total time: 10 *minutes*

Soaking time: 2 *hours (only if using sabja seeds)*

Servings: 6 *(8 oz. glasses)*

Ingredients

- 1 cup plain yogurt, whole
- 1 cup milk, whole
- 16 oz. can mango pulp
- 2 mangoes, diced (optional)
- 4 teaspoons sugar, or to taste
- 2 teaspoons sabja seeds or sweet basil seeds (optional)
- 1 teaspoon green cardamom, ground (save some for garnish if desired)
- few strands of saffron (save some for garnish if desired)
- ice cubes

Process

1. Soak sabja seeds in 4 teaspoons of water for 2 hours.
2. Put ice, mango pulp, yogurt, milk, sugar, cardamom, and saffron into a blender and blend till smooth.
3. Add the soaked sabja seeds and the diced mangoes. They create a texture to the lassi. Mix and pour into individual glasses.
4. Sprinkle cardamom powder and saffron as garnish on top.
5. The lassi drink can be kept refrigerated for up to 24 hours.

Aam ka Panna

A refreshing sweet tangy drink enjoyed on a hot summer day

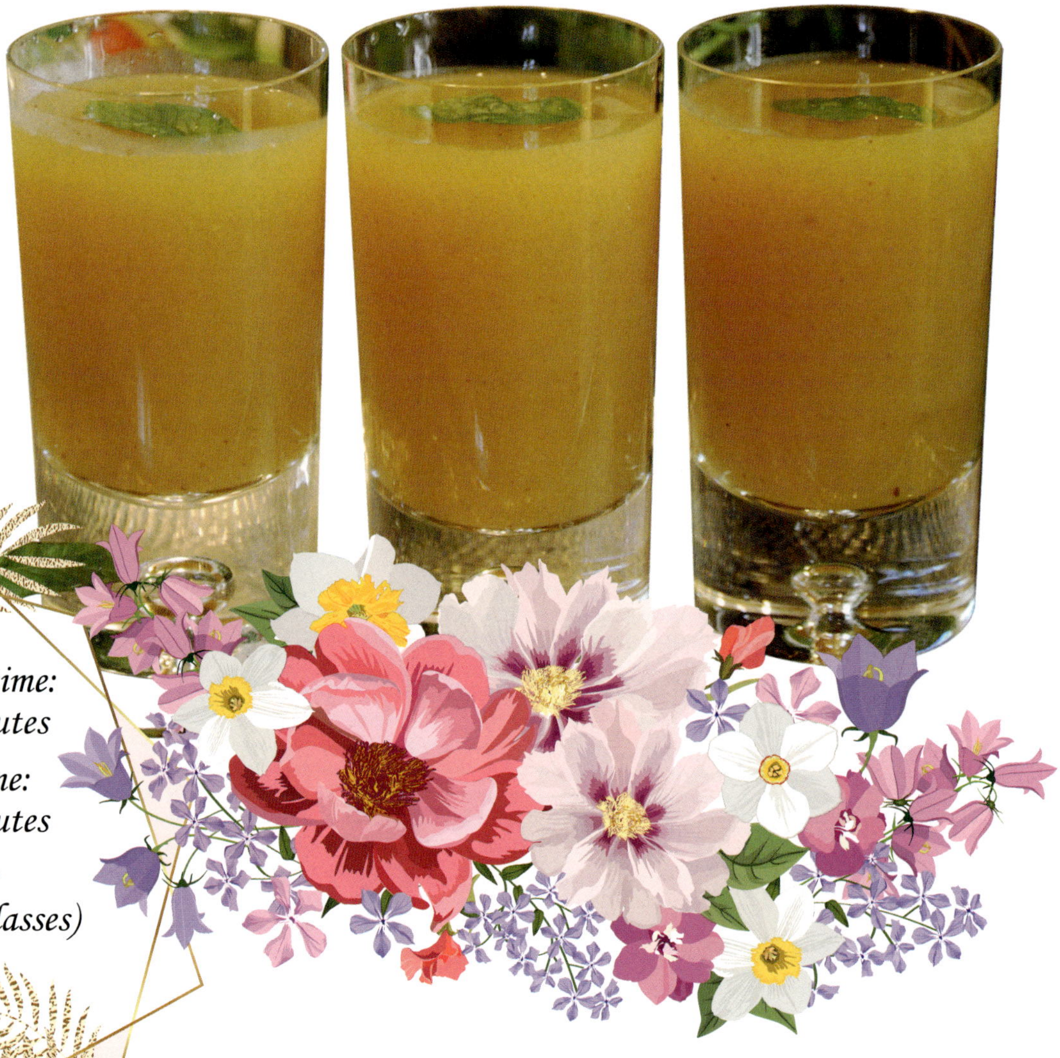

Preparation time:
10 *minutes*

Cooking time:
20 *minutes*

Servings:
3 *(6 oz. glasses)*

Ingredients

- 1 medium size raw mango, peeled and chopped
- ¼ tsp roasted cumin seeds powder
- 2-3 tablespoons sugar
- ½ teaspoon salt
- ½ teaspoon black salt
- ½ teaspoon black pepper
- 1 cup water to cook the mango
- 1 cup chilled water and few ice cubes
- 3-4 mint leaves for garnishing

Process

1. In a pressure cooker, add the mangoes and approximately 1 cup of water and pressure cook until soft (4-5 whistles).
2. Cool and blend the mixture.
3. Add roasted cumin seeds and black pepper powder, sugar, salt and black salt and stir well.
4. Add chilled water and ice cubes and mix.
5. Pour and serve chilled in glasses topped with mint.

Optional note: Crushed mint leaves may be mixed to the aam ka panna if a minty taste is preferred. Also, the color of panna varies based on the raw mangoes used.

Apple Cider

A cold weather soothing warm drink with an aroma of spices

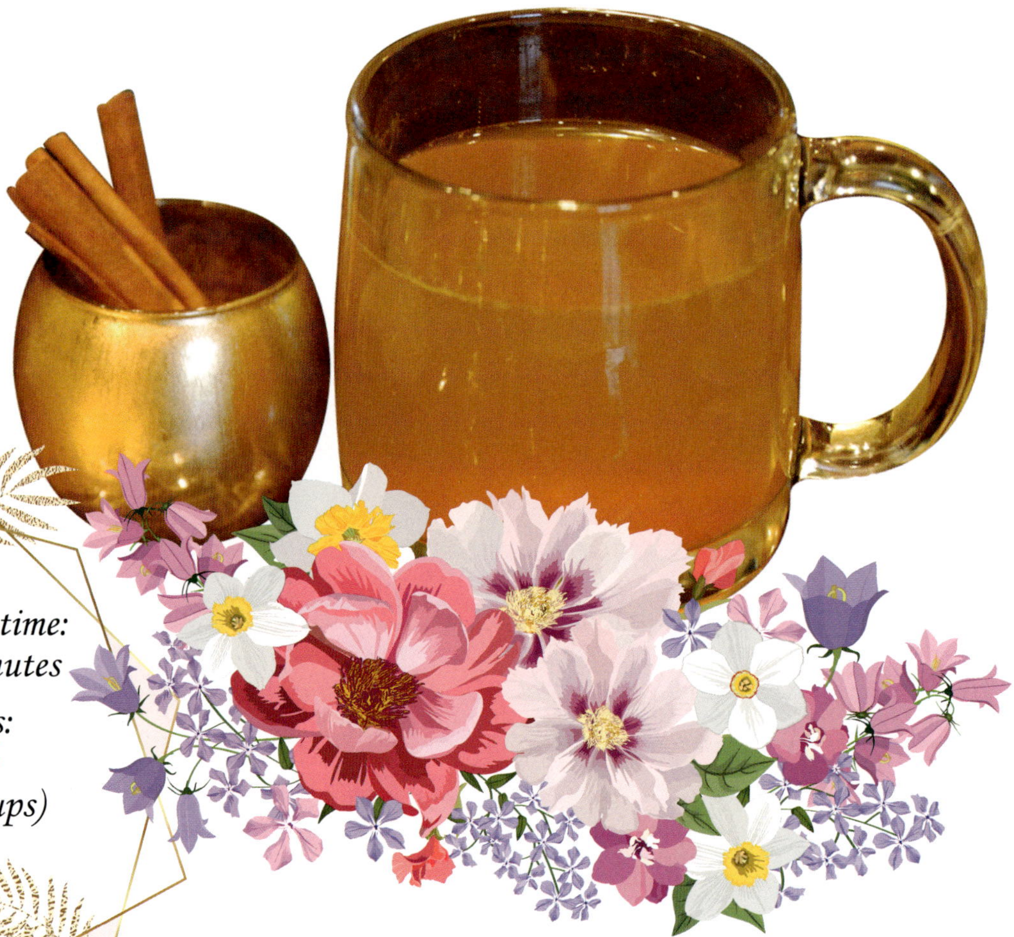

Preparation time:
30 *minutes*

Servings:
5-16
(5-6 oz. cups)

Ingredients

- 1-gallon apple cider or apple juice
- ¼ cup light brown sugar
- 2-3 cinnamon sticks
- 2-3 cloves
- 4-5 green cardamom crushed
- few strands of saffron

Process

1. Heat the apple cider or apple juice in a large pot. Add the brown sugar until dissolved and bring it to a low boil. Now add the cinnamon sticks, cloves, cardamom and saffron.
2. Cover and simmer over low heat for 20 minutes.
3. Strain and serve warm, in mugs.

Herbal Drink

Soothing relief for alleviating cold and cough symptoms

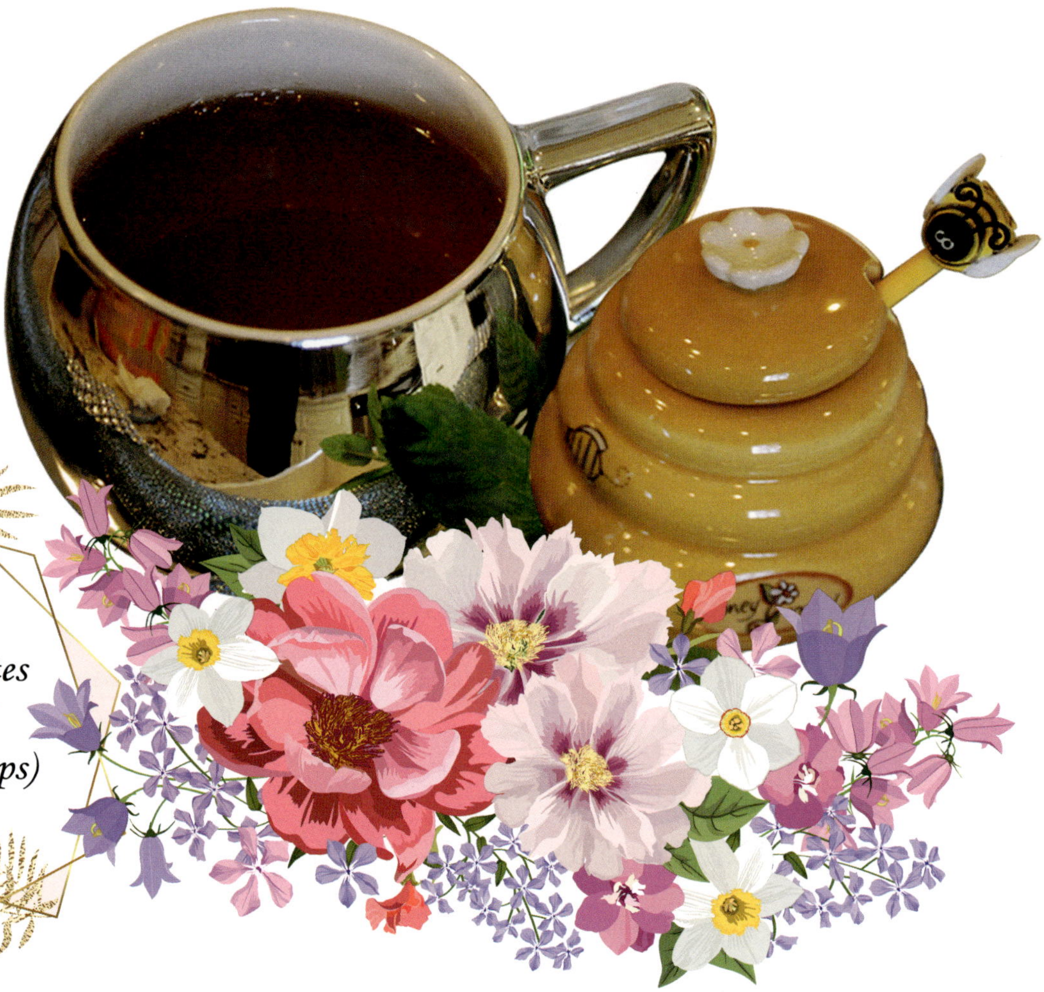

Total time: *15 minutes*

Servings: 1 *(8 oz. cups)*

Ingredients

- 2 cups water
- 1-inch ginger, grated
- 14 tulsi leaves (holy basil)
- 1 tablespoon lemongrass
- 10 mint leaves
- 1 cinnamon stick
- 8 black peppercorns
- 1 clove
- ½ teaspoon honey

Process

1. In a small pan heat water. Add grated ginger, tulsi, mint, lemongrass, cinnamon, peppercorns and clove.
2. Continue boiling till the water is reduced to half.
3. Now add the honey and stir it well.
4. Strain and serve hot.

Alternate option: Dry basil may be used if fresh tulsi leaves are unavailable.

Soups and Salads

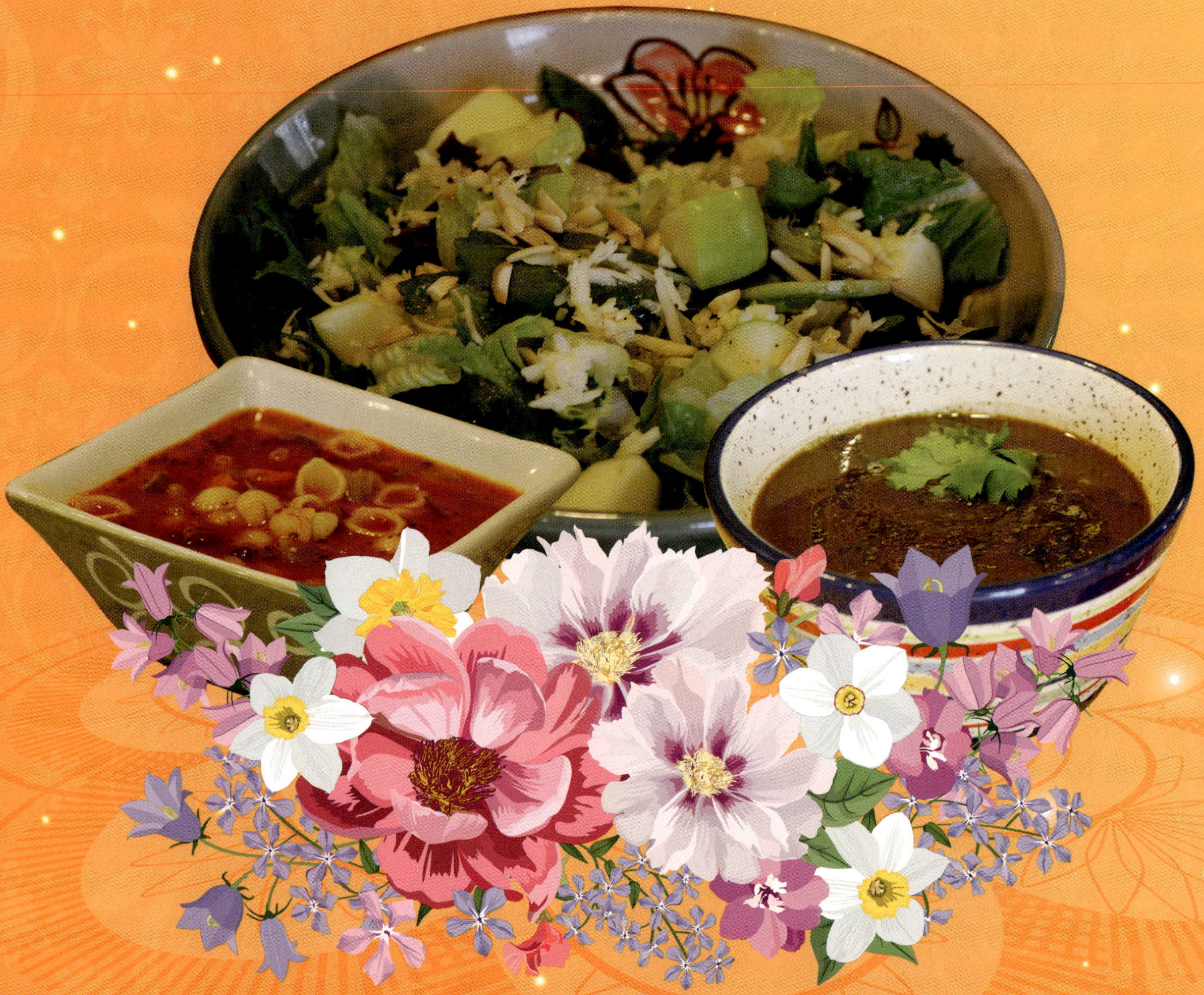

This collection of soups and salads includes fusion recipes drawn from various cuisines - Thai, Italian, Chinese, Indian and Mexican.

The comforting warmth of soups during cold winter months is uplifting to the soul! Soups can be served as light meal starters or as complete meals. *Clear, tomato, rasam thai and hot and sour* are good choices as meal starter soups whereas *minestrone* and *mixed bean* served with a slice of bread, sandwich, salad or just by themselves are a satisfying and a nourishing complete meal.

Salads too may be served as a meal starter, side or as a meal. The *dhokla salad* is a variation of a popular snack. The *quinoa* and *couscous salads* use nutritious grains as their base. The *spicy taco salad* with beans is a southern taste and the *toasted almond apple salad* is a typical salad made with greens drizzled with dressing. Loaded with fruits, vegetables, nuts they are all packed with goodness of nature. A combined meal of soup and salad and perhaps a sandwich, makes a great lunch option.

1. Clear Vegetable Soup
2. Tomato Soup
3. Rasam Thai Soup
4. Minestrone Soup
5. Black Bean Soup
6. Mixed Bean Soup
7. Hot and Sour Soup
8. Dhokla Salad
9. Couscous Salad
10. Quinoa Salad
11. Spicy Taco Salad
12. Toasted Almond Apple Salad

Clear Vegetable Soup

Light soothing soup with the crunch of vegetables

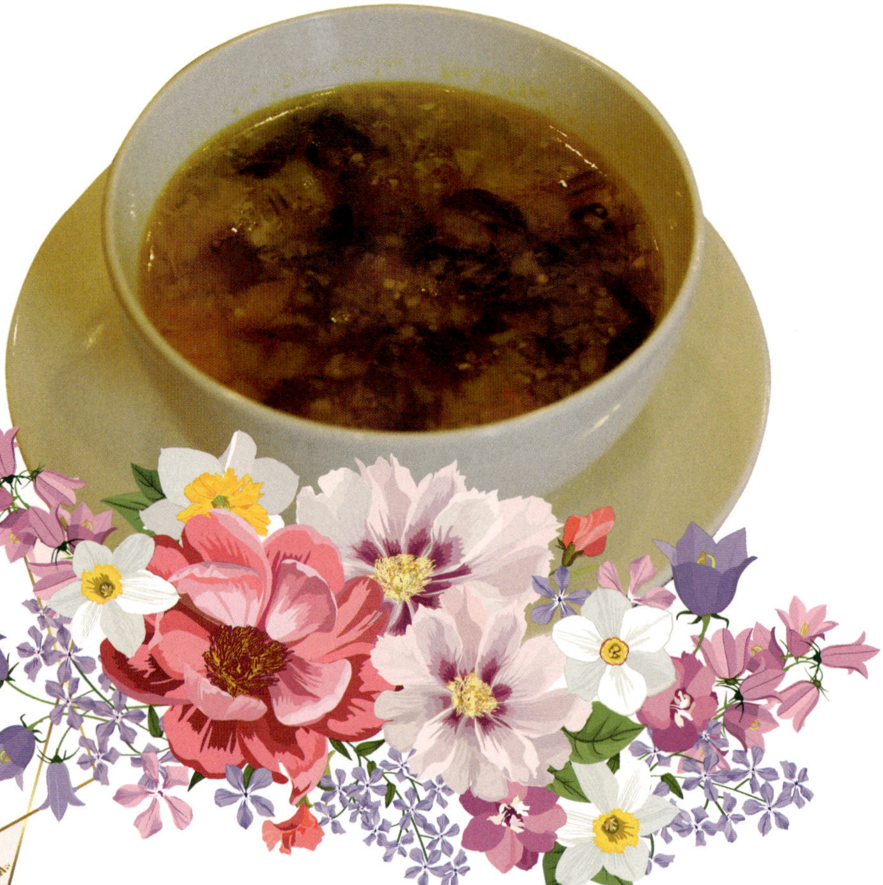

Preparation time: 25 *minutes*

Cooking time: 15 *minutes*

Servings: 10 *medium soup bowls*

Ingredients

- 1 cup cabbage, thinly sliced
- 1 cup multi-color peppers, chopped
- ½ cup spinach, chopped
- ½ cup carrots, finely cut
- ½ cup celery, chopped
- ½ cup French beans, finely chopped
- ½ cup spring onions, chopped (optional)
- ½ teaspoon garlic, finely chopped (optional)
- ½ teaspoon ginger, finely chopped
- ½ teaspoon crushed pepper
- 1 tablespoon olive oil
- 1 tablespoon lemon juice
- 5 cups vegetable stock or water
- salt to taste

Process

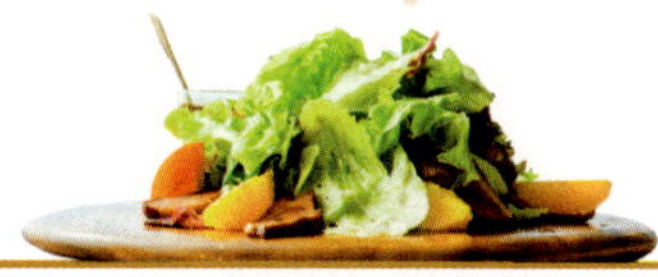

1. In a deep pot heat olive oil, and sauté chopped garlic and ginger, until the raw smell of garlic and ginger goes away.
2. Then add all chopped vegetables, except spring onion.
3. Sauté for few minutes and then add 5 cups of stock or water. Bring to a boil taking care not to overcook the vegetables. They need to remain crunchy.
4. Season with salt, pepper and lemon juice.
5. Garnish with spring onions (if using) and serve hot for best flavors and taste.

Nutrition tip: Adding sprouts will make this soup even more nutritious.

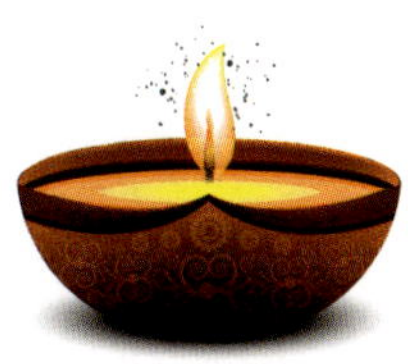

Tomato Soup

A classic soul satisfying soup, also a nutritional powerhouse

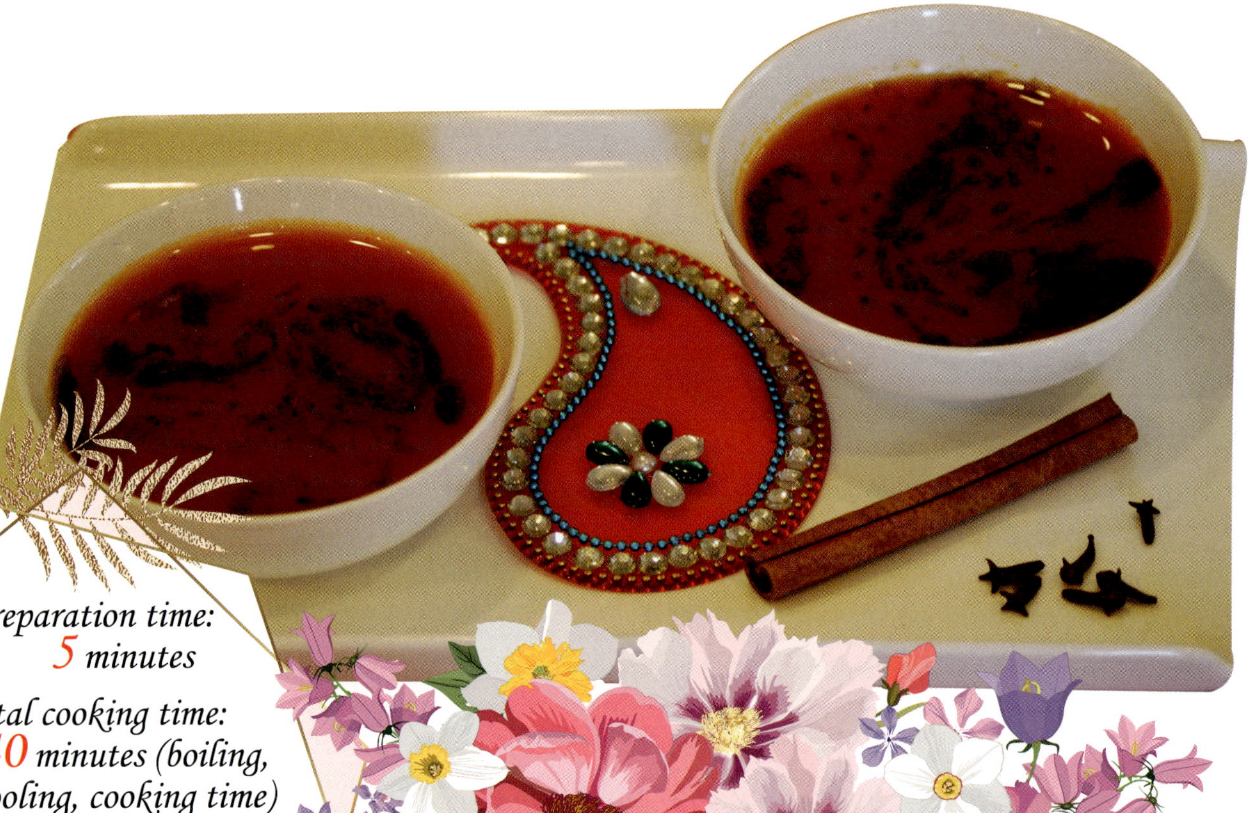

Preparation time: 5 *minutes*

Total cooking time: 40 *minutes (boiling, cooling, cooking time)*

Servings: 6 *medium size bowls*

Ingredients

- 6 fresh medium/large ripe tomatoes, round and juicy
- 1 tablespoon fresh cilantro, finely chopped
- 1 tablespoon brown sugar
- 1 teaspoon black pepper powder
- 3 cups water
- 1 tablespoon salt, or to taste

For tempering

- 1 tablespoon ghee
- 1 stick cinnamon
- 3 cloves
- 1 tablespoon roasted cumin powder

Process

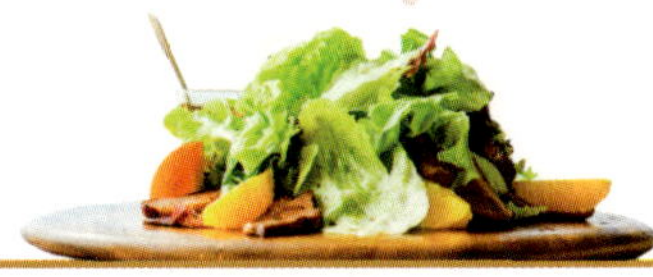

1. In a deep pot boil 3 cups of water.
2. Add the full tomatoes and boil for 8-10 minutes until they become tender and the skin starts separating from the tomatoes.
3. Cool the tomatoes and crush them in a blender to make a fine purée. This can be further strained to remove the seeds and skin.
4. Add brown sugar, pepper and salt to the puréed tomatoes and boil the purée.
5. Prepare tempering by heating ghee in a small vessel. Add cinnamon stick, cloves and cumin powder and heat till they are fragrant. Pour over the boiling soup.
6. Simmer for another 5 minutes and serve hot.

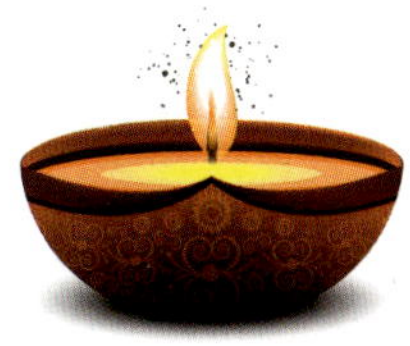

Rasam Thai Soup

A fusion tangy, spicy heartwarming soup

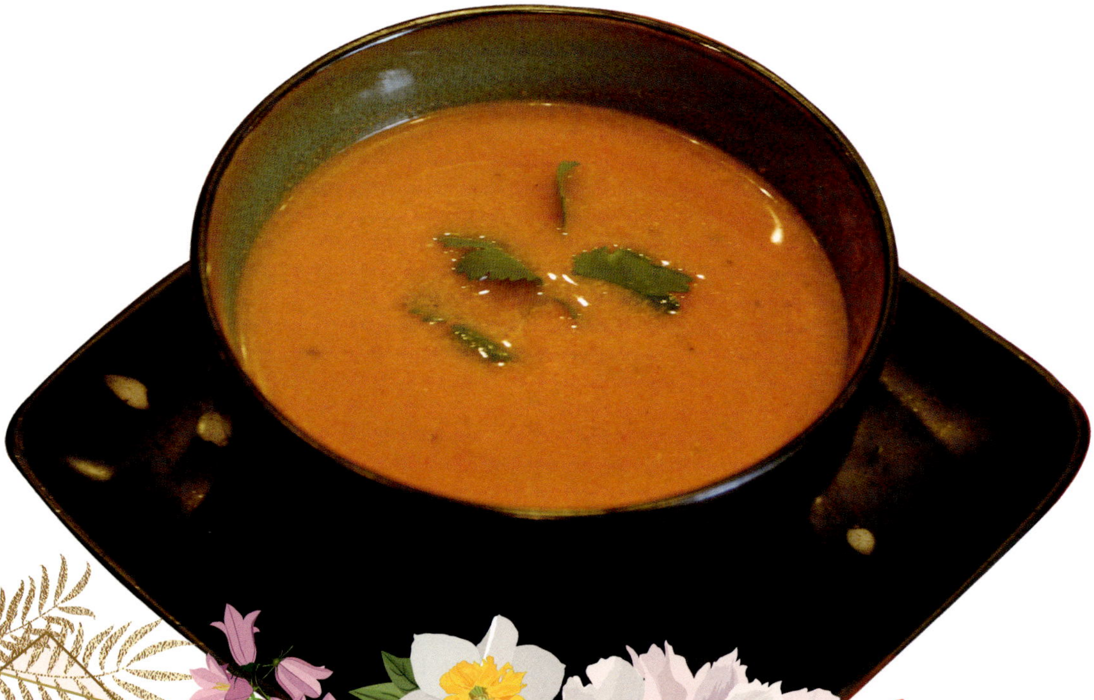

Preparation time: 10 *minutes*

Cooking time: 50 *minutes*

Servings: 4 *medium bowls*

Ingredients

- 16 oz. can of tomato sauce (Hunt's)
- 8 oz. can coconut milk
- 1 ½ cups water
- 3 teaspoons rasam powder
- pinch of red chilli powder
- 10-12 curry leaves
- bunch of minced cilantro leaves
- 2 teaspoons lemon juice
- salt and black pepper to taste

Process

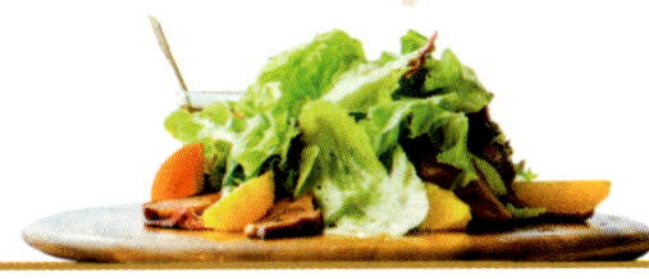

1. Add all these ingredients to a 5-quart crockpot.
2. Mix these up and cook on high for 20 minutes or till it comes to boil.
3. Let it simmer on low heat in a crockpot for ½ hour.
4. Rasam Thai Soup may be served hot as a starter with crackers or focaccia bread.

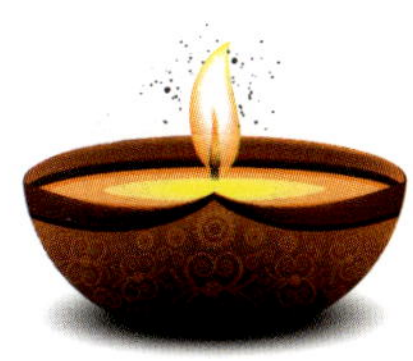

Minestrone Soup

Hearty Italian soup with seasonal vegetables

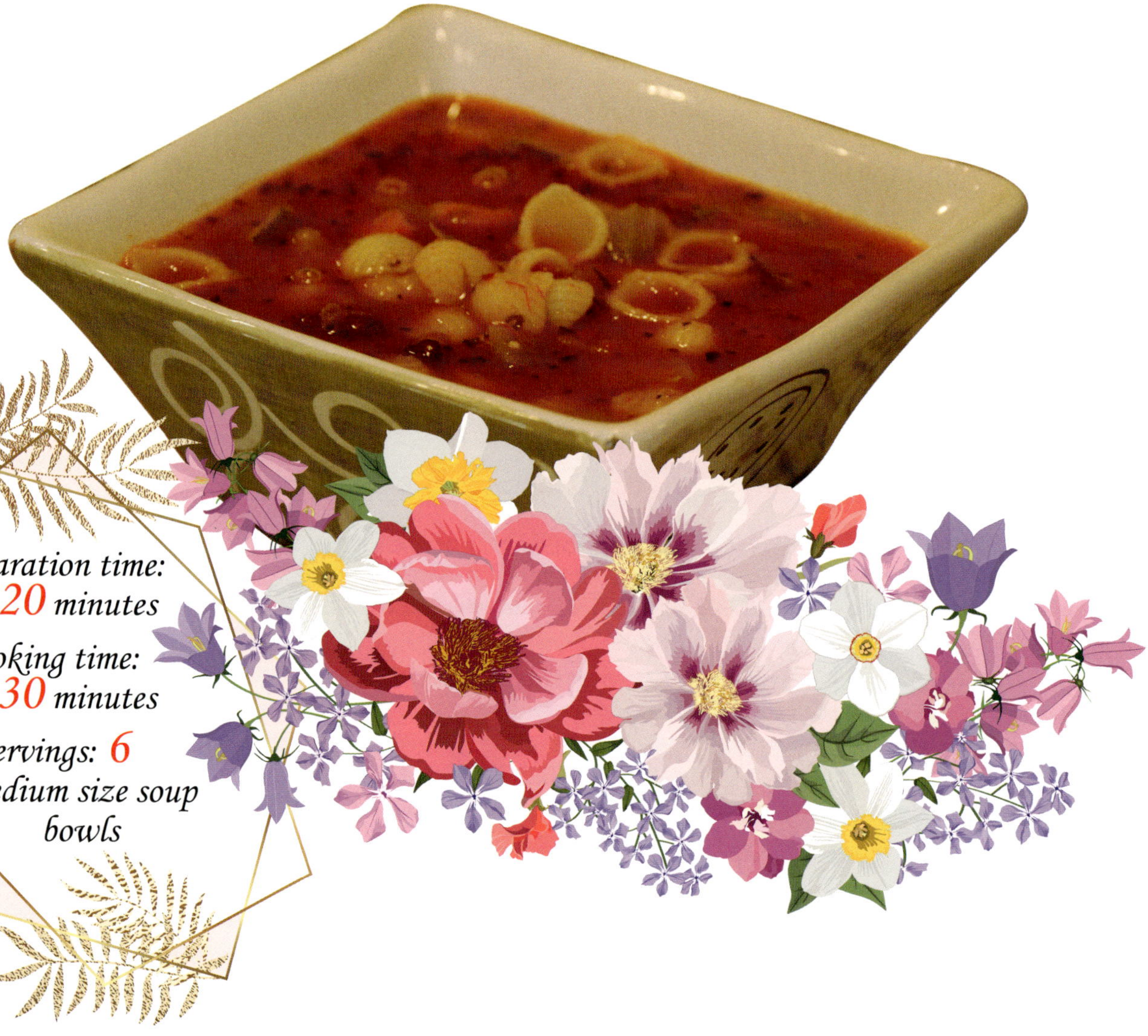

Preparation time: 20 *minutes*

Cooking time: 30 *minutes*

Servings: 6 *medium size soup bowls*

Ingredients

- 1 can red kidney beans
- 8 oz. can crushed tomatoes
- 1 cup small shell pasta, uncooked
- 5 cups vegetable broth, or plain water
- 1 medium onion, finely chopped (optional)
- 1 cup celery, chopped in small cubes
- 1 cup zucchini, chopped in small cubes
- 1 cup squash, chopped in small cubes
- 1 cup carrots, chopped in small cubes
- 1 tablespoon fresh basil leaves, chopped
- 3 medium sized garlic cloves, chopped (optional)
- 1 tablespoon dried Italian seasoning
- 1 tablespoon oregano powder
- 1 teaspoon crushed red pepper
- 2 tablespoons olive oil
- salt and black pepper to taste

Process

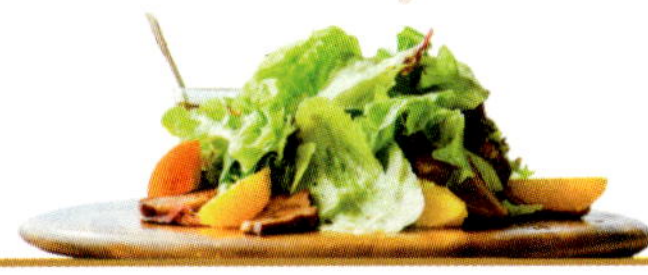

1. In a medium soup pot heat oil and sauté onion (if using) for a few minutes and then add garlic (if using) and sauté for another minute.
2. Add carrots, zucchini, squash, celery, crushed tomatoes and the broth. Add salt and black pepper to it and bring to boil.
3. Reduce to low heat and simmer for 10-12 minutes until vegetables are tender.
4. Finally, add the beans and pasta and simmer for another 5 to 9 minutes for all the flavors to get absorbed.
5. Season with oregano powder, Italian seasoning, crushed red pepper and fresh herbs. Serve hot.

Optional tip: The mix of vegetables and beans may be varied in this soup.

Black Bean Soup

A low-calorie, protein rich soup

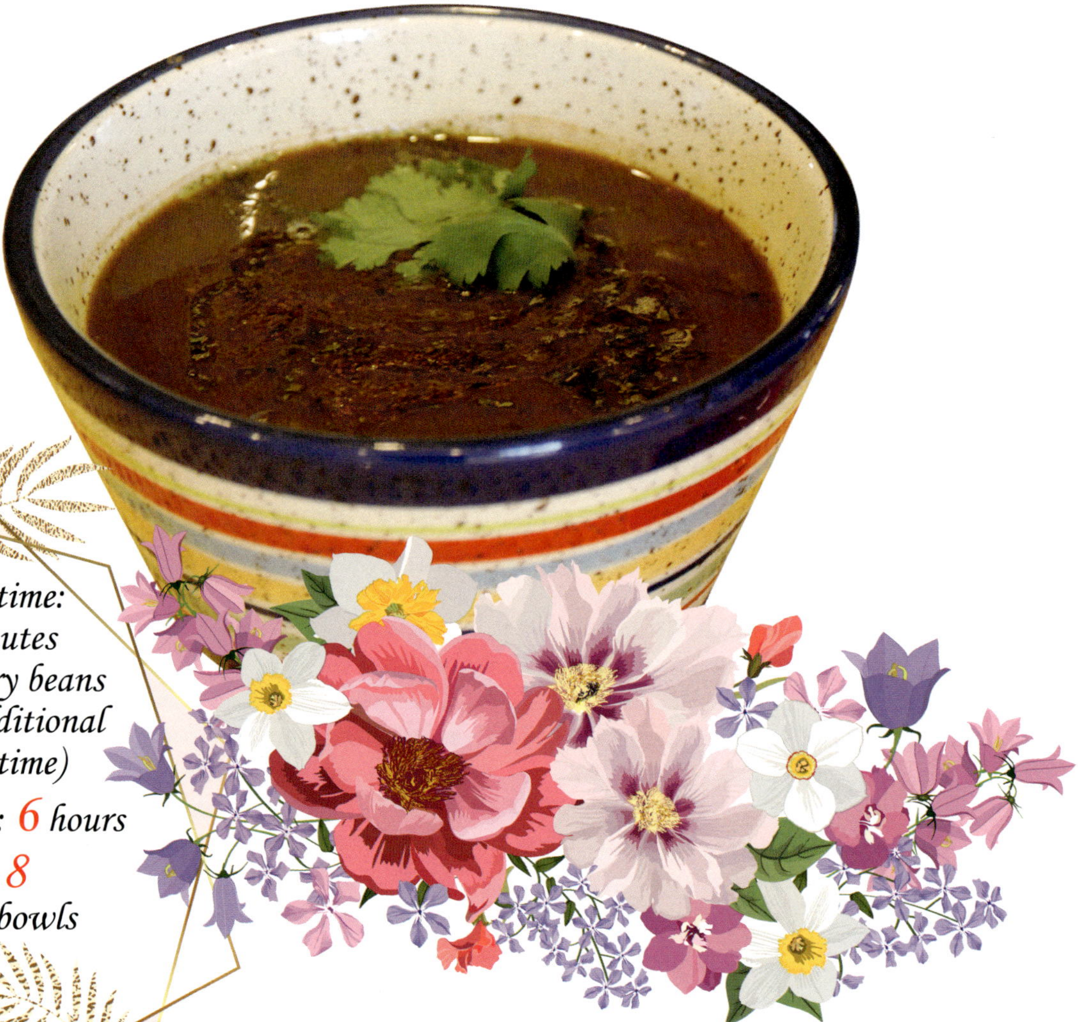

Preparation time:
20 minutes
(If using dry beans
6 hours additional
soaking time)

Cooking time: 6 hours

Servings: 8
medium bowls

Ingredients

- 1 cup dry black beans, or 2 cans (15 oz.) of black beans
- 4 cups vegetable broth or water
- 2 medium tomatoes, finely diced
- 1 red bell pepper, finely chopped
- 1 celery stalk, finely chopped without ribs
- 1 onion, finely chopped (optional)
- 2 garlic cloves (optional)
- 2 jalapeños, finely chopped
- 1 cup cilantro, chopped
- 1 tablespoon ground cumin powder
- 1 teaspoon ground black pepper
- ½ teaspoon dry oregano leaves
- 2 teaspoons kosher salt

For tempering

- 1 tablespoon olive oil
- 1 teaspoon cumin powder
- 1 teaspoon oregano powder

Process

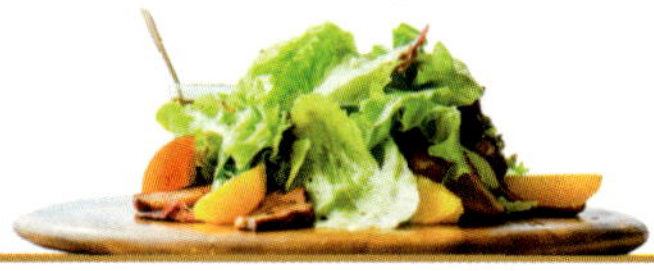

1. Soak the dry beans for 5 to 6 hours in warm water. Drain and rinse the beans. Skip this step if using cans.
2. In a 4-quart crock pot place beans, broth/water, tomatoes, peppers, celery, onion and garlic (optional), jalapeños, cilantro, cumin, black pepper, oregano and salt. Stir with a wooden spatula.
3. Cook on high for 6 hours, until beans are completely cooked.
4. With a hand blender blend the soup partially, just a few churns, so that the soup has a chunky texture.
5. For the tempering, warm olive oil and add oregano and cumin powder. When fragrant pour over the soup.
6. Garnish with cilantro and serve warm.

Cooking note: If canned beans are used then the cooking time would be reduced to 1 hour.

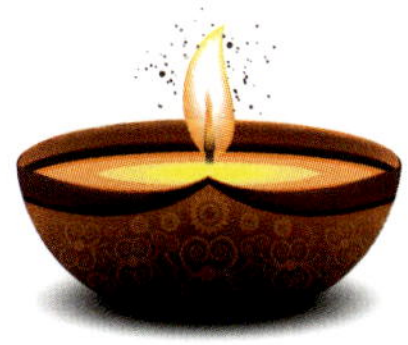

Mixed Beans Soup

A simple soup that is filling and flavorful

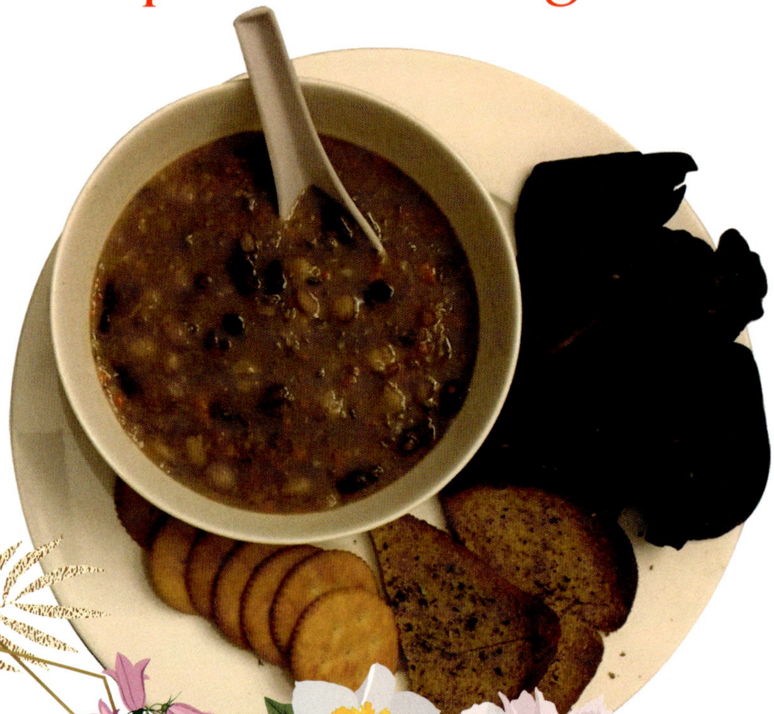

Preparation time:
15 minutes (additional 6-7 hours soaking time)

Cooking time:
40 minutes

Servings:
8-10 medium size bowls

Ingredients

- 1 cup of mixed dry beans (black, pinto, lima, kidney, chickpeas, black-eyed peas)
- ½ cup of mixed dry lentils (split chana, toor, whole green moong)
- 1 carrot, peeled and chopped
- ½ green pepper, chopped
- 2-3 sticks of celery, chopped
- 4-5 garlic cloves, minced (optional)
- 1 small piece of ginger, minced
- 3-4 cups of water
- 3-4 teaspoons vegetable oil
- salt and black pepper to taste

Process

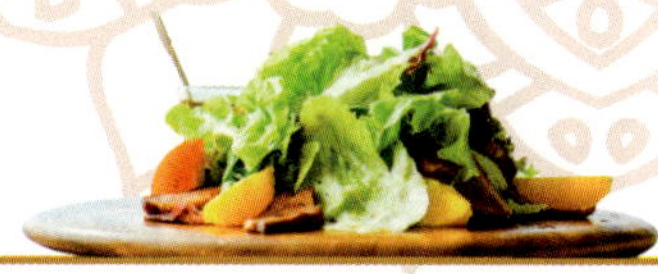

1. Mix the beans and lentils in large bowl with 4-5 cups of water. Soak for at least 6-7 hours, preferably overnight.
2. Drain the water and thoroughly wash the beans-lentil mix. Pressure cook this beans-lentil mix with 3-4 cups of water and salt.
3. Cook at medium-high heat until the first whistle. Then lower the heat and continue cooking for approximately 15 more minutes. Turn off the heat and let the pressure release from the cooker (about 10-15 minutes).
4. In a pan, heat oil and sauté ginger and garlic (optional) for 1 minute until lightly brown. Add the carrots, pepper and celery. Cook for a few minutes until the vegetables are tender.
5. Now, open the pressure cooker and check that the beans are well-cooked. Mix in the sautéed vegetables. Mash everything together to a preferred consistency.
6. If the soup is too thick, simply add boiled water and heat for a few minutes (without the lid).
7. Sprinkle some black pepper and serve hot.

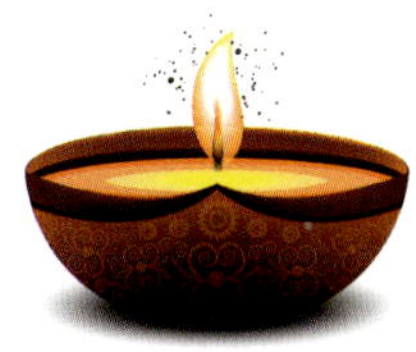

Hot and Sour Soup

Tangy, traditional, appetizing Chinese soup made with vegetables

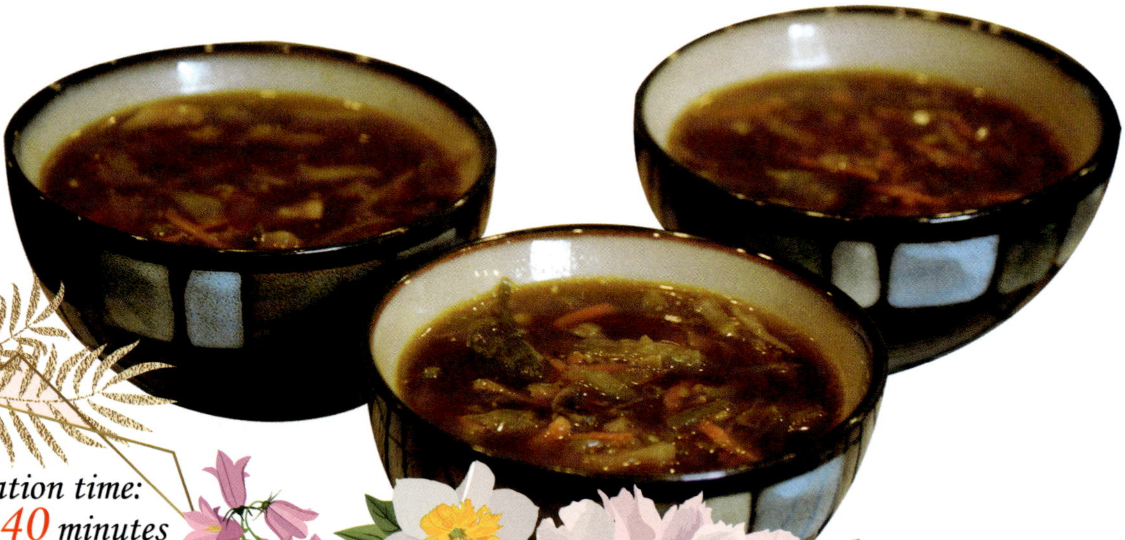

Preparation time: **30-40** *minutes*

Cooking time: **30** *minutes*

Servings: **6-8** *medium bowls*

Ingredients

- 5 cups vegetable broth or water
- 1 cup carrots, fine julienne cut
- 1 cup French beans, fine julienne cut
- 1 cup cabbage, thinly sliced
- ¼ cup button mushrooms, thinly sliced
- ½ cup green spring onions, coarsely sliced (optional)
- 1 cup bell pepper, fine julienne cut
- ¼ cup bean sprouts
- 1 small green chilli, finely chopped
- 1 teaspoon garlic, minced (optional)
- 1 teaspoon ginger, minced
- 2 to 3 tablespoons cornstarch, mixed with ½ cup cold water
- 2 tablespoons vinegar
- 3 tablespoons soy sauce or as per taste
- 1 tablespoon red chilli sauce, or as per taste
- 1 tablespoon vegetable oil
- salt and black pepper to taste

Process

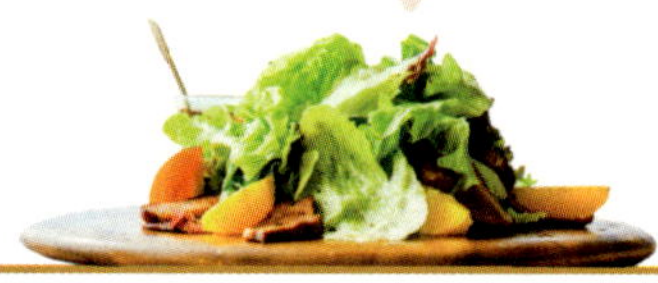

1. In a medium size wok, heat oil till it smokes. Add ginger and garlic and sauté for few minutes.
2. Add carrots, French beans, cabbage, bell peppers and green chilli. Sauté for another 1-2 minutes.
3. Now add vegetable broth, salt and black pepper. Bring mixture to a boil and add mushrooms and bean sprouts. Simmer until all vegetables are cooked (slightly undercooked) for 3 to 4 minutes.
4. Add chilli sauce, soy sauce and vinegar and let it boil. Then add the corn starch mixed with water gradually to the soup and bring to boil on low heat. Take it off the heat.
5. Garnish with spring onions, if using, and serve hot.

Ingredient tip: Thin slices of tofu may also be added to this soup.

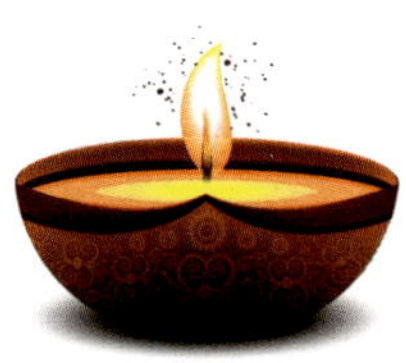

Colorful Dhokla Salad

A delectable twist to a traditional recipe!

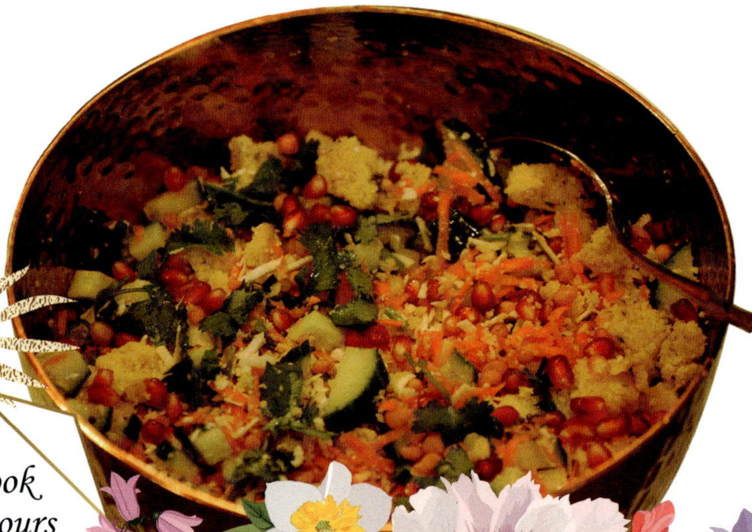

Cooking time:
30 minutes to cook dhokla, plus few hours refrigeration time for dhokla or these can be made a day in advance

Assembling time:
30 minutes

Servings: 6-8
(8 oz. bowls)

Ingredients

- 6 oz. or 1 packet khaman dhokla mix
- 1 cup salted dry boondi
- 1 cup coconut, freshly grated
- 1 cup cucumbers, finely cubed
- 1 cup carrots, very finely cubed
- 1 cup fresh pomegranate kernels
- ½ cup cilantro, chopped
- ½ teaspoon green chillies, finely chopped (optional)
- 1 tablespoon fresh lemon juice
- ½ teaspoon mustard seeds
- 1 tablespoon cooking oil
- salt to taste

Process

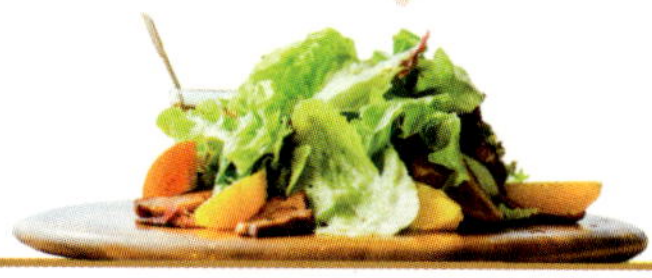

1. Make dhokla as per packet instructions. Do not temper the dhoklas.
2. Cool the dhoklas by refrigerating for a couple of hours or can even make them a day ahead.
3. In a food processor gently pulse the cooled dhoklas so you get tiny pieces but not a powder. Transfer the pulsed dhokla pieces into a large mixing bowl.
4. Add cucumber, carrots, grated coconut, green chillies, and pomegranate kernels. Add lemon juice and salt according to taste. Gently toss salad.
5. Make a tempering with oil and mustard seeds and pour on the salad.
6. Transfer the salad into a serving bowls. Garnish with salted boondi and cilantro leaves and serve immediately.

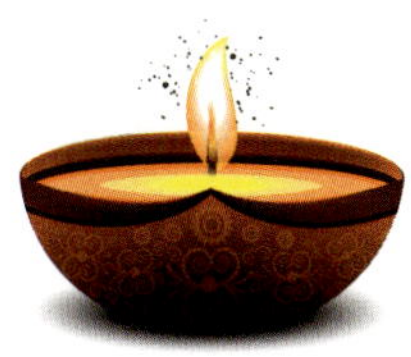

Couscous Salad

A quick n easy, and refreshing Mediterranean salad

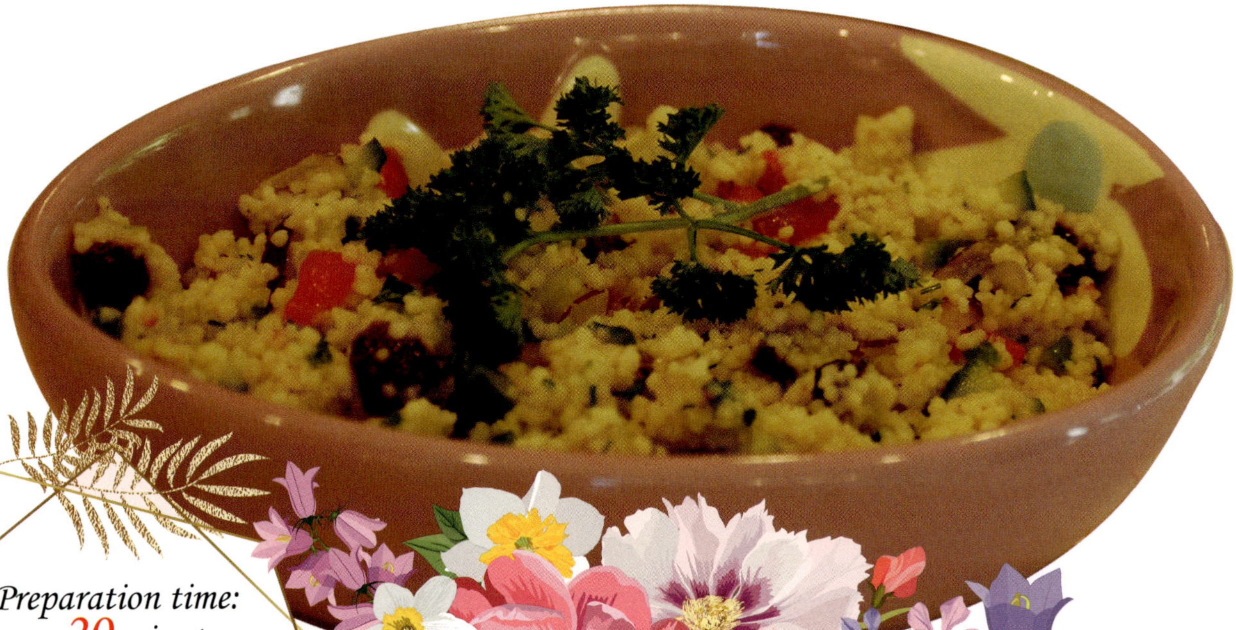

Preparation time: 20 *minutes*

Chilling time: 15 *minutes*

Servings: 6 *small bowls*

Ingredients

- 1½ cups Israeli couscous, cooked
- 1 small cucumber, finely chopped
- 10-12 cherry tomatoes, chopped
- 1-2 tablespoon or more red onions, sliced (optional)
- 1 tablespoon lemon zest
- 1-2 tablespoons orange zest
- 3 tablespoons (or according to taste) orange juice
- 1-2 tablespoons lemon juice
- 1 green chilli, finely chopped
- coriander leaves or dill leaves, finely chopped (a few sprigs)
- 1-2 tablespoons olive oil
- ½ cup walnuts, cranberries and golden raisins
- salt and black pepper to taste

Process

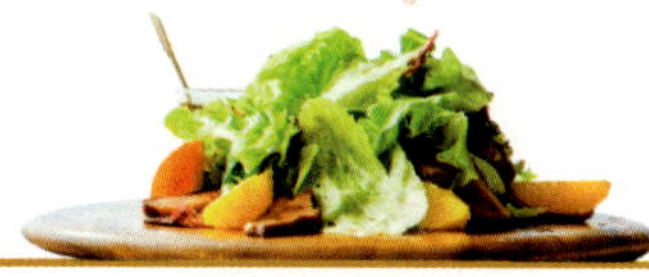

1. To the couscous, add 2 cups of boiling water and cook for 10 minutes. Drain and run cold water.
2. Transfer couscous to a mixing bowl. To this add cucumber, tomatoes, onions, lemon zest, orange zest, orange juice, lemon juice, chillies, coriander or dill, olive oil, walnuts, cranberries, raisins, salt, pepper, and stir.
3. Chill the salad in the refrigerator for 15 minutes and serve.

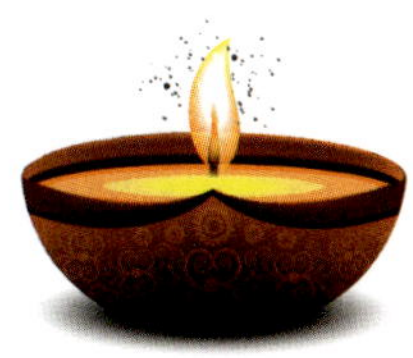

Quinoa Salad

Great tasting powerhouse of proteins and vitamins

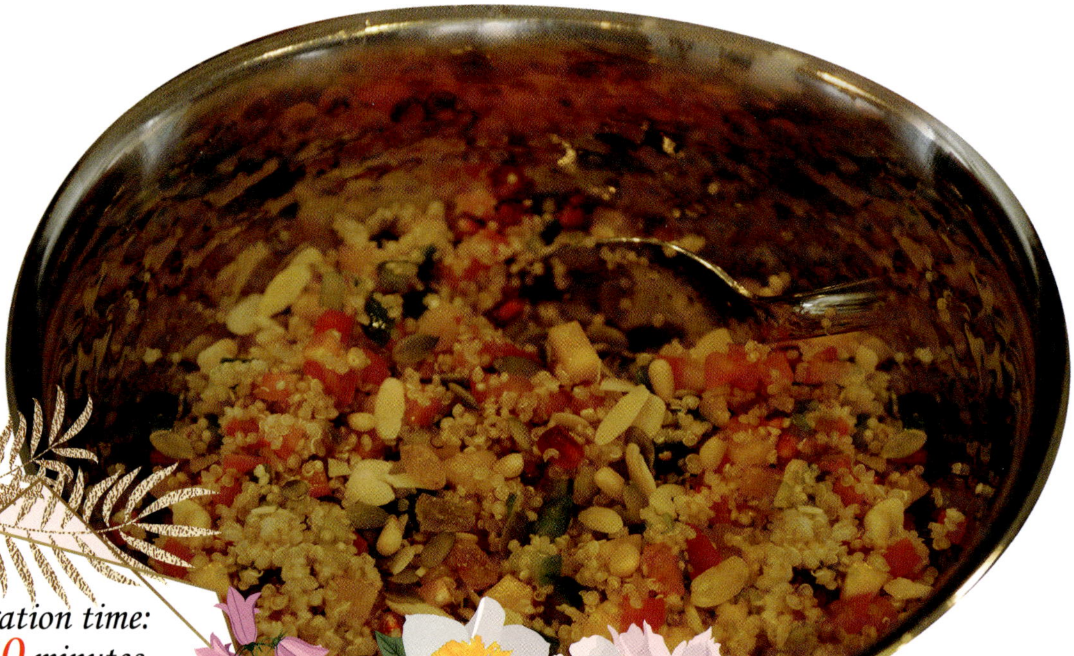

Preparation time:
20 *minutes*
(additional time for overnight refrigeration)

Cooking time:
15 *minutes*

Servings:
5 *salad plates*

Ingredients

For the salad

- 1 cup raw quinoa (3 cups cooked and chilled)
- 1 carrot, peeled and grated
- 1 English cucumber, finely chopped
- 1 green bell pepper, finely chopped
- 1 floret broccoli, finely chopped
- 1 ripe mango, finely chopped
- 3 strawberries, finely chopped
- 1/4 cup cilantro, freshly chopped
- 2 tablespoons mint, freshly chopped
- 1 tablespoon pine nuts
- 1 tablespoon walnuts, chopped
- 1 tablespoon almonds, sliced
- 1 tablespoon cranberries
- 1/4 teaspoon crushed pepper
- 1/2 teaspoon salt

For the dressing

- 1 lime, freshly squeezed lime juice
- 1/2 tablespoon olive oil
- 1 teaspoon red wine vinaigrette (optional)

Process

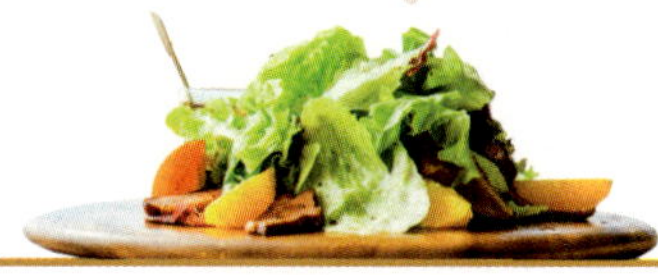

1. In a medium saucepan, add washed quinoa, salt and 2 cups water. Bring to a boil and then reduce heat to low, cover, and cook for 15 minutes, until the quinoa is cooked. Drain the excess water with a strainer. Transfer to a serving bowl and let it cool in the refrigerator overnight.
2. To the cooled quinoa add carrot, cucumber, bell pepper, broccoli, mango, strawberries, fresh herbs, nuts and the dressing.
3. Toss well, taste and add lime juice if necessary.
4. Chill in the refrigerator until ready to serve.

Spicy Taco Salad

A salad that features a tangy, refreshing taste of the Southwest

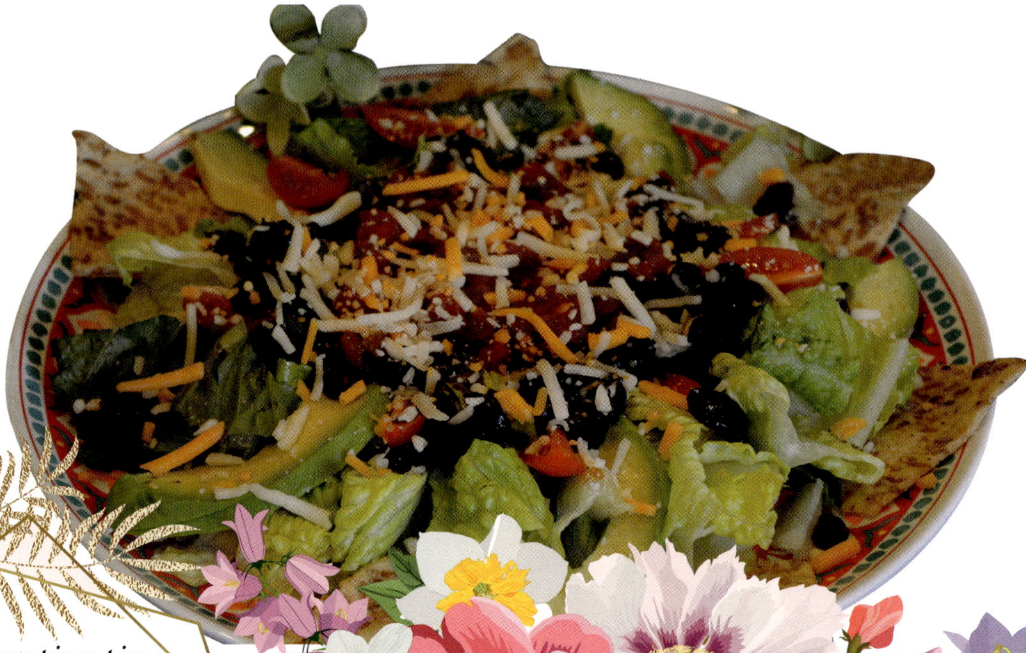

Preparation time:
20 *minutes*

Cooking time:
about 7-12 *minutes*

Servings:
4 *salad plates*
(or, 4 medium bowls)

Ingredients

- 1 can (16 oz.) black beans, (no or less salt), rinsed and drained
- 4 cups romaine lettuce, chopped
- 12 cherry tomatoes, halved or 3-4 tomatoes chopped
- 1 avocado, sliced
- 1 onion, chopped (optional)
- 1 tablespoon green chillies or jalapeños, finely chopped
- ½ cup dried cranberries
- ½ cup grated Mexican 3-cheese
- 1 cup hot/medium salsa (low sodium)
- 1 tablespoon canola oil

Process

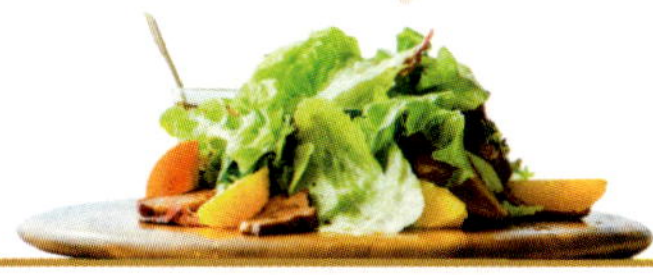

1. Heat the oil in a large pan over medium heat. If using onions, add the chopped onions and cook for about 3-4 minutes or until they soften.
2. Add beans and green chillies/jalapeños. Cook for 5-7 minutes, stirring frequently.
3. Divide lettuce among 4 salad plates/bowls.
4. On each plate, top the lettuce with the onion-beans mixture and tomatoes.
5. Add cheese, avocado, cranberries and salsa.

Serving tip: Serve with whole grain baked tortilla chips.

Toasted Almond Apple Salad

A tasty crunchy mix of apples, almonds and greens topped with honey-mustard dressing

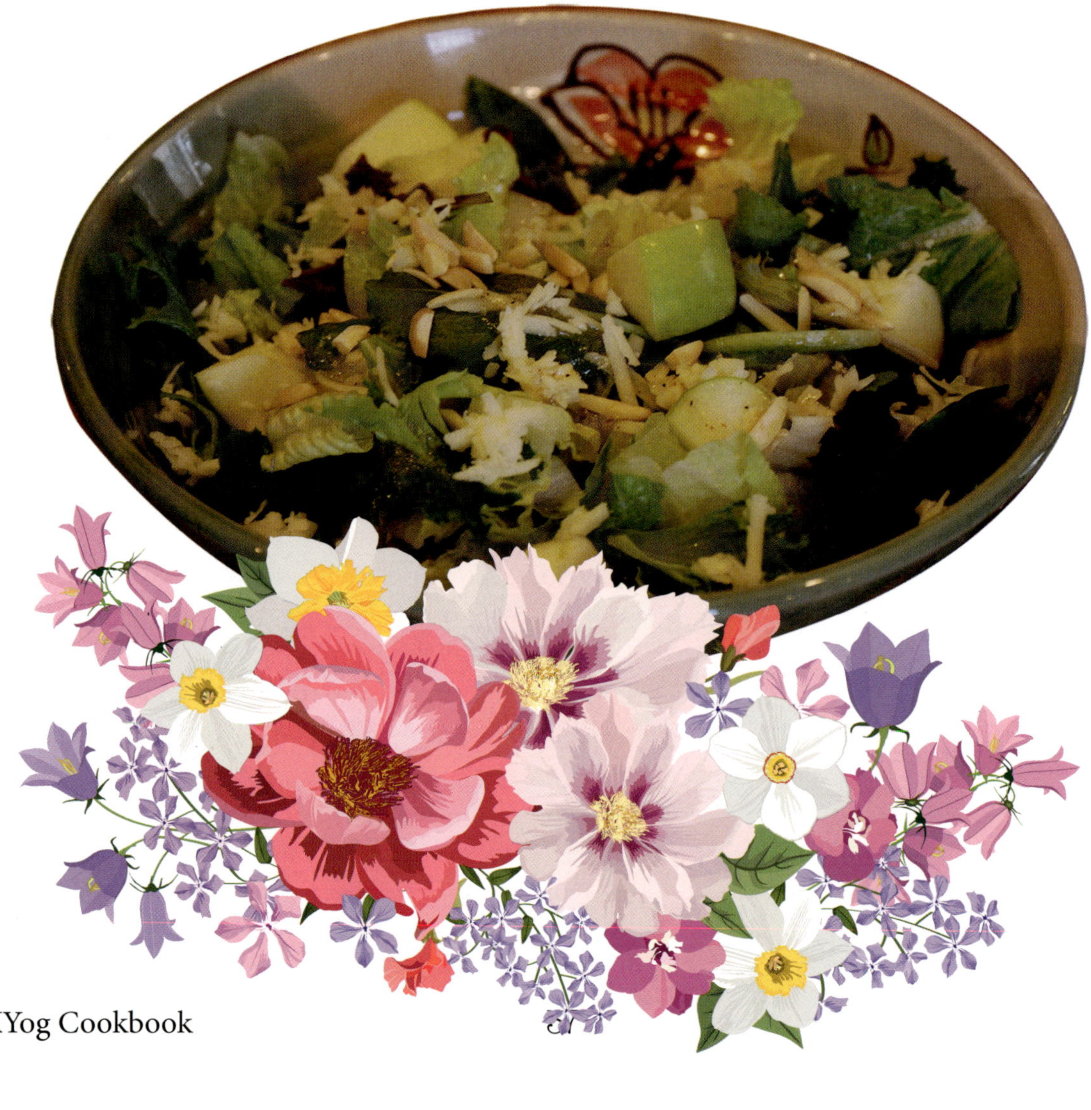

Ingredients

For the salad

- ½ cup slivered almonds, toasted
- 3 golden delicious apples, cut into small cubes
- 6 oz. romaine lettuce
- 6 oz. mixed spring greens
- 6 to 7 oz. of white sharp cheddar cheese, shaved or grated

For the dressing

- 1 tablespoon mustard
- 1 tablespoon honey
- ⅓ cup of vegetable or canola oil
- 1 tablespoon apple cider vinegar
- salt and black pepper to taste

Process

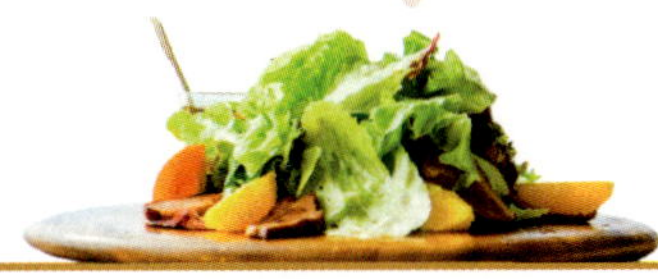

For the salad

1. Pre-heat oven to 350 degrees.
2. Toast almonds for a few minutes until light brown.
3. Mix romaine lettuce, mixed greens and apples in a bowl.
4. Add cheese and toasted almond just before serving.

For the dressing

5. Whisk all ingredients in a small bowl. Pour over the salad just before serving.

Optional note: For the dressing the apple cider vinegar may be substituted with red vine vinaigrette or lemon juice.

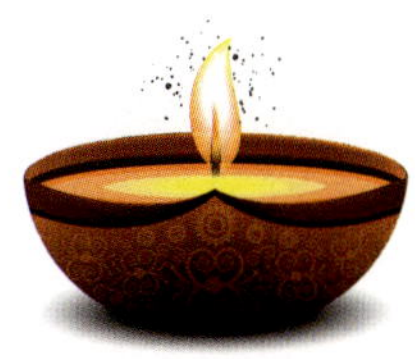

Snacks – Appetizers

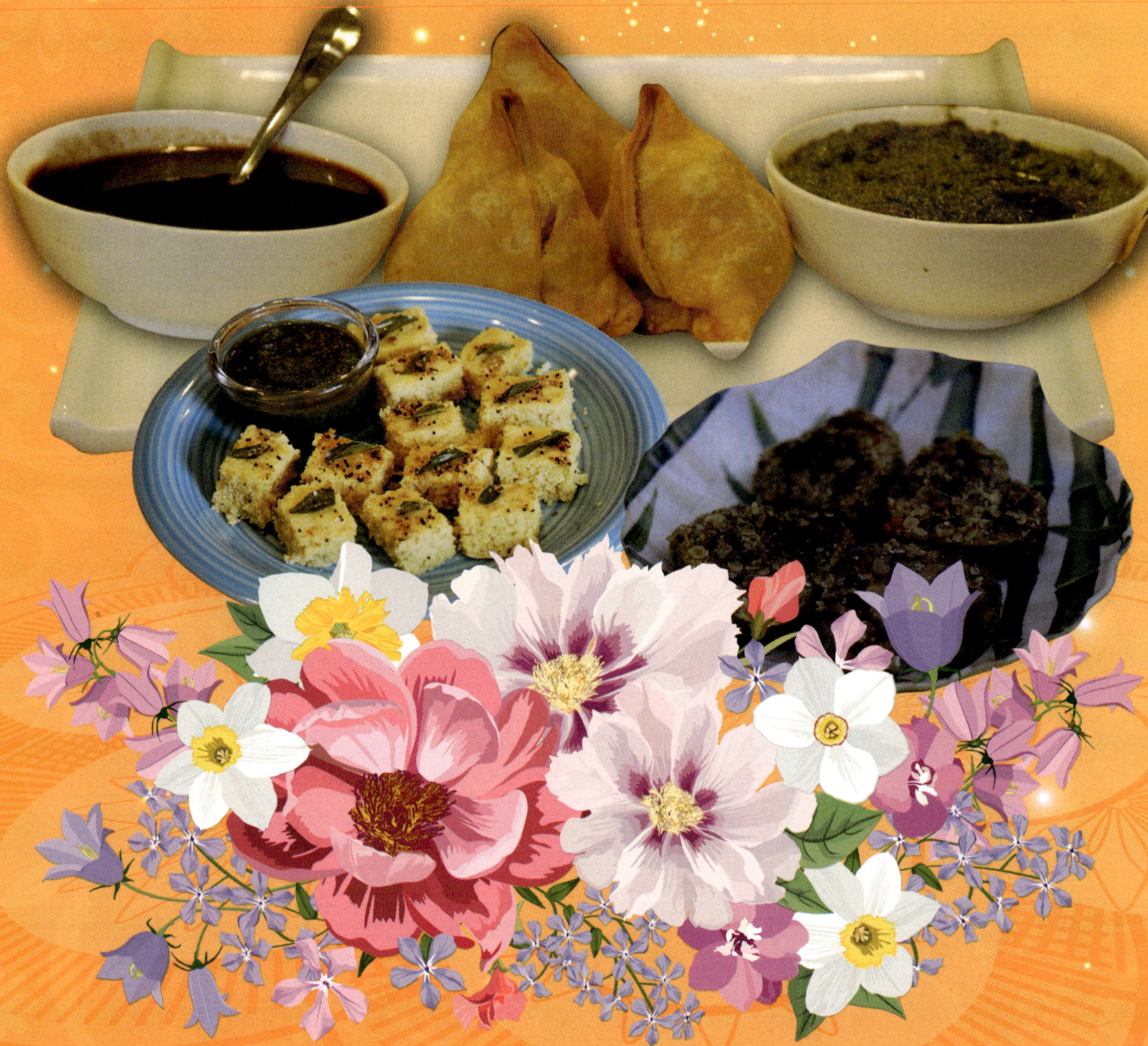

Indian cuisine offers an array of preparations that can be served as snacks and appetizers and many are popular street foods too. This chapter includes recipes that are mostly served as snacks and appetizers or can even be light breakfast or lunch box options. Others that can also become mini meal options have been presented in the next chapter.

Dhoklas, idlis and vadas are popular healthy choices even though making them requires pre-planning in terms of soaking, fermenting and grinding. *Masala rava idli* is an easier option to prepare. *Oats tikki, vegetable bean cutlets, kale pakoras* and *albeli chaat* are healthier versions of the traditional recipes. *Samosas*, an all-time favorite is a popular choice. *Paneer chilli* from Indo-Chinese cuisine is another well-liked starter option.

Preparing these snacks employs various cooking methods such as fermenting, steaming, shallow frying, deep frying and baking. The methods have been explained in detail here but cooking times can be drastically reduced by using alternate methods or buying fresh batters from stores.

1. Lentil Dhokla
2. Buckwheat Dhokla
3. Masala Rava Idli
4. Masala Oats Idli
5. Oats Healthy Tikki
6. Vegetable Bean Cutlet
7. Kale Pakoras
8. Chana Dal Vada
9. Sabudana Vada
10. Samosa
11. Paneer Chilli
12. Albeli Chaat

Lentil Dhokla

A traditional Gujarati preparation made with mixed lentils and rice

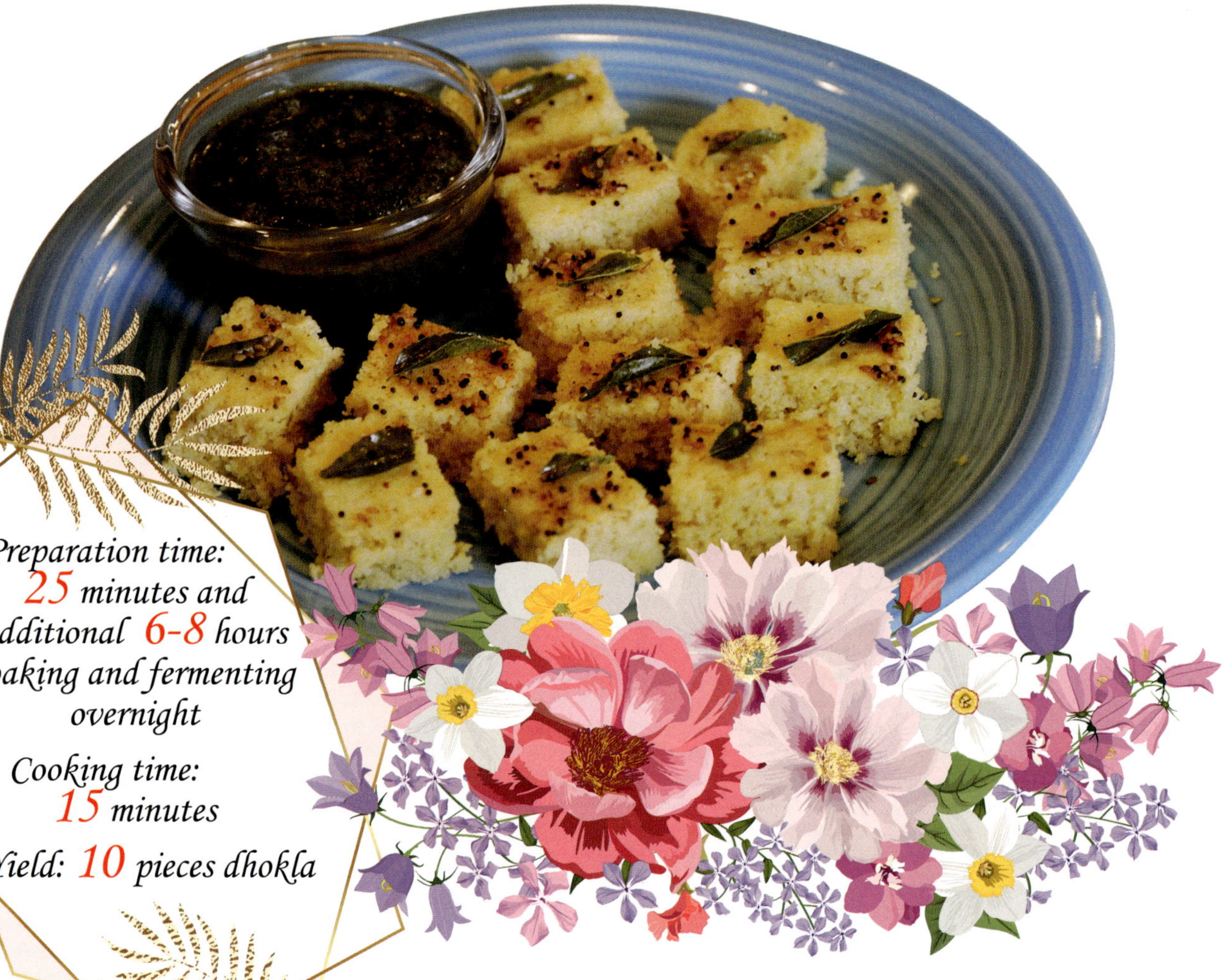

Preparation time: 25 *minutes and additional* 6-8 *hours soaking and fermenting overnight*

Cooking time: 15 *minutes*

Yield: 10 *pieces dhokla*

Ingredients

- 1½ cups chana dal (gram dal)
- ½ cup urad dal (split black dal)
- 1 cup rice
- ½ cup yogurt
- 2 green chillies
- 1 small piece of ginger
- 2 tablespoons grated coconut (for garnishing)
- ¼ teaspoon roasted sesame seeds (for garnishing)
- 2 tablespoons chopped cilantro (for garnishing)
- 2 teaspoons baking soda or 2 teaspoons Eno salts
- ¼ teaspoon chilli powder
- 3 tablespoons vegetable oil
- salt to taste

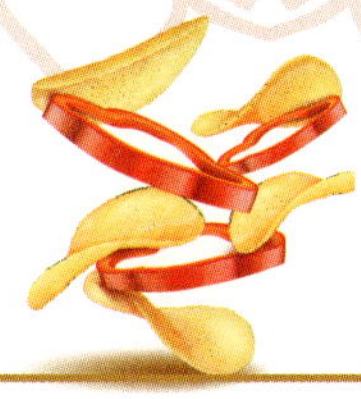

Process

1. Wash chana, urad dal, and rice and soak them together in approximately double water for 6 hours.
2. Drain well and grind the soaked lentils and rice in a food processor with little water to make a smooth mixture.
3. Grind green chillies and ginger along with it. The batter should be of the same consistency as idli batter, on the thicker side, not watery.
4. Mix yogurt into the batter and keep batter covered overnight to ferment.
5. For preparing dhoklas, first grease a big thali (big steel plate with lips)/ or dhokla steamer trays with little oil.
6. Just before steaming add oil and baking soda or Eno salts to the batter and mix in, not overdoing it as the batter is immediately activated.

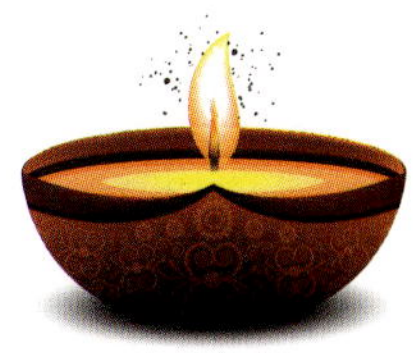

Note: If using a big thali add the 2 teaspoons of baking powder or Eno salts all at once but if using a small one and cooking in 2 batches, mix only half.

7. Pour the batter on a greased thali/plate and put the them in the steamer. A pressure cooker without a whistle may be used in place of a steamer too.
8. Cover and steam for 20 minutes on medium heat.
9. Take off heat, cool for 5 minutes and then remove the dhoklas still slightly warm. Slice them in 15-20 minutes to get clean cut pieces.
10. Garnish by sprinkling red chilli powder, coconut, cilantro and roasted sesame seed on top and serve hot with green chutney.

Alternate tip: Tempering made with mustard seeds may also be added in the end or mustard seeds may be added to the batter before steaming.

Buckwheat Dhokla

A healthier spin on the basic Gujarati dhokla and a quick to prepare fasting food

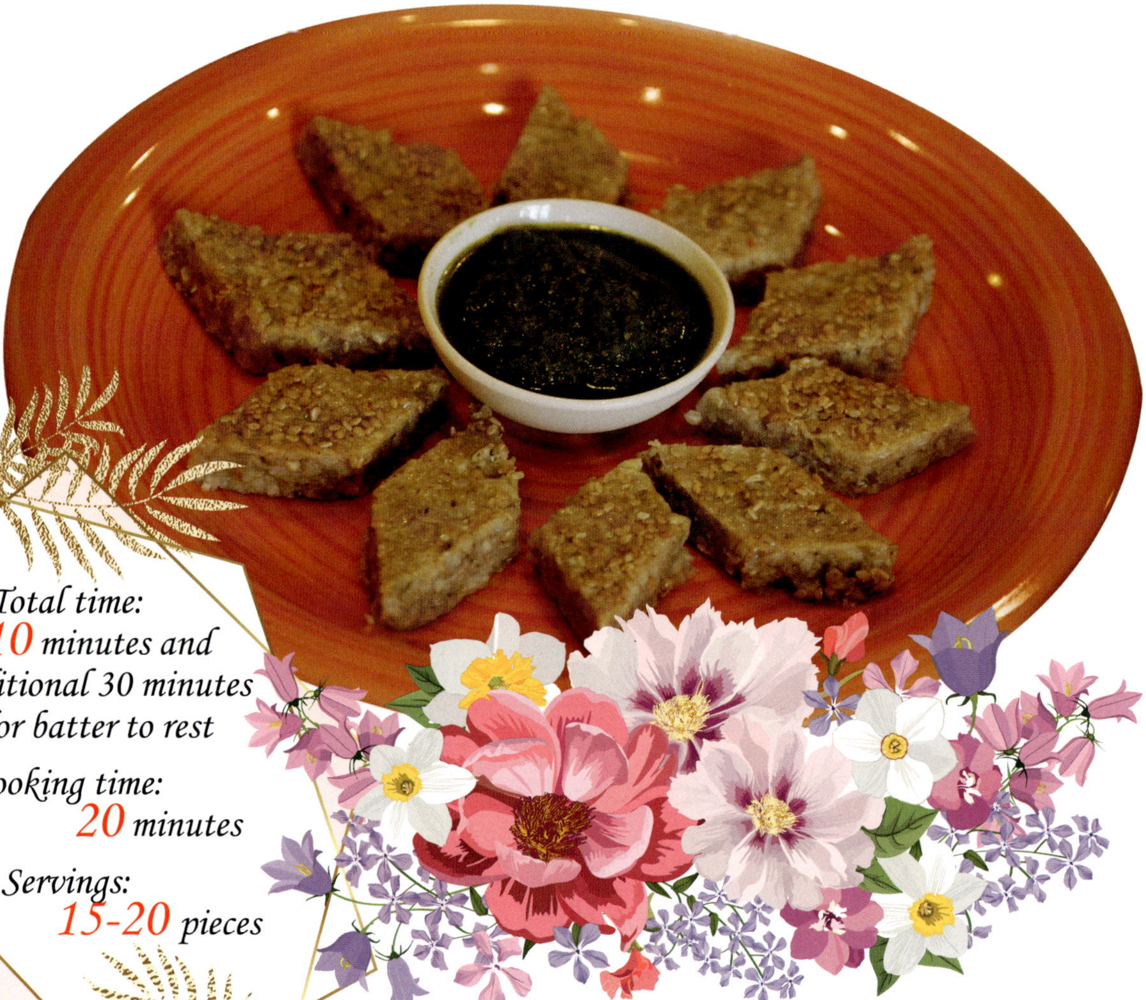

Total time:
10 minutes and additional 30 minutes for batter to rest

Cooking time:
20 minutes

Servings:
15-20 pieces

Ingredients

- 1 cup of coarse buckwheat (Red Mills Organic brand)
- 1 cup of plain yogurt (sour is preferred)
- 1 teaspoon ginger, grated
- 1 teaspoon green chilli, chopped
- 1 teaspoon coriander chopped for garnish
- ¼ teaspoon oil for greasing
- ½ teaspoon ENO fruit salt
- ½ teaspoon pepper
- salt to taste

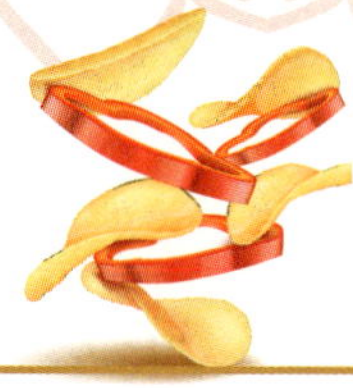

Process

1. Wash the buckwheat and add yogurt. Mix well. Let it rest for 30 minutes.
2. Add ginger chilli and salt to the mixture. Mix well to make a dhokla batter consistency.
3. Just before steaming add the fruit salt to the batter and sprinkle a little water over it so that it forms bubbles. Mix it in quickly.
4. Pour the batter on a greased pan/plate and put that in the steamer. In place of a steamer, a pressure cooker without the whistle may be used too.
5. Sprinkle coarse pepper evenly on it.
6. Steam for 15 to 20 minutes till the dhokla is cooked well.
7. Cool and cut into square pieces.
8. Garnish with coriander and serve.

Serving tip: This recipe without tempering in the end, or just using roasted sesame seeds makes this a good choice for serving as a fasting food.

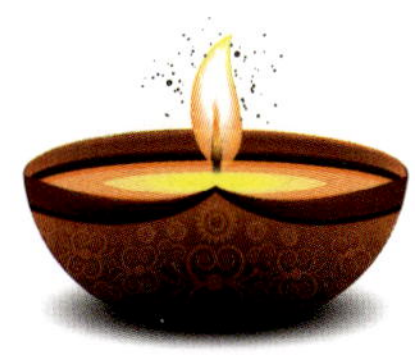

Masala Rava Idli

A low-calorie light snack that is easy to digest – also a lunchbox and snack option for kids

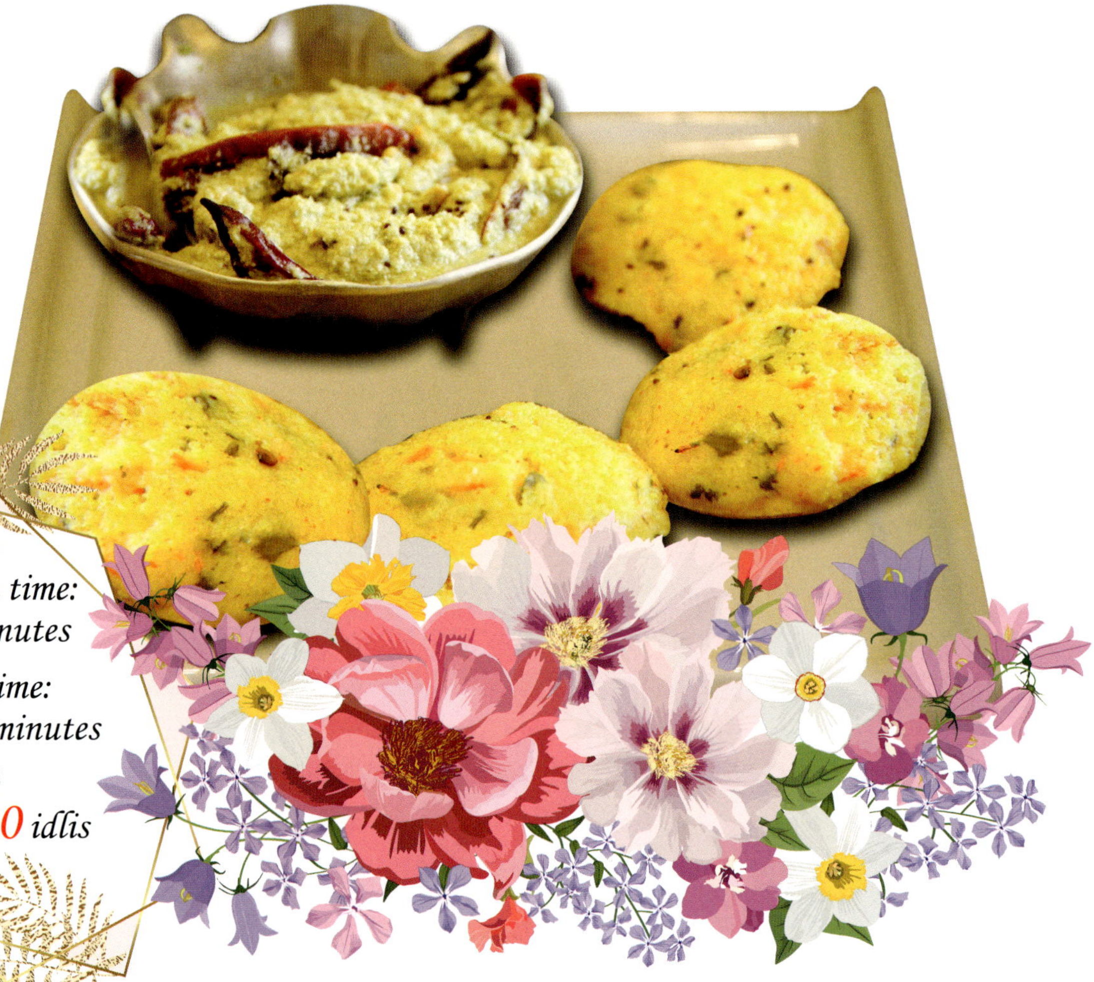

Preparation time:
30 *minutes*

Cooking time:
20 *minutes*

Yield:
20 *idlis*

Ingredients

- 2 cups sooji, coarse (cream of wheat/ semolina)
- 1 cup sour curd
- 1 cup water
- 1 teaspoon ginger, finely grated
- 3 sprigs curry leaves
- 2 green chillies, finely chopped
- 1 tablespoon cilantro, finely chopped
- 1 tablespoon cashews, broken
- 1 teaspoon turmeric
- 2 teaspoons ENO fruit salts
- 3 teaspoons salt, or to taste

For the tempering

- 1 teaspoon mustard seeds
- ⅓ teaspoon asafoetida
- 1 whole red chilli
- 1 teaspoon chana dal
- 1 teaspoon urad dal
- 2 teaspoons ghee/oil for tempering and some oil for greasing plates/trays

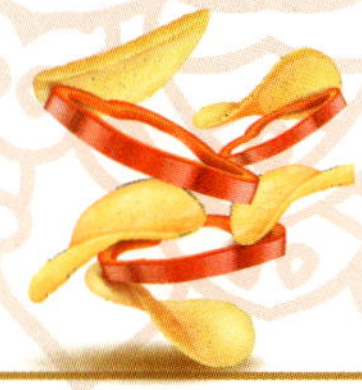

Process

1. In a medium pan, heat the ghee/oil saving enough for greasing the trays. To this add mustard seeds and when they pop, add asafoetida, whole red chilli, chana dal and urad dal. When the dal turns brown add the sooji and roast it along with the previously added ingredients till it becomes light brown. Let it cool for 10 minutes.
2. In another small bowl mix yogurt with curry leaves, green chillies, cilantro, ginger, turmeric and salt. Mix it all well.
3. To the yogurt mix add the roasted sooji mix and mix well till there are no lumps. Add water and let it rest for 15 minutes. The batter should be of idli like consistency. More water can be added if required.
4. Prepare the idli steamer by pre-heating the water and grease the idli trays with ghee/ oil.
5. Now mix in ENO salts to the batter and it becomes very light. Immediately pour it in idli trays and steam for 15 minutes on medium heat.
6. Cool the idlis for 7-8 minutes. Then remove idlis with a spoon and serve hot with sambar, coconut or almond chutneys.

Time-saver tip: A large batch of sooji mix may be prepared ahead of time and stored in the refrigerator to save idli preparation time.

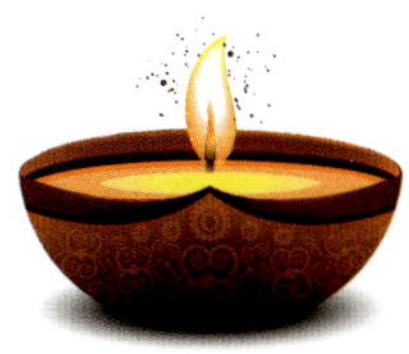

Masala Oats Idlis

A tasty low calorie and nutritious food option

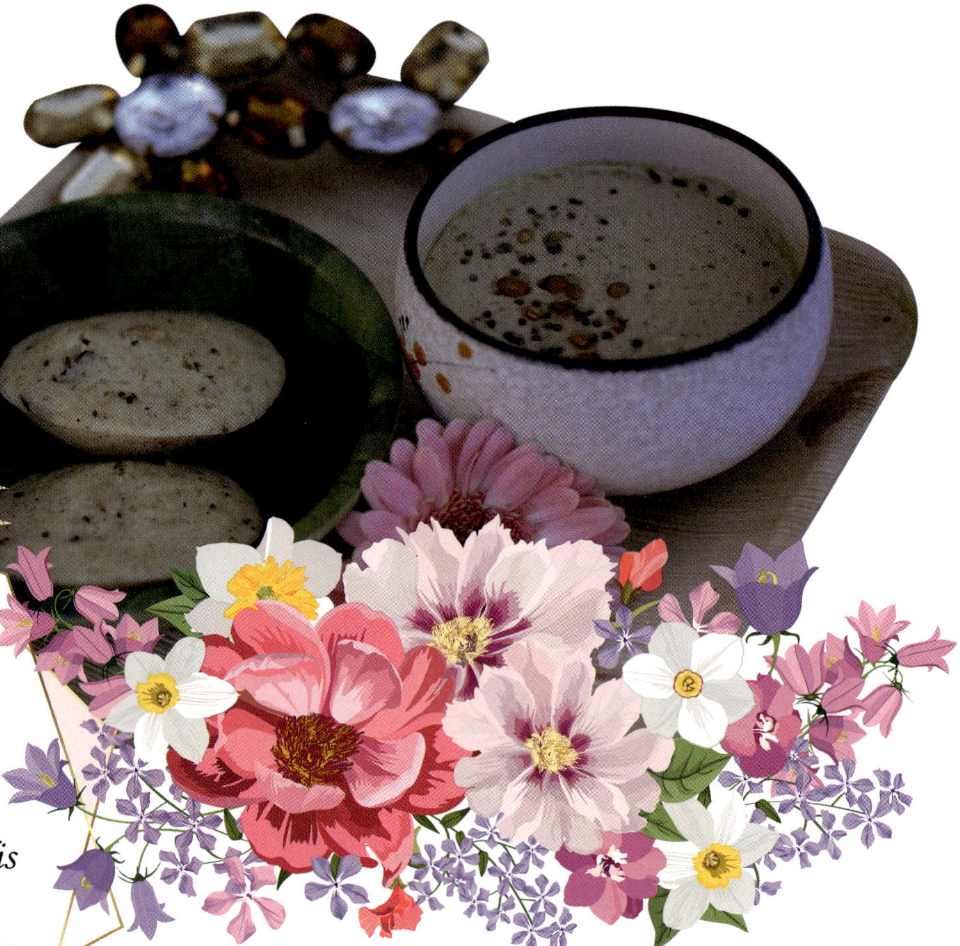

Preparation time: 25 *minutes*

Cooking time: 30 *minutes*

Yield: 16-20 *idlis*

Ingredients

For idli batter

- 1 cup coarse sooji
- 2 cup powdered oats, coarsely ground instant oats
- 1 cup plain yogurt
- ½ cup shredded carrots
- 1 teaspoon green chillies, finely chopped
- 1 teaspoon ginger, minced
- 2 teaspoons Eno fruit salts
- ½ teaspoon flax seed powder
- 1 cup water or maybe more to get a thicker idli consistency
- 1 teaspoon salt
- 1 cup water for idli steamer
- oil for greasing idli mold trays

For tempering

- ½ teaspoon mustard seeds
- 1 teaspoon chana dal
- 1 teaspoon urad dal
- ¼ cup cashew nuts, broken
- sprig of curry leaves
- 2 tablespoons vegetable oil

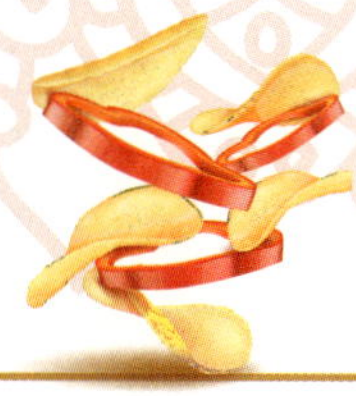

Process

1. To prepare the idli batter, in a mixing bowl combine sooji, oats and salt. Add yogurt and mix it well. Keep aside for 15 minutes.
2. To prepare the tempering for the batter, heat oil in a pan on medium heat and add mustard seeds. Whey they crackle, add urad and chana dal. Once they are cooked add the cashew nuts. Roast until light brown and turn off the heat. Add curry leaves now. Once they are cooked pour this tempering over the idli batter prepared in step 1.
3. Then mix other ingredients in the idli batter - shredded carrots, green chillies, minced ginger and flax seed powder ensuring everything is mixed well.
4. Now, prepare the idli pot for steaming idlis. Heat a cup of water in the steamer and grease idli mold trays.
5. If sooji batter is too thick, ½ cup to ¾ cups of water can be added to get the right idli batter consistency.
6. Just when ready to steam, mix in the Eno fruit salts to the idli batter, and pour the batter into the mold trays. Steam for about 12-15 minutes on medium heat.
7. Let them cool for a few minutes and then using a spoon remove the idlis from the molds. Serve with sambar and chutney.

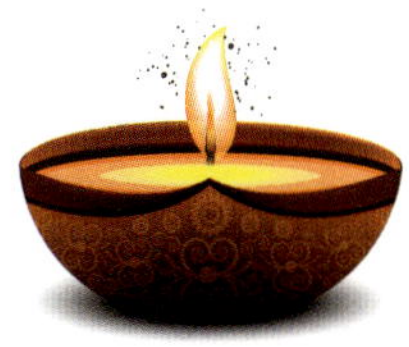

Oats Healthy Tikki

Tasty and crunchy, enriched with the goodness of oats

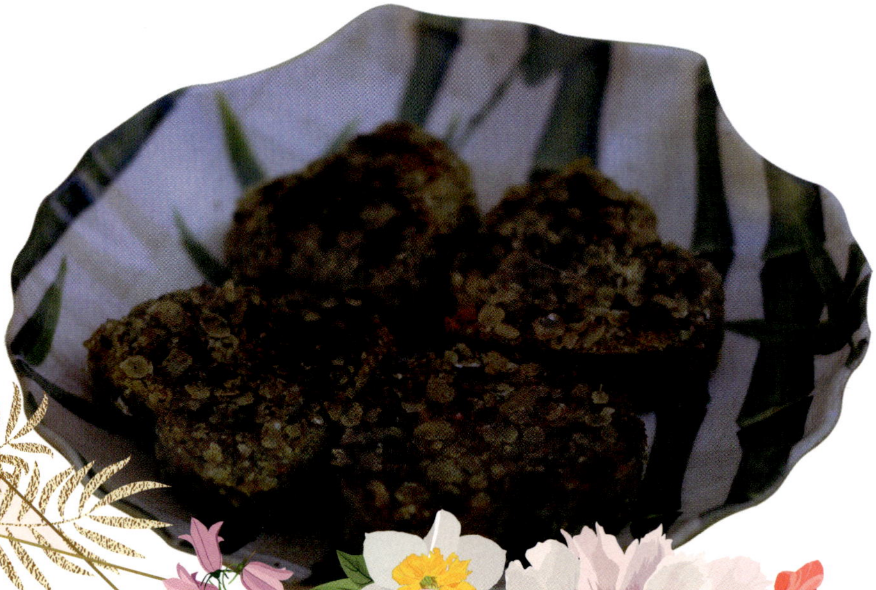

Preparation time: 50 *minutes*

Cooking time: 10-12 *minutes per batch*

Yield: 12 *tikkis*

Ingredients

- 1 cup instant cooking rolled oats
- 1 cup boiled potato, mashed
- ¼ cup grated paneer
- ¼ cup grated carrot
- ¼ cup boiled peas
- 2 tablespoons cilantro, finely chopped
- 1 teaspoon lemon juice
- ½ teaspoon ginger paste
- 1 teaspoon crushed or chopped green chilli
- ½ teaspoon garam masala
- 1 teaspoon dried mango powder (amchur)
- 1 teaspoon turmeric powder
- 1 teaspoon sesame seed
- salt to taste

Other Ingredients:

- ¼ cup water
- ½ cup bread crumbs for coating
- 1 ½ teaspoons oil for greasing and cooking

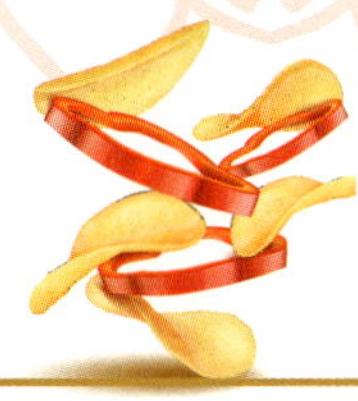

Process

1. Combine all the ingredients in a deep bowl and mix well.
2. Divide the mixture into 12 equal parts and press slightly with both hands to make a tikki shape.
3. Dip each tikki in the water and roll them in bread crumbs.
4. Heat a non-stick griddle/tawa and grease it with oil.
5. On medium heat, cook a batch of tikkis until they turn golden brown on both sides. Depending on the size of the griddle they can be cooked in 2 or more batches.
6. Serve tikkis hot with green chutney.

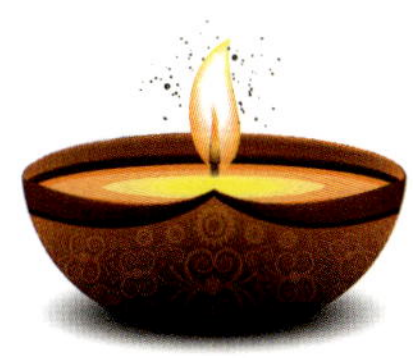

Vegetable Bean Cutlet

A delicious and healthy protein appetizer enjoyed with chutneys or ketchup

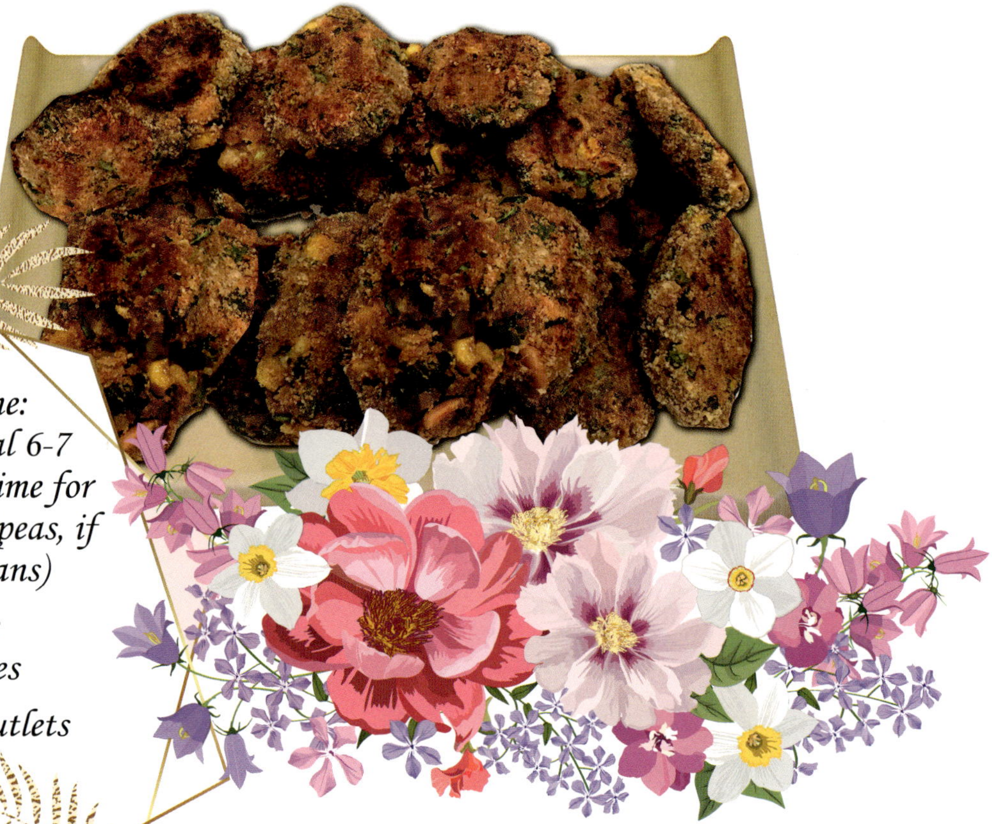

Preparation time: 30 *(additional 6-7 hours soaking time for beans and chickpeas, if using dry beans)*

Cooking time: 20 *minutes*

Yield: 20 *cutlets*

Ingredients

- 2 medium size sweet potatoes, boiled, mashed or finely chopped
- 1 bunch spinach, finely chopped and boiled
- 1 medium size green pepper, finely chopped
- 1 can black beans, boiled and mashed or ¼ cup dry beans
- ½ can chickpeas, boiled and mashed, or ⅛ cup chickpeas (kabuli chana)
- 2 green chillies, finely chopped
- 1-inch ginger, finely chopped
- ½ cup cilantro, finely chopped
- ½ cup (or more) breadcrumbs (as required for binding)
- 1 teaspoon turmeric powder
- 2 teaspoons garam masala or as per taste
- red chilli powder as per taste (optional)
- vegetable oil for frying
- salt to taste

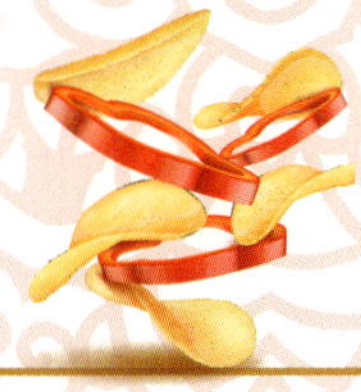

Process

1. Soak black beans and chickpeas for 6-7 hours and pressure cook them for 15 minutes. Once cooked, drain excess water and allow it to cool. If using canned beans, boil them for 10 minutes, drain the water and allow to cool. Mash the black beans and chickpeas.
2. Boil sweet potatoes in a pressure cooker or regular pan until cooked and soft. Once cooled peel the skin and finely chop or mash them.
3. Wash, chop and boil spinach, for 5 minutes
4. In a big mixing bowl add boiled sweet potatoes (either mashed or finely chopped).
5. Then, add the cooked spinach, mashed black beans and chickpeas, green pepper, chillies, ginger and cilantro.
6. Add turmeric powder, garam masala, red chilli powder and salt.
7. Mix all these ingredients gently in the bowl. Add bread crumbs to the mixture to absorb any extra water from mixture and prepare a soft dough. Let it rest for 20 minutes.
8. Make small balls for making cutlet. Take extra bread crumbs in plate. Roll the balls into this bread crumbs mixture and make cutlets of your desired shape.
9. Shallow fry in a frying pan until golden brown. Place on a paper towel to remove the excess oil.
10. Serve warm with chilli tomato sauce, other chutneys or tomato ketchup.

Alternate serving tip: These may be served inside a burger making it a more filling meal.

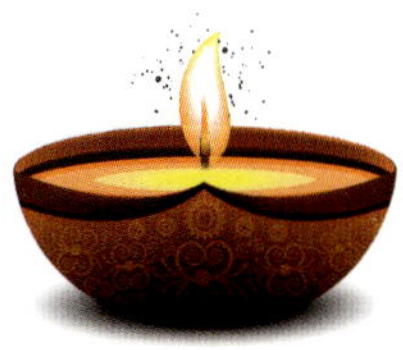

Kale Pakoras

A healthier and crispier twist to traditional pakoras

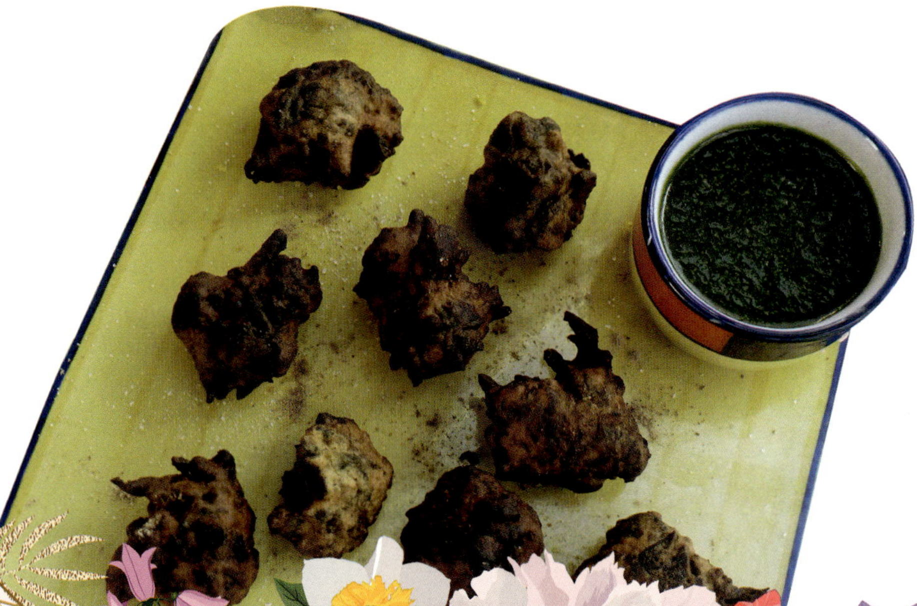

Preparation time: 20 *minutes*

Cooking time: 20 *minutes*

Servings: 20-25 *pakora pieces*

Ingredients

- 2 ½ cups gram flour (besan)
- 3-4 tablespoons rice flour
- 1 bunch kale, remove the thick stems from the leaves and chop coarsely
- 1 cup potatoes, chopped in small cubes
- 1 cup onions, finely chopped (optional)
- 1 teaspoon fresh ginger, minced
- 1 teaspoon garlic salt or 1 teaspoon minced fresh garlic (optional)
- 2 tablespoons cilantro, finely chopped
- lettuce leaves for serving (optional)
- 2 teaspoons garam masala
- 2 teaspoons turmeric
- 1 teaspoon red chilli powder
- red pepper flakes to taste (optional)
- pinch of baking soda
- water to make batter
- canola or vegetable oil for deep frying
- 2 teaspoons salt or to taste if using garlic salt

Process

1. In a bowl, mix the gram flour, rice flour, turmeric, garam masala, red pepper flakes, red chilli powder and baking soda together.
2. Add cilantro, ginger and garlic. Gradually add a small amount of water mixing until the mixture is a bit of a thick consistency. Add in the kale, potatoes, onion and mix well to coat all the vegetables.
3. Heat oil on medium heat in a skillet or wok.
4. Add salt to the batter before frying. Mix well.
5. Carefully place (using hand or spoon) the batter into the skillet/wok and cook on either side for about 3 minutes, or until the pakodas are crispy and brown.
6. Remove from heat and place on a paper towel to remove the excess oil.
7. Serve 2-3 pakoras in lettuce leaves with cilantro chutney.

Chana Dal Vada

A crunchy delight loved by kids

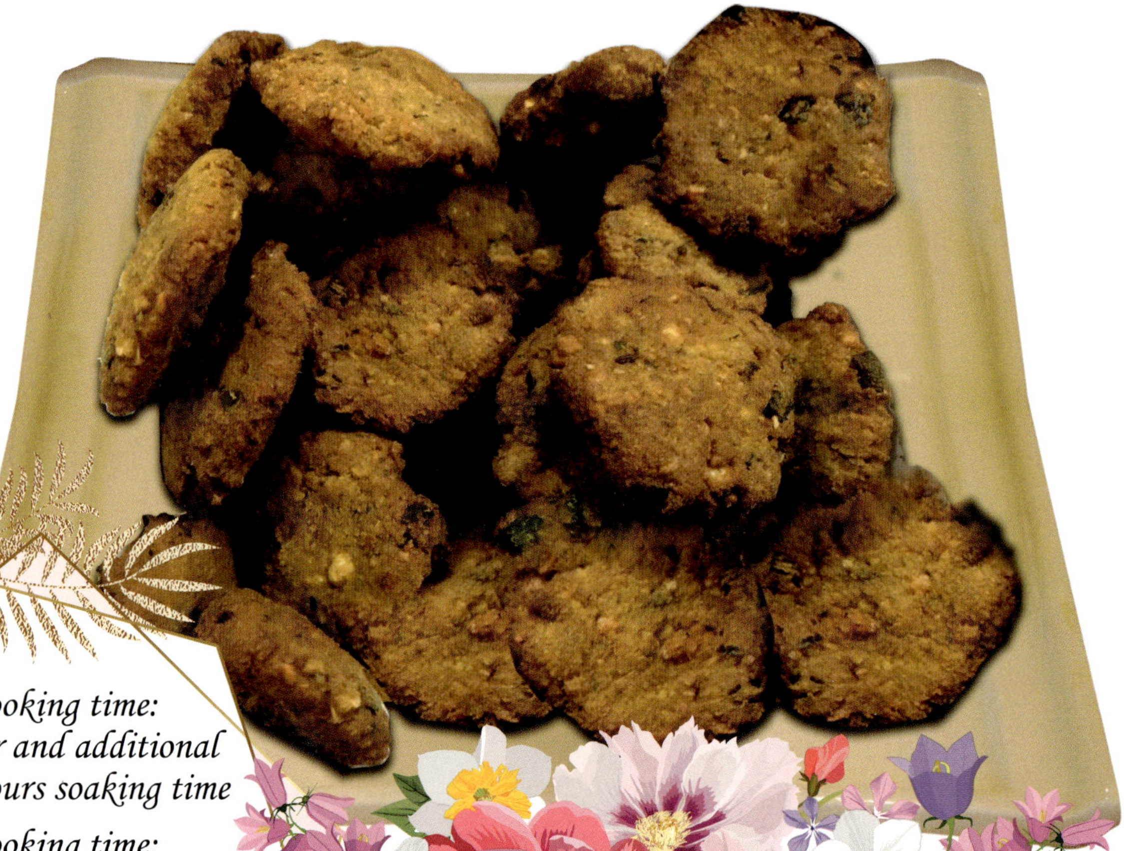

Cooking time:
1 hour and additional
5-6 hours soaking time

Cooking time:
1 hour

Servings:
15-20 vadas

Ingredients

- 2 cups chana dal
- 1 onion, chopped (optional)
- 1-inch ginger, grated
- 3 green chillies, or to taste
- 1 stalk curry leaves
- ½ cup mint leaves
- 1 cup cilantro, chopped
- ½ cup coconut, shredded, fresh or frozen
- few pinches asafoetida
- vegetable or peanut oil for frying
- salt to taste

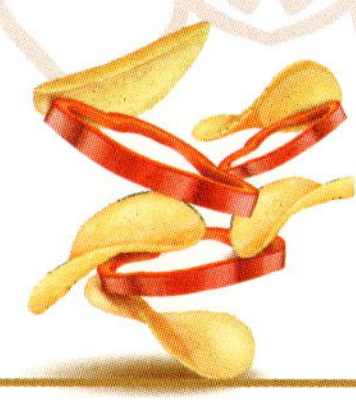

Process

1. Soak 2 cups of chana dal for 5-6 hours. Drain the water afterwards.
2. Grind dal coarsely along with cilantro, green chilli, ginger, coconut and salt with minimal water to make a thick batter.
3. Add chopped onion (if using) and mint leaves to the ground dal and mix well. Add the curry leaves and asafoetida.
4. Make small flattened balls of the mixture.
5. Heat oil in a pan (kadai/or a pan for frying) and keep on a medium flame.
6. Fry the vadas until brown. Remove from heat and place on a paper towel to remove the excess oil.
7. Serve hot with any coconut or pudina chutney.

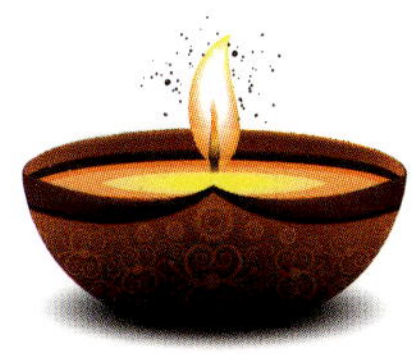

Sabudana Vada

A deep-fried teatime snack, a popular fasting food option and a kids' favorite

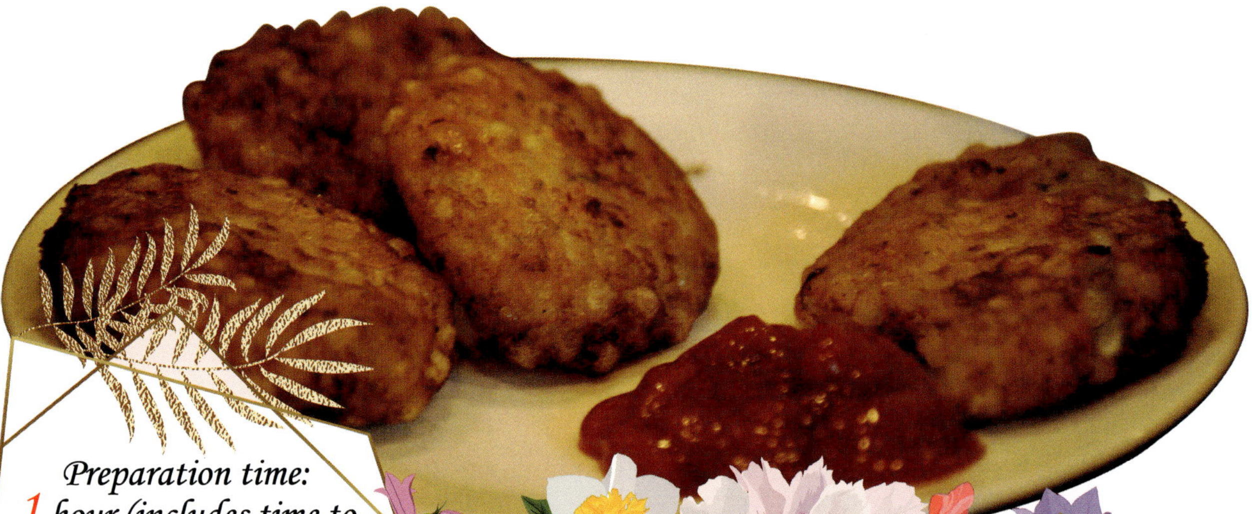

Preparation time:
1 hour (includes time to boil and mash potatoes. Additional 5-6 hours are required for presoaking the sabudana)

Cooking time:
45 minutes for frying

Yield: 30-35 vadas

Ingredients

- 1 ½ cups sabudana
- 4 medium potatoes, boiled and mashed
- ¼ cup roasted peanuts
- 2 teaspoons green chilli paste
- 2 teaspoons ginger paste
- 2 tablespoons cilantro leaves, chopped
- ½ teaspoon cumin seeds
- 1 teaspoon sesame seeds
- 1 teaspoon sugar
- 2 teaspoons lemon juice
- salt to taste

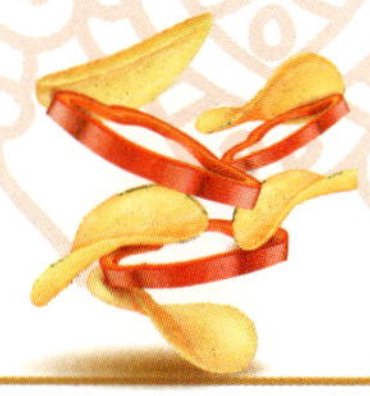

Process

1. Wash and soak sabudana for 5 to 6 hours.
   Note: Soak sabudana completely submerged in water for the first half an hour. Then drain excess water and continue soaking for another 5 hours. You will observe that the sabudana will double in size, each piece separate and can easily be pressed between fingers.
2. Roast peanuts and powder them coarsely.
3. Boil potatoes and mash them.
4. Mix together sabudana, mashed potato, roasted peanuts, green chilli paste, ginger paste, cilantro, cumin, sesame and salt. Add lemon juice and sugar and mix them all together to a dough like consistency.
5. Make 30 to 35 balls with hands and then flatten them with your palms to shape them like mini size flat patties – about 1.5-inch diameter.
6. Deep fry in hot oil until golden brown color.
7. Drain excess oil on paper towels and serve them hot with mint chutney or ketchup.

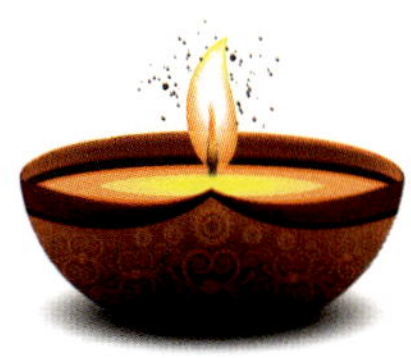

Samosa

Triangular crusty pastries filled with potatoes, peas and spices–an evergreen snack

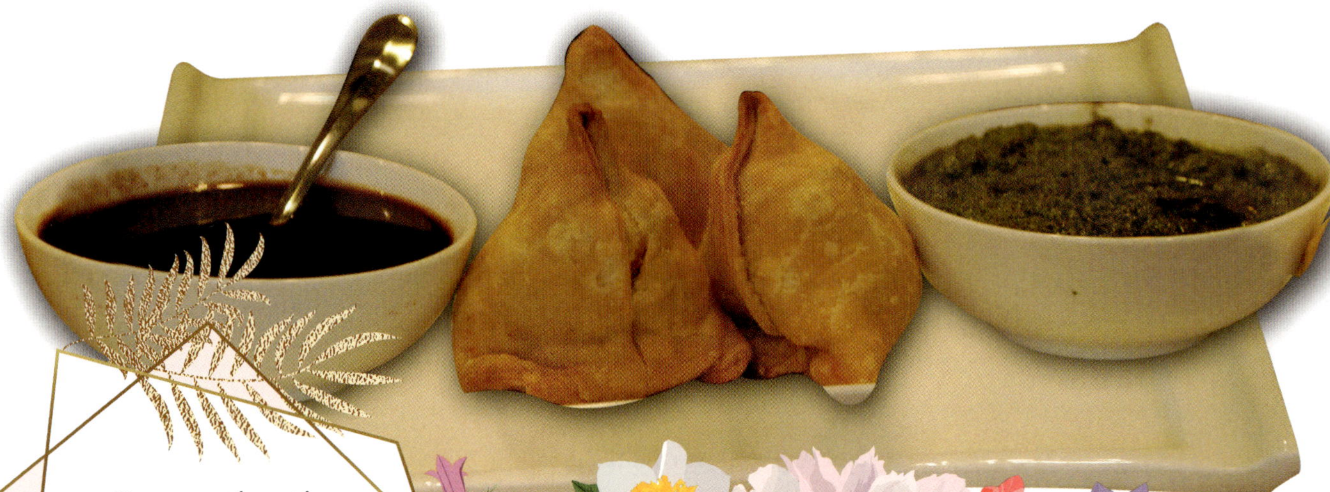

Preparation time:
20 minutes (additional time for boiling and cooling potatoes, and ½ hour for resting dough)

Cooking time:
30 minutes

Yield: 30 samosas

Ingredients

For filling

- 6 medium potatoes, boiled
- ½ cup green peas, boiled

For tempering

- 1 tablespoon olive oil
- 1 teaspoon mustard seeds
- 1 teaspoon cumin seeds
- 1 teaspoon coriander seeds
- 1 teaspoon fennel seeds
- ½ teaspoon asafoetida
- 1 teaspoon dry mango powder (amchur powder)
- 1 teaspoon turmeric powder
- 1 teaspoon garam masala powder
- 1 small bay leaf
- 1 dry red chilli
- 1 teaspoon green chilli, crushed
- 1 teaspoon ginger, crushed
- 5 to 6 curry leaves
- salt to taste

For the crust

- 2 ½ cups all-purpose flour (maida)
- 4 tablespoons ghee
- ½ cup water
- 1 teaspoon carom seeds
- 1 teaspoon salt

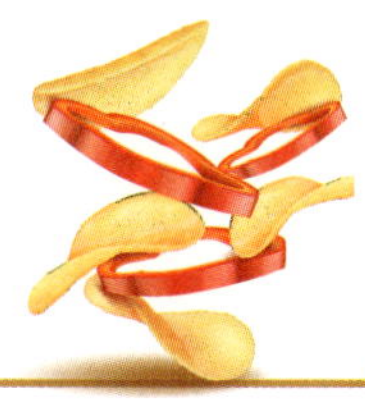

Process

For samosa crust dough

1. Mix all-purpose flour, ghee, carom seeds and salt together. Rub the flour well with two hands so that the fat is worked well into the flour.
2. Then add water little by little and make a stiff dough.
3. Cover with a muslin cloth or keep in airtight container and let it rest for half an hour.

For samosa filling

4. In a deep bowl, take boiled potatoes, green peas and crumble them coarsely. Keep aside.

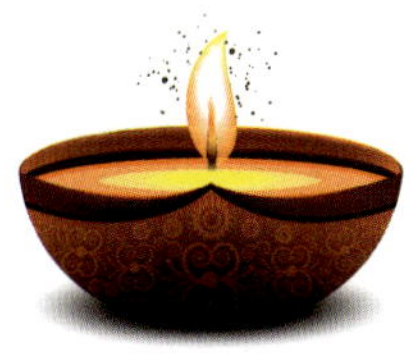

5. In a small vessel heat oil for tempering. Add mustard, cumin, fennel and coriander seeds and let them pop, keeping low-medium heat so that the tempering does not get burned.
6. Then add asafoetida, bay leaf, curry leaves, red chilli, ginger paste, green chilli paste, turmeric, amchur powder, garam masala and salt.
7. Pour the tempering over the crumbled potatoes and peas and mix them well. Let this filling cool down.

Making samosas

8. Once again, knead the dough and make about 15 balls of equal size.
9. Roll out each ball into a round shape, like a thin poorie/or pastry of about 5-inch diameter.
10. Cut from the middle to make two halves.
11. Moisten the straight edges of the cut half with water and make a cone shape by pressing the edges together. Fill the cone with samosa filling and tightly seal the open edges of the samosa with water.
12. Repeat for rest of the balls.
13. Heat oil in a deep pan/kadai for deep frying the samosas.
14. On medium heat fry the samosas in batches of 5-6 depending on the pan/kadai size, and ensuring that all sides are golden in color. Remove from oil and drain the excess oil on paper towels.
15. Serve warm with tamarind-date chutney, mint-coriander chutney or just tomato ketchup.

Time-saver tip: Half cooked frozen wheat rotis sold at Indian stores/or tortillas can be used for the samosa crust, stuffing them with samosa filling, and having samosas ready in no time.

Albeli Chaat

A unique chaat presented in a criss-cross potato basket

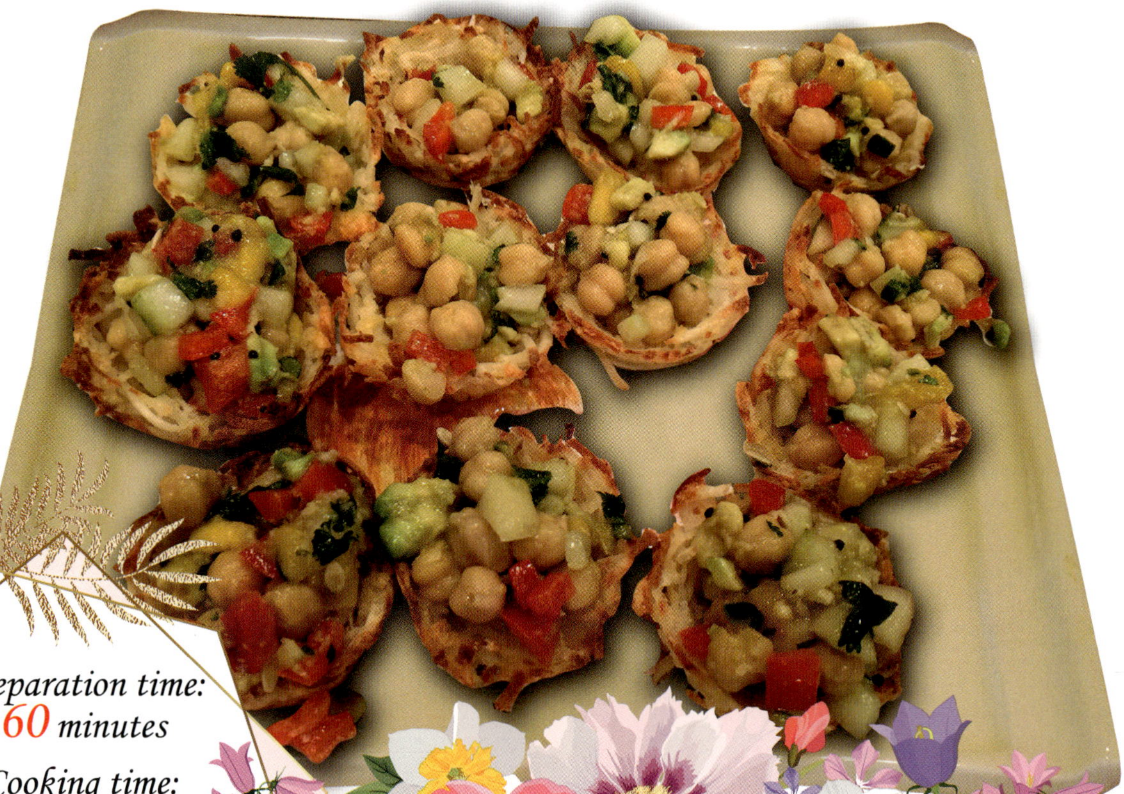

Preparation time: **60** *minutes*

Cooking time: **30** *minutes*

Servings: **20** *cups*

Ingredients

For the potato basket/cups

- 8-10 small julienned potatoes
- 1 teaspoon melted butter

For the filling

- 1 red bell pepper, finely diced
- 1 cucumber, finely diced
- 1 avocado, finely diced
- ½ cup moong sprouts
- 2 green chillies, finely diced
- 1 lemon
- 3 tablespoons cilantro, chopped
- 1 teaspoon mustard seeds
- 1 teaspoon vegetable oil
- salt to taste

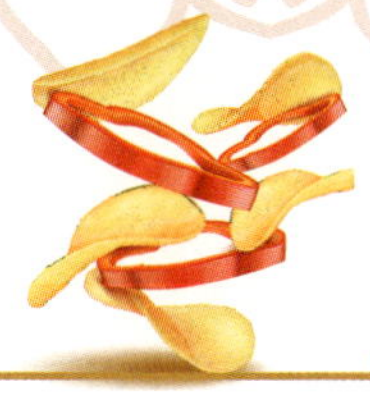

Process

For potato baskets/cups

1. Coat 20 cups in a 3.5" non-stick muffin pan with butter.
2. Evenly distribute a layer of julienned potatoes inside the cups.
3. Bake the layered potatoes in the muffin pan for 30 minutes at 425°F, until potatoes are golden brown. Remove pan from oven and allow it to cool before removing these potato cups.

For filling

4. To prepare the filling for the potato cups, mix red bell pepper, cucumber, avocado and moong sprouts in a bowl. Add green chilli, lemon juice and salt to taste.
5. Heat oil in a small pan and add mustard seeds. Once the seeds start popping transfer to the bowl above and mix again.
6. Remove potato cups from muffin pan and add filling to each cup.
7. Decorate with cilantro and serve with tamarind or cilantro chutney.

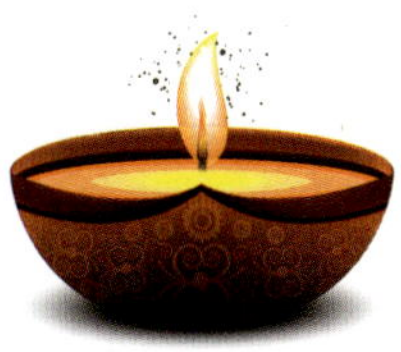

Paneer Chilli

A spicy starter of Chinese origin, now a popular menu option in Indian cuisine

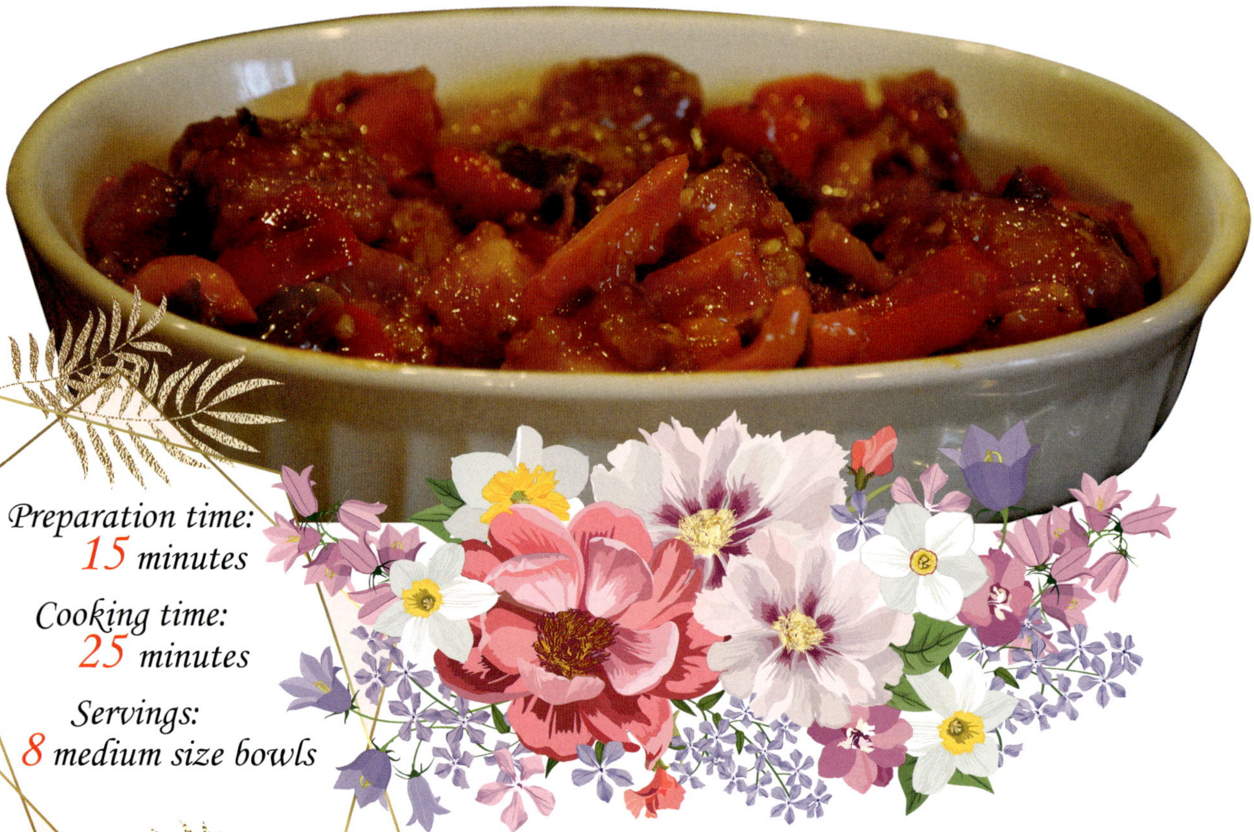

Preparation time:
15 minutes

Cooking time:
25 minutes

Servings:
8 medium size bowls

Ingredients

For frying paneer

- 16 oz. block of paneer or 2 cups paneer, cut into cubes
- 2 tablespoons all-purpose flour
- 2 tablespoons corn flour
- 1 tablespoon ginger garlic paste
- 1 tablespoon soy sauce
- 1 tablespoon white vinegar
- 3 tablespoons water
- 2 tablespoons oil for shallow frying
- 1 teaspoon salt

For chilli paneer

- 1 cup onions, chopped in big paneer size pieces (optional)
- 2 cups multi-color peppers (red, orange, yellow), chopped in big pieces
- 1 cup green bell pepper, chopped in big pieces
- 2 teaspoons garlic, finely chopped (optional)
- 2 teaspoons ginger, finely chopped
- 1 green chilli, finely chopped
- ¼ cup spring onions, finely chopped for garnishing
- 2 tablespoons soy sauce
- 2 teaspoons white vinegar
- 2 tablespoons tomato ketchup
- 2 tablespoons red chilli sauce
- 2 tablespoons vegetable oil (canola, corn, sunflower)
- 1 teaspoon salt, or to taste

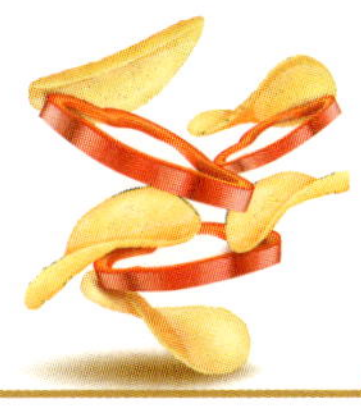

Process

For frying paneer

1. In a shallow bowl add paneer, all-purpose flour, corn flour, ginger garlic paste, vinegar, soy sauce and salt. Sprinkle some water if the batter is dry.
2. Mix paneer with the help of a fork coating all sides of the paneer cubes with the batter.
3. Heat 2 tablespoons oil in a nonstick medium shallow pan. Shallow fry the paneer till all sides are golden brown.
4. Remove the paneer to a plate and keep aside.

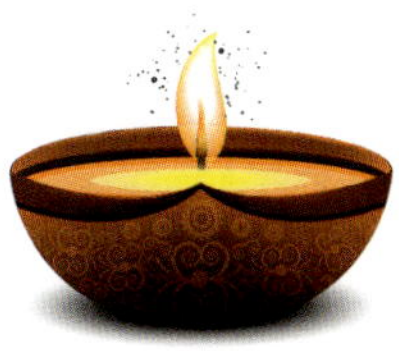

For making chilli paneer

5. In a small mixing bowl, mix together soy sauce, ketchup, red chilli sauce, vinegar and salt for the sauce and keep it aside.
6. Heat 2 tablespoons oil in the paneer frying pan over medium heat. Add chopped garlic, ginger and green chillies. Sauté for a minute or more, till the raw smell goes away.
7. Then add onions and sauté for 2 minutes, followed by peppers for another 2 minutes. The vegetables need to remain crunchy and under-done, not soft and cooked.
8. To these add the sauce mixture from step 5 above and mix it in well.
9. Once the sauce is heated up, add fried paneer. Mix well and heat up everything well.
10. Garnish with spring onions and serve immediately as a starter or can even be served in a wrap.

Snacks – Mini Meals

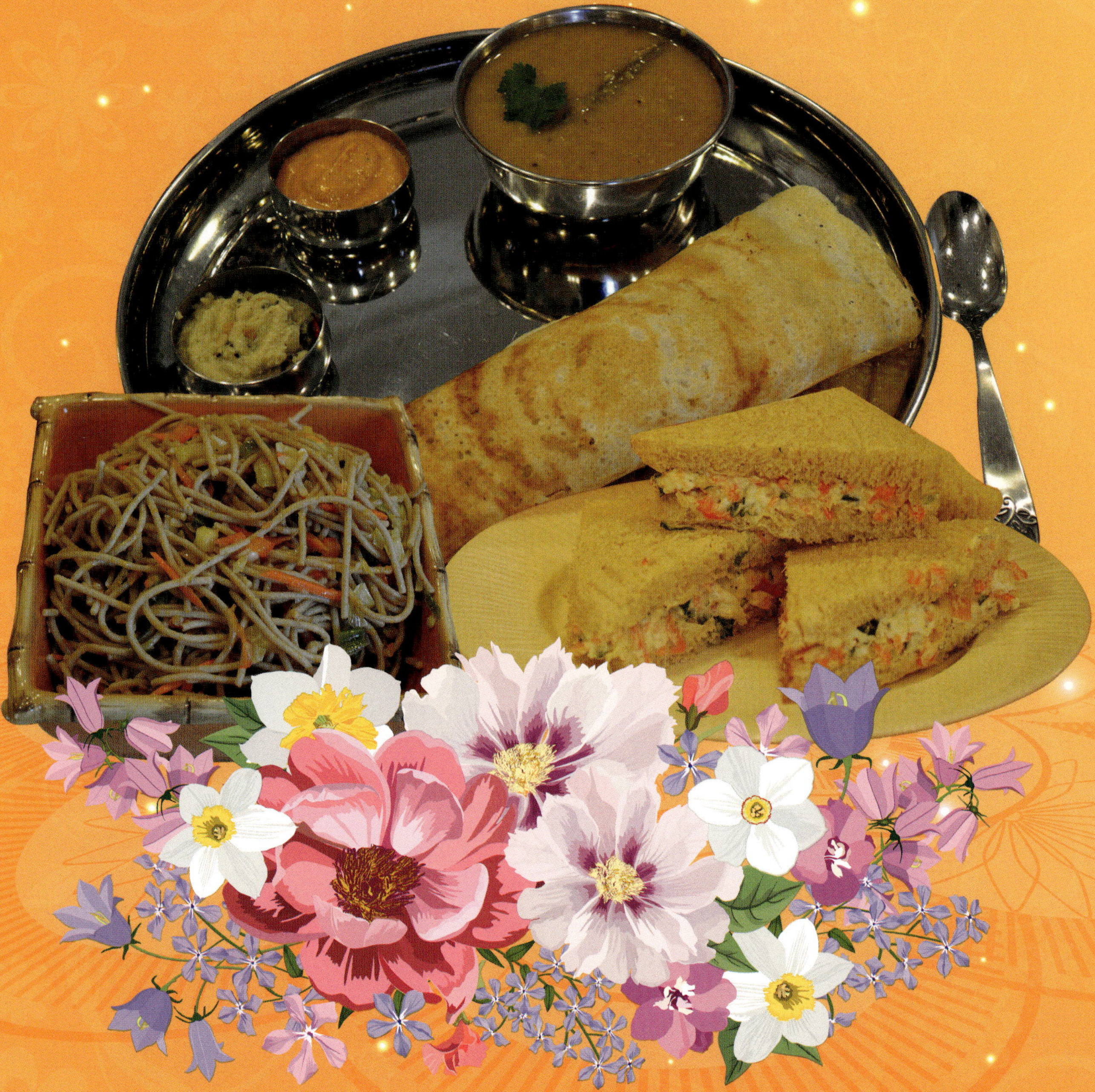

The choices presented in this chapter offer alternate options to pick from when a quick, filling, or an alternate meal is preferred to a typical Indian meal. Some of the very popular recipes selected here are drawn from Mexican cuisine (*avocado sandwich* made with guacamole), Italian (*pizza and pasta in white sauce*) and Chinese (*Hakka noodles*). South Indian popular meals of *dosa* and *uttapam*–lentil-rice crepes/pancakes are also included. The sandwiches and bread toasts are not just filling but quick and easy to prepare. They are excellent lunch box options too. The *healthy cereal chivda* made with an interesting mix of puffed grains and makhanas provides a light and tasty munching option.

Some of these recipes are made with ingredients rich in nutrients and vitamins such as avocadoes, buckwheat flour, makhanas and *dosa* made with a variety for lentils, *pizza* made with whole wheat flour and a variety of vegetables used in various recipes.

1. Avocado Sandwich
2. Cream Cheese Sandwich
3. Chilli Cheese Toast
4. Sooji Toast
5. Buckwheat Chilla
6. Uttapam
7. Mixed Lentil Masala Dosa
8. Healthy Cereal Chivda
9. Pizza
10. Pasta
11. Hakka Noodles

Avocado Sandwich

A healthy grilled sandwich made with guacamole

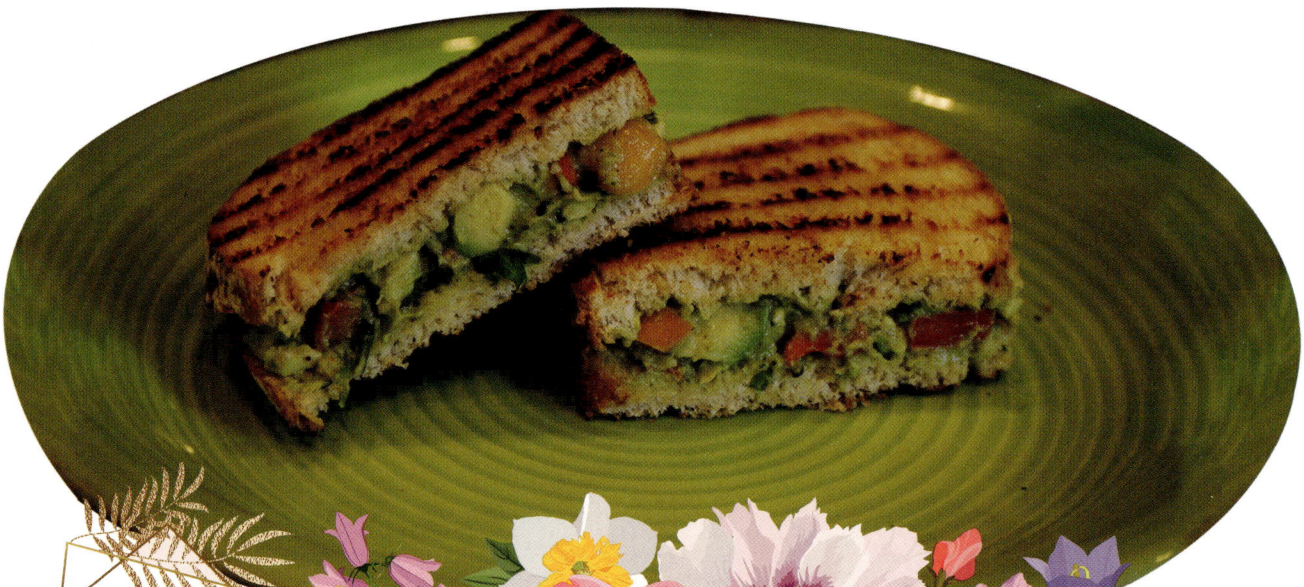

Total time: 30 *minutes*

Servings: 4 *sandwiches*

Ingredients

For sandwich filling (guacamole)

- 2 ripe avocadoes, diced, slightly mashed
- 1 small tomato, finely chopped
- 3-5 mini multi-color peppers, finely chopped
- 1 green chilli, finely chopped
- 7-8 sprigs of cilantro, finely chopped
- 1 tablespoon lemon juice
- 1 teaspoon Italian seasoning
- 1 teaspoon black sesame seed (optional)
- salt and black pepper to taste

For sandwich

- 8 slices sourdough or Italian bread
- 2 tablespoons olive oil or to taste

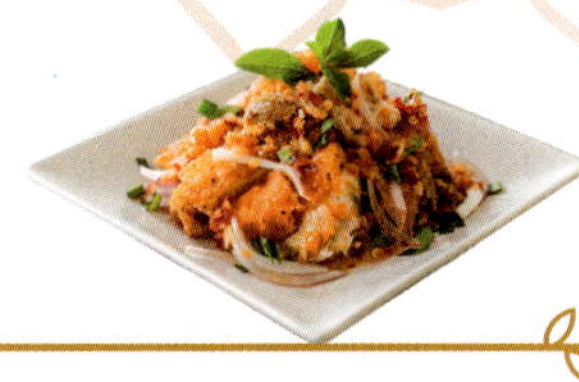

Process

Making sandwich filling (guacamole)

1. Dice the avocadoes and slightly mash them to keep a chunkier texture.
2. Add the finely cut tomatoes, peppers, chilli and cilantro. Also, add in the seasonings, sesame seed, lemon juice, salt and pepper and mix them in well.

Sandwich preparation

3. Apply olive oil on bread slices and grill these on a heated skillet. The bread can also be toasted in a toaster and olive oil applied afterwards.
4. Spread the guacamole filling on four slices of bread. Close the sandwich with the remaining slices.
5. Cut the sandwiches in half and serve them with hot sauce or ketchup.

Optional tip: Coconut oil or butter can be used instead of olive oil if preferred.

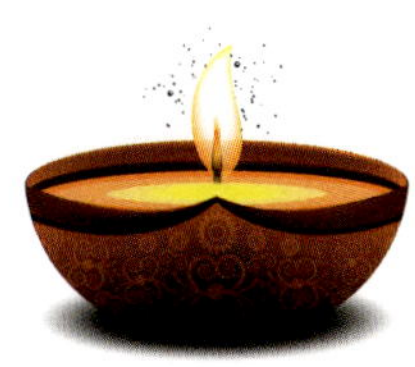

Cream Cheese Sandwich

A perfect snack or lunchbox staple

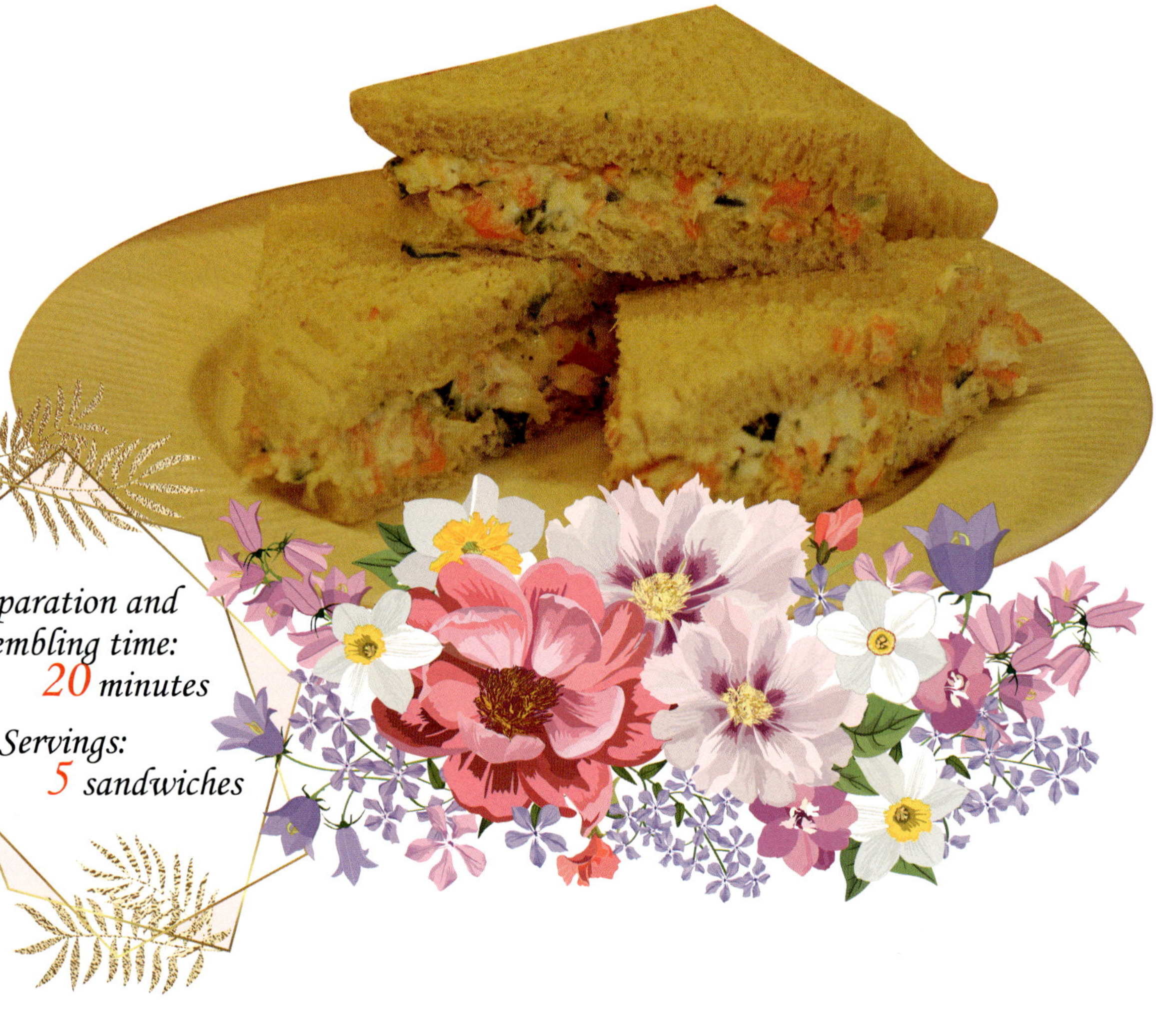

Preparation and assembling time: 20 *minutes*

Servings: 5 *sandwiches*

Ingredients

- 10 slices of sourdough bread or a plain sandwich bread
- 8 oz. cream cheese
- 1 cup medium-size English cucumber, shredded
- ¼ cup multi-color peppers, finely chopped
- 1 cup carrot, shredded
- 1 teaspoon ginger, finely shredded
- 1 teaspoon green chilli, finely chopped
- 2 tablespoons cilantro (optional)
- 1 tablespoon breadcrumbs (they help soak off any water released by vegetables, if sandwiches are packed in a lunchbox or kept for some time)
- ⅛ teaspoon black pepper powder
- ¼ teaspoon salt

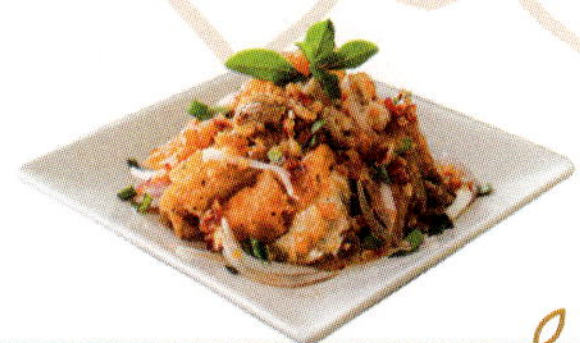

Process

1. Shred cucumbers and carrots and squeeze out the water.
2. Cut the bell pepper into very small pieces and pat them dry with a paper towel.
3. In a mixing bowl, mix together all the ingredients, cream cheese, cucumber, peppers, carrot, ginger, green chili, cilantro, seasonings and breadcrumbs to make a thick spread.
4. Spread this cheese vegetable mix on five slices of bread and close with the remaining slices of bread.
5. Trim the crust. For clean-cut keep the sandwiches aside and slice them after about half an hour.
6. Serve these sandwiches as a snack, or they are great for lunch boxes or picnics.

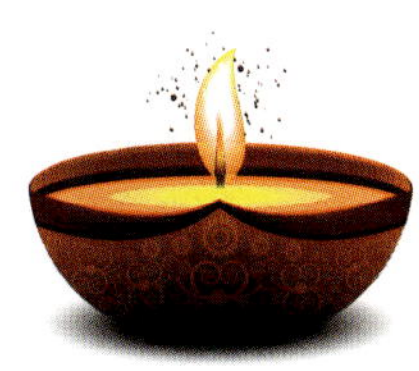

Chilli Cheese Toast

A perfect breakfast or snack time favorite

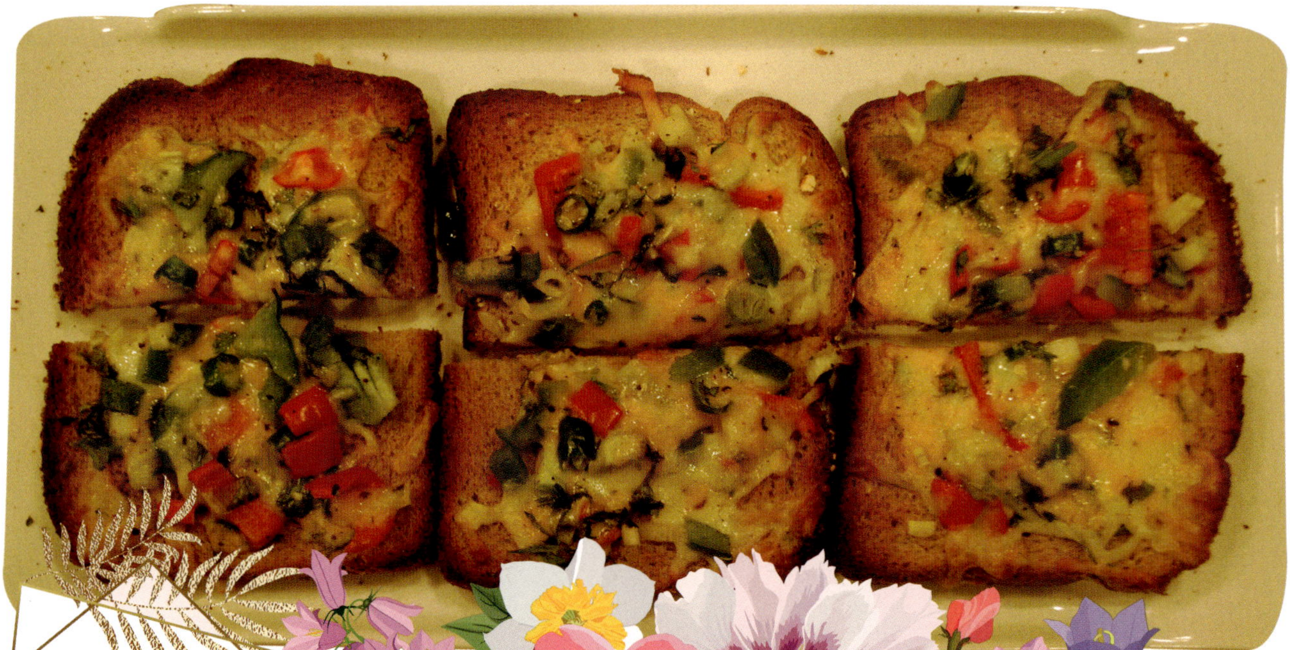

Preparation time:
20 *minutes*

Cooking time:
10 *minutes*

Servings: **4**
(8 quarter toast pieces)

Ingredients

- 8 slices of sourdough bread
- ¼ cup green peppers, finely chopped
- ¼ cup red peppers, finely chopped
- ¼ cup red onions, finely chopped (optional)
- 1 green chilli, finely chopped
- 2 tablespoons cilantro, finely chopped
- 1 cup of grated cheese (cheddar, mozzarella, any kind of cheese)
- salt and black pepper to taste

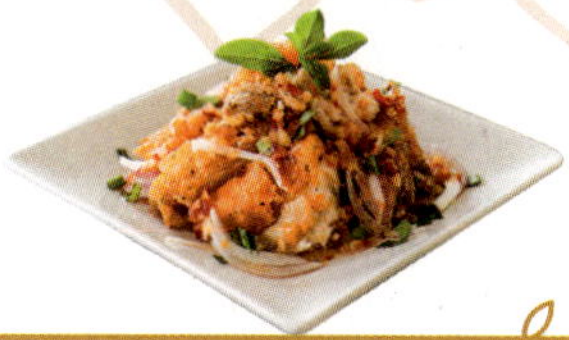

Process

1. Preheat the oven to 400°F.
2. Keep a baking sheet ready, lined with aluminum foil or a silpat.
3. For the sandwich filling, mix the peppers, onions, green chilli, cilantro and grated cheese together in a bowl.
4. Arrange all the bread slices on the tray and toast until they are golden brown (approximately 5 minutes but also depends on oven).
5. Spread the mixture evenly in between two slices of toasted bread.
6. Bake in the oven for 8 to 10 minutes, or until the cheese melts and the bread becomes crisp.
7. Remove from oven and once it has cooled slightly, cut each slice into 4 pieces and serve with spicy chutney or ketchup.

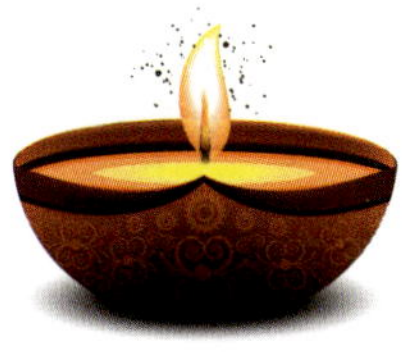

Sooji Toast

A quick n easy savory bread snack

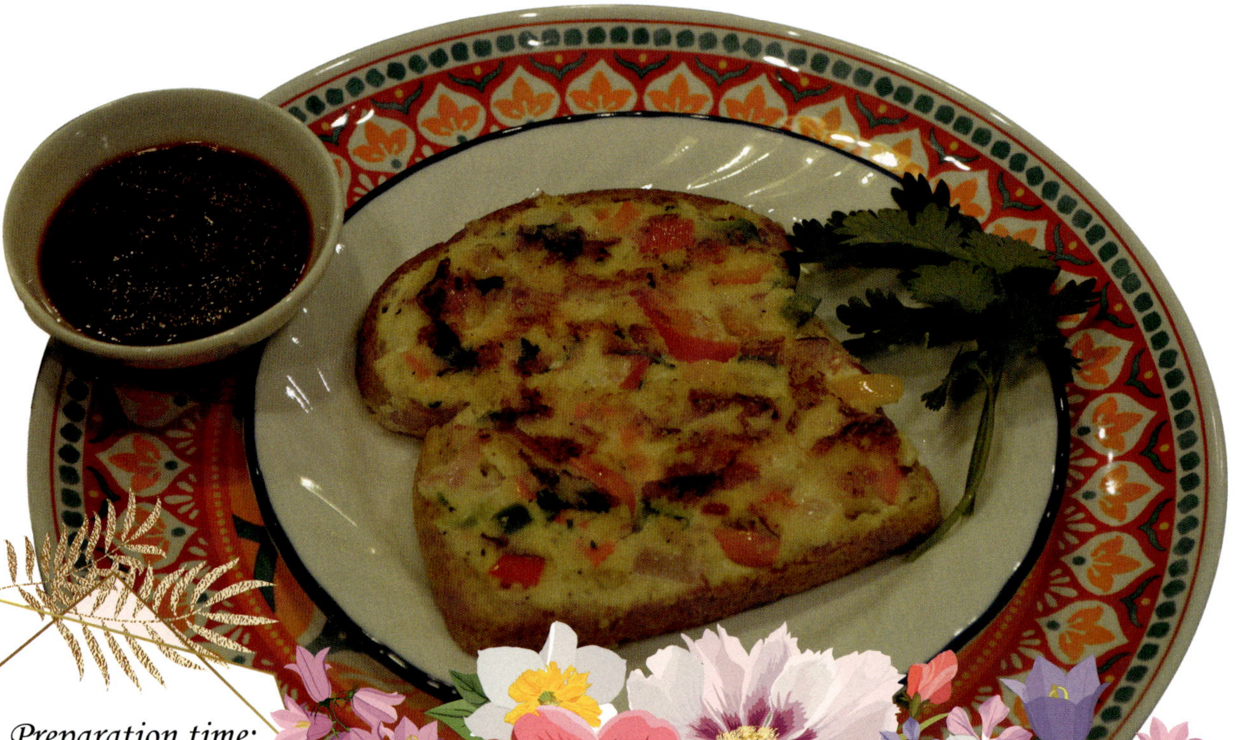

Preparation time:
10 *minutes*

Cooking time:
20 *minutes*

Servings: **6** *to* **8**
bread slices

Ingredients

- 6 to 8 bread slices, Italian bread or Sourdough bread
- 1 cup fine sooji (semolina)
- 1 cup yogurt
- 1 small onion, finely chopped (optional)
- 1 small tomato, finely chopped
- 4-5 mini multi-color peppers, finely chopped
- 1 small green chilli, finely chopped
- 1 teaspoon ginger, grated
- 1/8 teaspoon black pepper, crushed
- 2 teaspoons olive oil for spreading on each slice of bread
- salt to taste

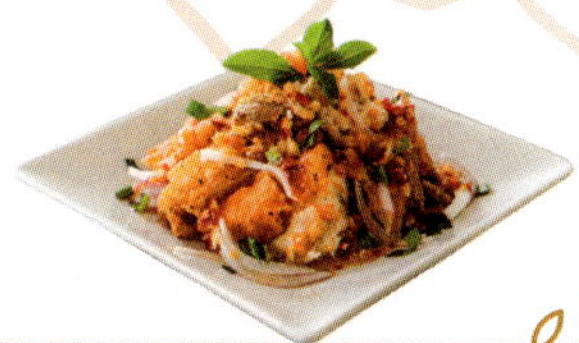

Process

1. In a medium size bowl mix all the ingredients (sooji, yogurt, chopped vegetables, chilli, ginger, salt and pepper) to prepare a thick spreadable mixture.
2. Using a spoon spread the mixture evenly on one side of a slice of bread.
3. Place the slice of bread on a heated and greased nonstick skillet (medium heat), with filling side down. Cook till it is golden brown on both sides.
4. Apply some oil on the top side. Now flip and toast this side.
5. Flip again and let it toast until it becomes light brown and crunchy.
6. Repeat steps 2-5 for all bread slices.
7. Serve warm with chutney.

Optional tip: Chutney can even be layered on the bread slice before spreading the sooji mixture to make the toast spicier.

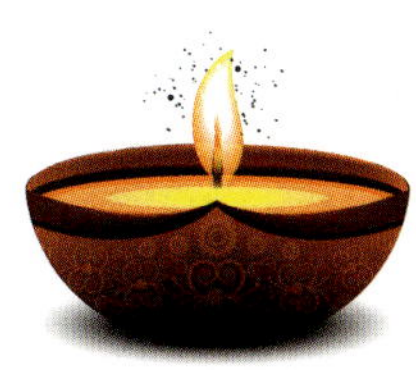

Buckwheat Chilla

Buckwheat chillas are a healthy iron and fiber-rich snack or breakfast meal

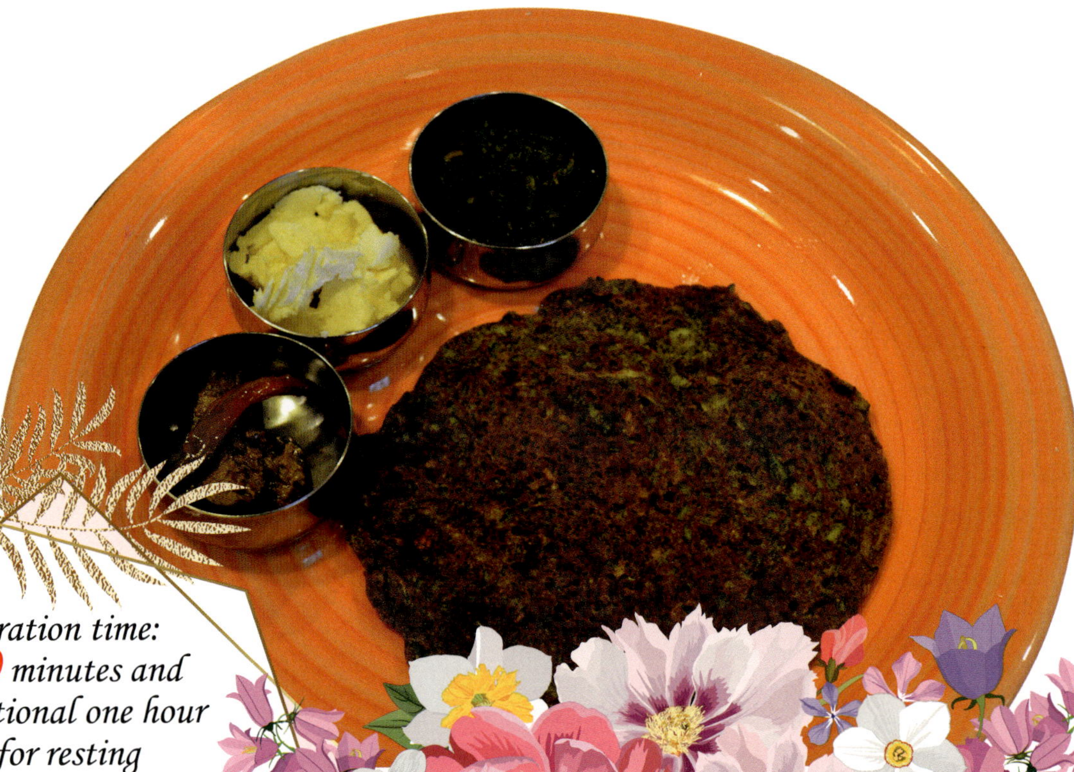

Preparation time:
30 *minutes and additional one hour for resting*

Cooking time:
10-15 *minutes*

Servings:
10 *chillas*

Ingredients

- 1 ¼ cups buckwheat flour (kuttu ka atta)
- ½ cup sour low-fat yogurt
- 1 tablespoon spinach, chopped
- ½ cup grated lauki, (bottle gourd/doodhi)
- 2 tablespoons cilantro, finely chopped
- 1 teaspoon ginger-green chilli paste
- pinch of asafoetida
- 1 teaspoon sesame seed
- 1 teaspoon cumin powder
- pinch of turmeric powder
- 3 teaspoons oil for greasing and cooking
- salt as per taste

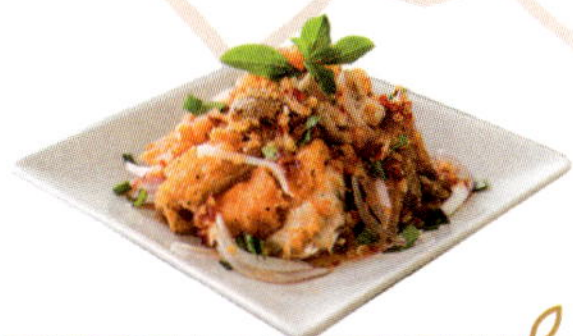

Process

1. Mix buckwheat flour and yogurt in a bowl, cover, and set aside for an hour.
2. Now, to the flour-yogurt mix add spinach, lauki, ginger-green chilli paste, cilantro, sesame seed, jeera powder, turmeric powder, asafoetida, salt and 1 tablespoon of water. Mix well and set aside for another 10 minutes for flavors to blend in.
3. Heat a non-stick skillet and grease it with a little oil. Pour a ladleful, ½ cup batter on it and spread it to make a thick circle.
4. Cook, until it is light brown on both sides.
5. Continue to make more chillas one at a time.
6. Serve with any chutney.

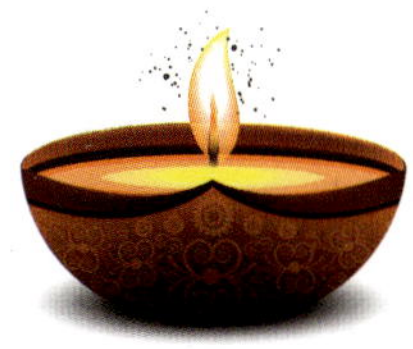

Uttapam

A South Indian dosa–like thick pancake made with idli batter and topped with vegetables

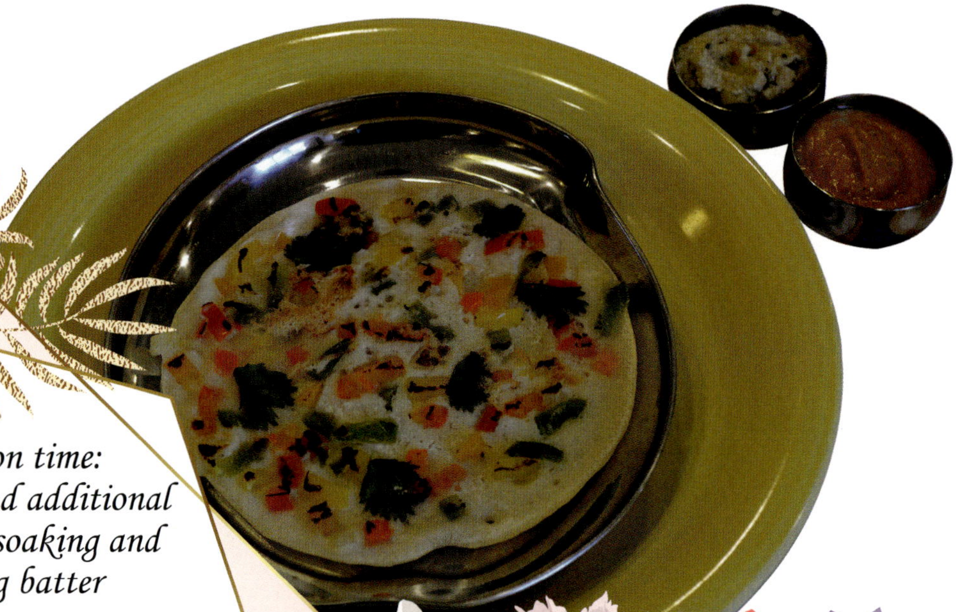

Preparation time:
25 *minutes and additional* 14 *hours for soaking and fermenting batter*

Cooking time:
1:15 *minutes*
(5 minutes per uttapam)

Makes about:
15 *uttapams*

Ingredients

For Idli batter

- 1 cup urad dal (polished split black lentils)
- 3 cup idli rice (or parboiled rice)
- 1 tablespoon fenugreek seeds (methi)
- 1 tablespoon salt

For Uttapam toppings

- ½ cup red onions, finely chopped
- ½ cup tomatoes, finely chopped
- ½ cup green and yellow peppers, finely chopped
- ½ cup carrots, shredded
- 2 green chillies, finely chopped
- ½ cup cilantro, chopped
- 2 tablespoons ghee

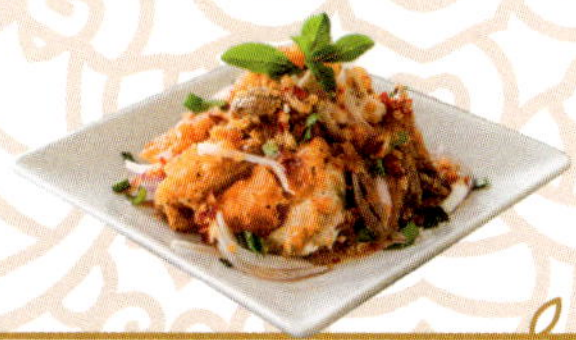

Process

For batter

1. In a medium bowl, wash and soak urad dal and fenugreek seeds in 4 cups water for 6 hours.
2. In another medium bowl, wash and soak idli rice in 9 cups water for 6 hours.
3. Drain the water from both and grind to a smooth thick batter in a high-speed blender with a little water at a time. Add salt and mix it in well.
4. Transfer the batter to a big container giving it space to rise and ferment for 8 hours or overnight.

For Uttapam

5. Stir the idli batter in a bowl. The batter needs to be medium thick, thicker than the dosa batter, but if too thick, some water may be added.
6. Keep all finely chopped vegetables ready.
7. Heat a non-stick pan and grease it with a brush dipped in ghee. Pour a ladleful of batter and spread it in a circular motion to form a 6-inch diameter. Unlike for the dosa, the layer needs to be medium thick and not too thin.
8. When you see small holes appearing on the surface, spread some chopped vegetables and coriander evenly on entire uttapam. Drizzle ghee around the edges and at the center.
9. Reduce the heat to medium, cover the pan and steam cook for a few seconds.
10. Once the vegetables are cooked and color changes to golden brown, flip to the other side and cook for a few minutes till it becomes golden brown. Approximately 2-3 minutes each side on medium heat.
11. Serve the vegetable uttapam with sambar and chutney.

Time-saver option: Store bought idli batters drastically reduce the preparation time to make uttapams.

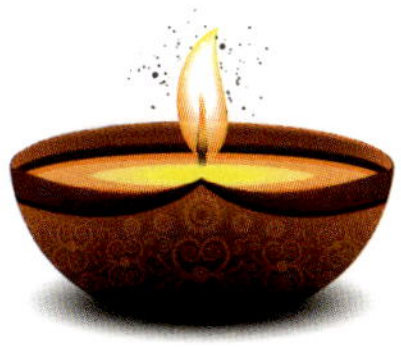

Mixed Lentil Masala Dosa

An all-time favorite South Indian taste–the popular rice and dal crepes withpotato filling

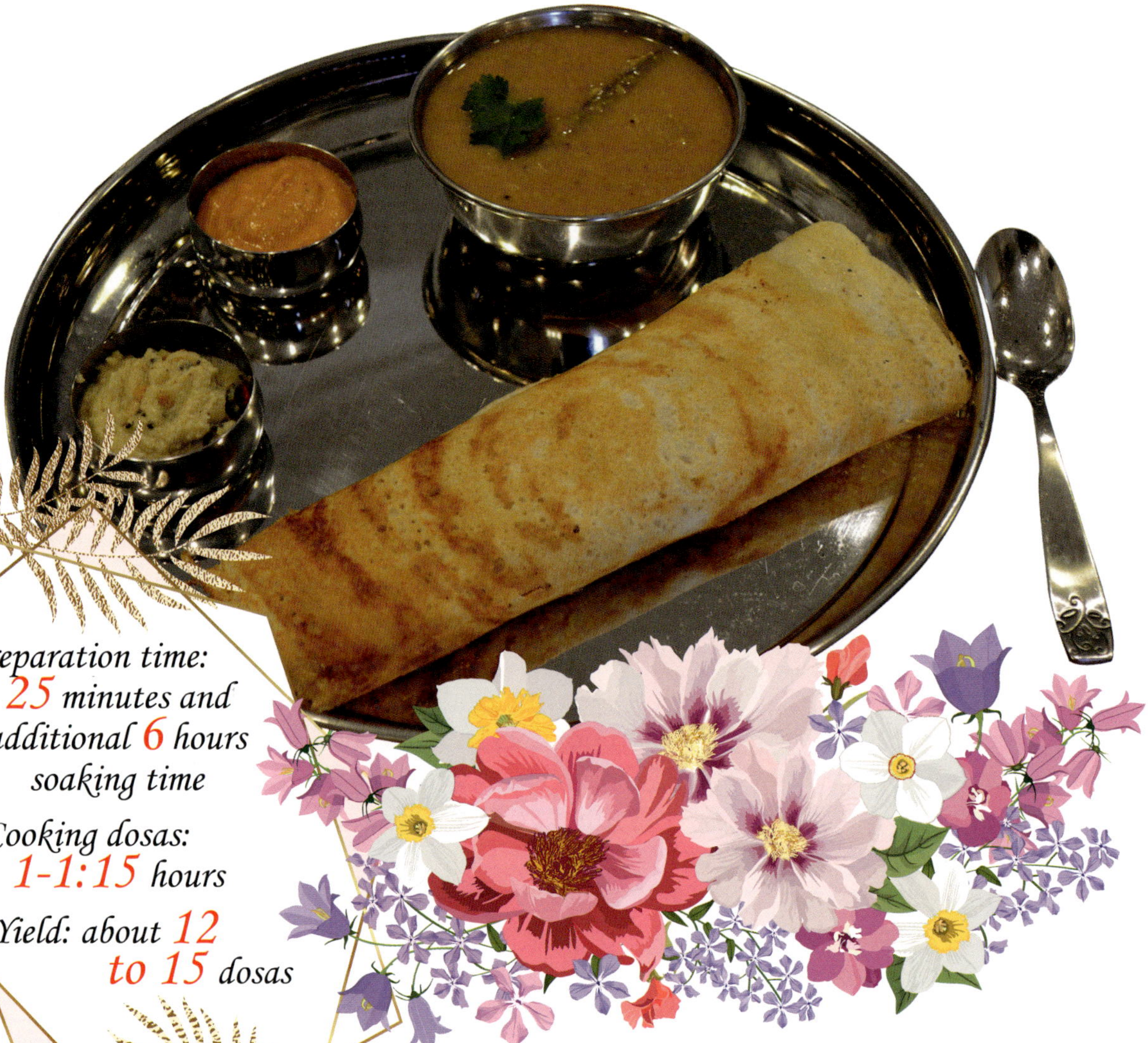

Preparation time:
25 minutes and additional 6 hours soaking time

Cooking dosas:
1-1:15 hours

Yield: about 12 to 15 dosas

Ingredients

For dosa batter

- 1 cup idli rice
- 1/3 cup urad dal
- 1/3 cup moong dal
- 1/3 cup chana dal
- 1 tablespoon fenugreek seeds
- 1 tablespoon salt

For potato filling

- 4 large potatoes, boiled and chopped
- 1 large onion, sliced
- 1 teaspoon mustard seeds
- 3 dry red chillies
- 1/2 teaspoon turmeric powder
- 1/4 teaspoon asofoetida
- 1 teaspoon urad dal
- 1 teaspoon chana dal
- 2 green chillies, sliced
- 6 to 8 curry leaves
- 2 tablespoons ghee plus extra ghee/butter to make dosas
- I tablespoon cilantro for garnishing
- 1 teaspoon salt

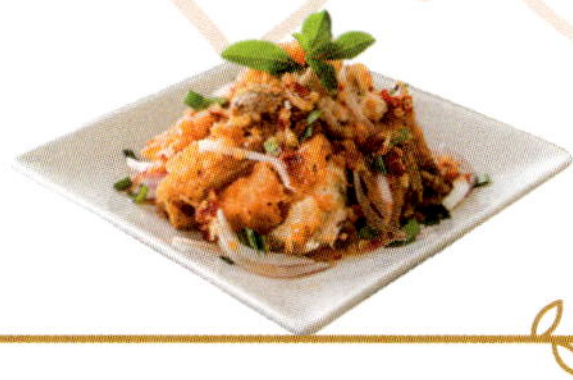

Process

Dosa batter

1. Wash and soak rice in a medium bowl with 4 cups water for at least 6 hours.
2. Wash and soak dals (urad, moong, chana) and fenugreek seeds together in a bigger bowl with 8 cups water for at least 6 hours.
3. Drain the water from rice and dals but saving enough to grind them all together with salt to a fine paste. Grinder should be high power.
4. More water may be added for grinding, but a little at a time as the batter needs to be thick.
5. Keep aside this batter in a large container in a warm place to ferment for at least 6 to 8 hours. The batter should fill only half or third of the container leaving enough room for it to rise.

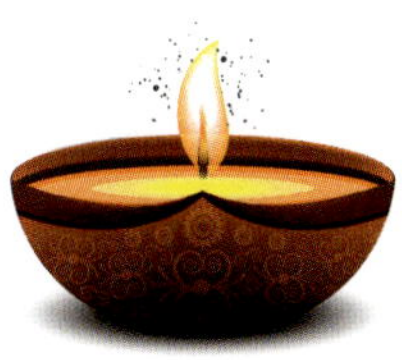

Potato filling

6. In a medium shallow frying pan heat ghee and then add mustard seeds. When they pop add green chillies, curry leaves, red chilli and asafoetida and cook for a minute or so.
7. Add onions (if using) and sauté until golden brown. Add turmeric powder and salt and cook a little.
8. Now add the boiled potatoes, chopped in medium size cubes.
9. Mix well and turn off the stove. Garnish with fresh coriander leaves.

Making dosas

10. Set a flat nonstick griddle (iron griddle) on a medium heat. Brush 1 teaspoon ghee to it. With the flat ladle pour ½ cup batter in the center of the griddle.
11. Using the bottom of the ladle, quickly spread the batter outwards in a circular motion to a round (6 to 7-inch diameter).
12. Lightly spread ghee with the brush along the edges and center. Cook the dosa till it becomes brown and the edges are cooked and can be lifted easily with a spatula.
13. Cook on one side only, and add ¼ cup dosa filling in the center of dosa and spread along the center.
14. With the spatula loosen the edge of dosa from one side and fold the sides of the dosa around the filling to make a cylindrical shape.
15. Dosas are cooked one at a time and served immediately, with sambar and any south Indian chutney.

Cooking tip: To make consistently good dosas, after cooking each dosa, wipe the griddle with a cloth or paper towel moistened with oil.

Healthy Cereal Chivda

A spiced light munchie made with some nutritious ingredients

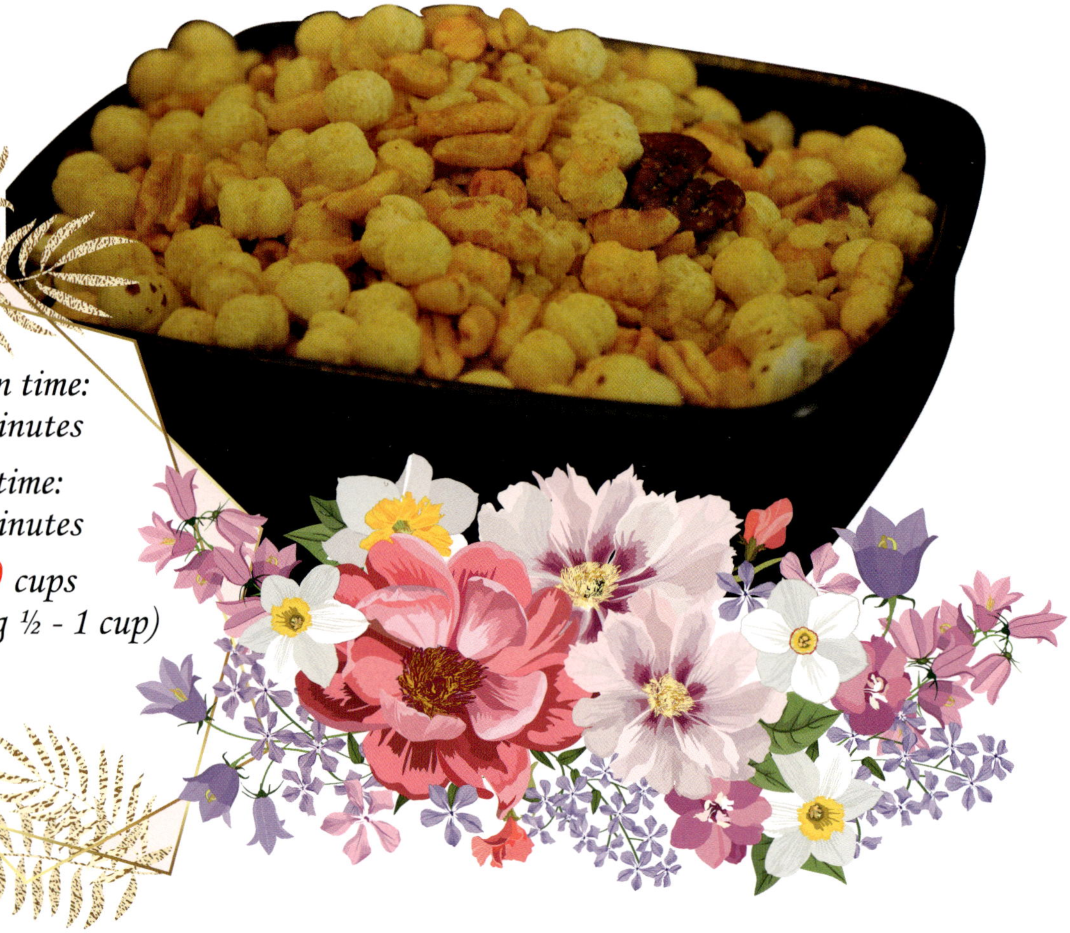

Preparation time:
10 *minutes*

Cooking time:
20 *minutes*

Yield: 10 *cups*
(one serving ½ - 1 cup)

Ingredients

- 2 cups organic puffed kamut cereal
- 2 cups sliced half makhana (fox nuts or lotus seed)
- 2 cups rice puffs
- 2 cups oat cheerios

For tempering

- 3 teaspoons vegetable oil
- ¼ teaspoon asafoetida
- 2 teaspoons mustard seeds
- ½ cup dalia (dry roasted chana dal)
- ½ cup nuts any type (almond, walnuts, cashews, pine nuts)
- ½ cup raw peanuts
- 1 teaspoon red chilli powder
- 1 teaspoon turmeric powder
- 2 red chillies dried
- 8 to 10 curry leaves
- 1 teaspoon salt
- ¼ teaspoon rock salt

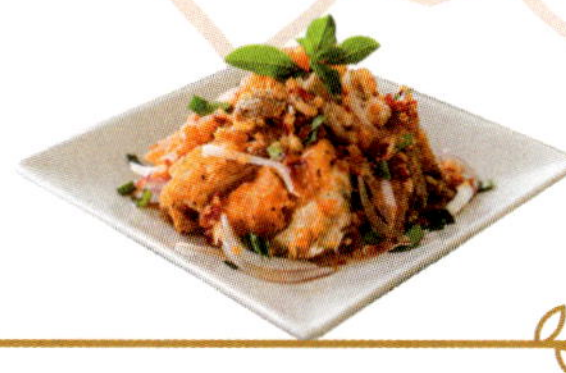

Process

1. In a large mixing bowl, mix together all four cereals.
2. In a large pan/kadai, heat oil on medium heat to prepare the tempering. First add mustard seeds to hot oil. When they pop add asafoetida. Next add curry leaves and cook till crisp. Now add peanuts and roast till slightly golden brown. Add dalia and all nuts and roast some.
3. To the above mix now add the dry red chillies and red chilli powder, turmeric powder, salt and rock salt. Mix everything and turn off the heat.
4. Immediately add cereal and toss for a few minutes until everything is mixed well.
5. Allow it to cool to room temperature and store in an air-tight container.

Alternate option: Other nuts and raisins may be added at the same time as peanuts.

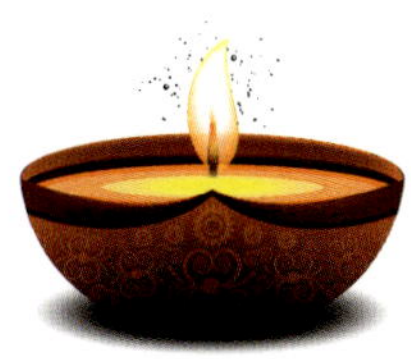

Pizza

A healthier whole wheat version of an all-time kids' favorite

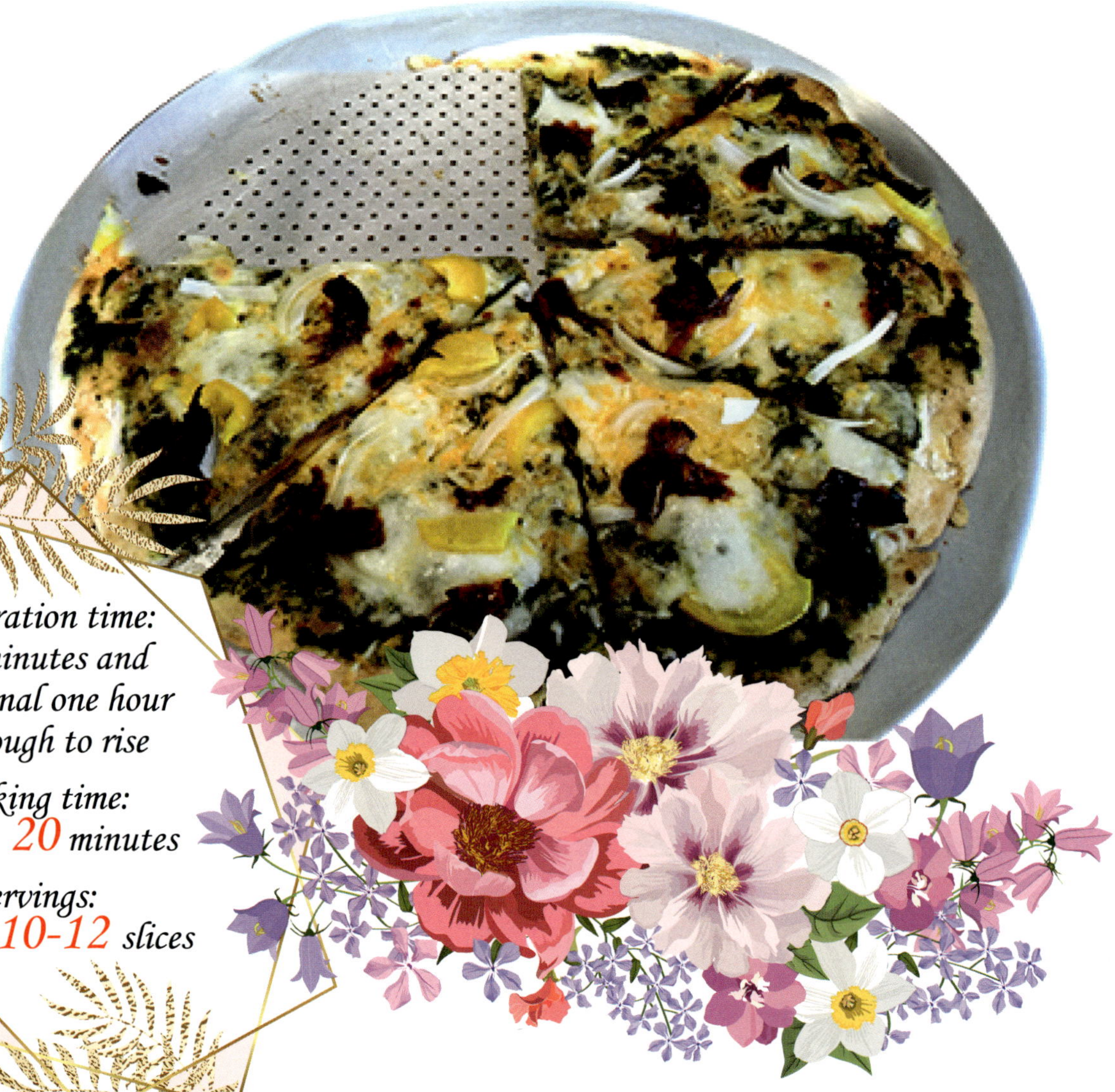

Preparation time:
30 minutes and additional one hour for dough to rise

Cooking time:
20 minutes

Servings:
10-12 slices

Ingredients

For dough

- 2 cups whole wheat flour
- 1 cup all-purpose flour (maida)
- 2 tablespoons oil
- 1 teaspoon sugar
- 1 tablespoon yeast
- 1 teaspoon salt
- warm water to knead dough

For sauce

- 6-7 medium tomatoes, finely chopped
- 2 cloves garlic, minced (optional)
- 1 tablespoon oregano
- 1 bay leaf
- 4-5 basil leaves, finely chopped
- salt and black pepper to taste
- 3 tablespoons olive oil

Cheese

- 2 cups or less, pizza cheeses (mozzarella, provolone, cheddar and parmesan), mixed in any preferred combination and ratio

Vegetable Toppings

- 1 cup spinach
- ½ cup bell pepper
- ½ cup onion (optional)
- $1/4^{th}$ cup sun dried tomatoes

Equipment: pizza stone or pizza pan

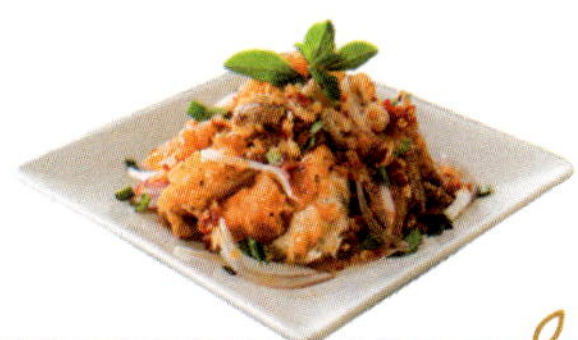

Process

For dough

1. Dissolve yeast in 4 tablespoons of warm water and sugar. Wait for it to get frothy.
2. Add the flour, oil, salt in a big mixing bowl. Mix everything together and make a dough with warm water.
3. Sprinkle with flour and put dough away for at least an hour to rise.
4. Roll the pizza base to whatever thickness is preferred.

For sauce

5. In a saucepan, heat olive oil. Add garlic, bay leaf, oregano and cook for a few minutes until the flavors are infused in the oil.

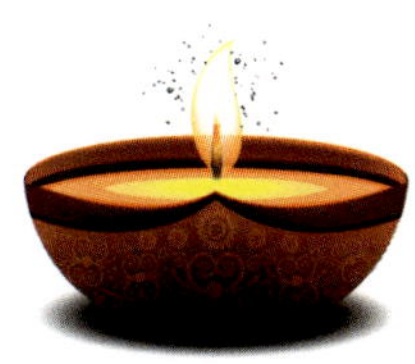

6. Add chopped tomatoes and cook for 10-15 minutes until it becomes a sauce like consistency.

Assembling of the Pizza

7. Preheat the oven at 400°F with pizza stone in middle rack. Using the pizza stone will ensure the crust is crisp. If using a pizza pan, place the rolled dough on the pan and follow the steps in #8 and 10.
8. Spread the sauce on the base and sprinkle the cheese. Add toppings as per taste.
9. Slide the pizza onto the stone carefully. You can use a wooden board to roll out the dough and slide onto the stone.
10. Bake in the oven for approximately 15-20 minutes until the base is crisp and the cheese has melted and is light brown in color.
11. Serve warm.

Note on cheese : If vegetarian cheese is preferred, then the Indian Amul cheese can be used for its flavor and taste. Sargento brand sold in the US is vegan friendly, or, made with non-animal rennet.

Alternate topping tips: Toppings may be roasted or sautéed, depending on personal preference.

Several other suggested combinations for toppings:

- Kale and Mushroom (1 cup kale chopped, 1 cup mushroom sliced)
- Corn, Green Pepper, Red Pepper and Cilantro (1 cup corn, 1 cup sliced green and red pepper, ½ cup chopped cilantro)
- Green Pepper, Mushrooms, Spinach (1 cup sliced green pepper, ½ cup mushrooms, ½ cup chopped spinach)

Pasta in White Sauce

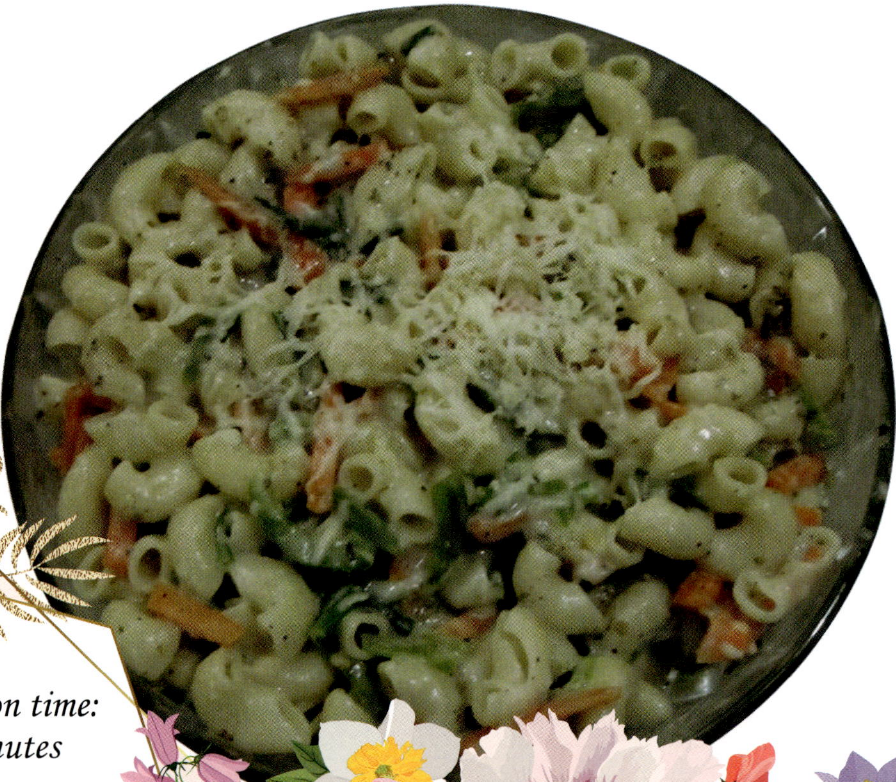

Preparation time: 45 *minutes*

Cooking time: 30 *minutes*

Servings: 4-5

Ingredients

For white sauce

- 3 tablespoons all-purpose flour (maida)
- 2 tablespoons butter
- 2 cups whole milk
- 1 teaspoon sugar
- black pepper powder to taste
- oregano to taste
- salt to taste

For pasta

- 3 cups of uncooked pasta, pipe rigate (elbow shells) or others like rigatoni, penne
- 1 bell pepper, sliced
- 2 carrots, julienne cut
- 1 cup mushrooms, sliced (optional)
- 1 cup broccoli florets (optional)
- 1 cup chopped kale or spinach (optional)
- 2-3 green chillies, diced
- ¼ cup mozzarella cheese, grated
- 2 tablespoons olive oil

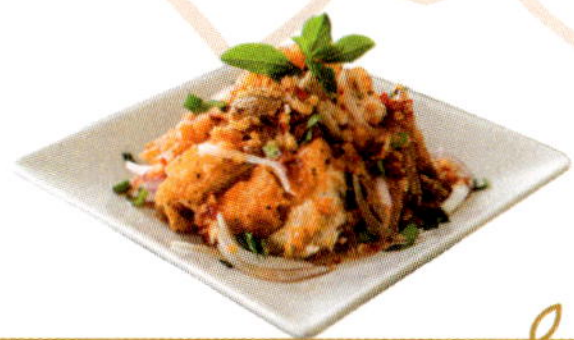

Process

For white sauce

1. Take a non-stick thick bottom pan and add butter.
2. Add the all-purpose flour. Sauté this mixture with spatula in low fire. When white flour changes color slightly, then switch off the heat.
3. Add milk in a separate bowl and boil it slightly. Add milk to the butter and flour in the pan. Continuously stir this mixture to dissolve the lumps. If required add some more milk or water to get sauce consistency. Keep it aside.

For pasta

4. Boil 6-8 cups of water in a big pan, and then add pasta in boiling water. Let it cook for 8-10 minutes (al dente, slightly less cooked). Add 1 teaspoon of salt and 1 teaspoon of oil to the pasta (so that pasta doesn't stick).

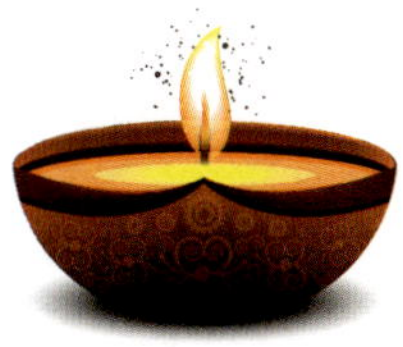

5. Once pasta is cooked, strain the water using a colander and keep aside.
6. *Preparing vegetables:* Heat 2 tablespoons of olive oil in a pan. Add all the vegetables and sauté them for 5 minutes or till the vegetables are half cooked.
7. Add salt, pepper powder and oregano to this.
8. Now add the cooked pasta to the vegetables and mix it well.
9. Add the white sauce and keep stirring the mixture in the pan for 2 minutes on low fire.
10. Top with grated cheese as seasoning and serve warm.

Vegetable Hakka Noodles

A popular favorite dish from Indo-Chinese cuisine

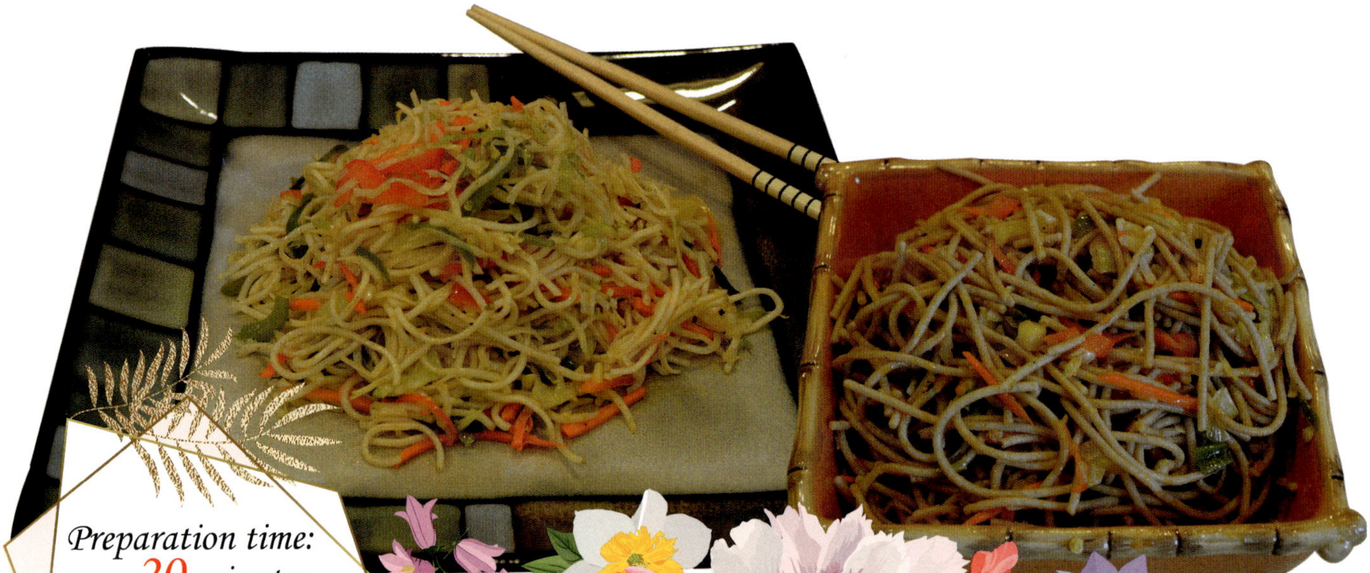

Preparation time: 20 *minutes*

Cooking time: 30 *minutes*

Servings: 5 *medium size bowls*

Ingredients

- 5.3 oz. Ching Secret Hakka noodles or similar brand (approx. 3 cups boiled noodles)
- ½ cup multi-color peppers, finely sliced
- ½ cup carrots, julienne sliced
- ½ cup French beans, finely sliced at an angle
- 1 cup cabbage, finely shredded
- ½ cup onion, finely sliced (optional)
- 1 tablespoon vinegar
- 1 teaspoon soy sauce
- 1 teaspoon red chilli sauce
- 3 tablespoons oil
- ½ cup spring onions, finely cut for garnishing
- pinch of black pepper powder
- salt to taste

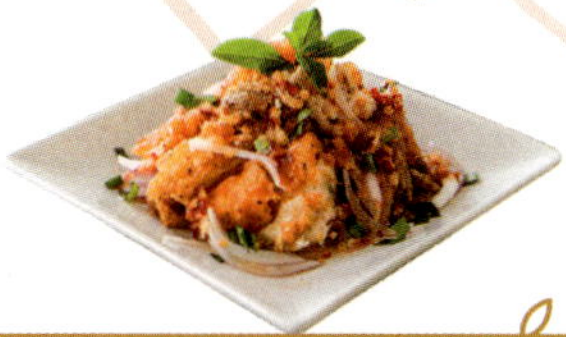

Process

1. Boil 6 cups of water with a little salt and one teaspoon oil in a deep pot. Then add the Hakka noodles.
2. Once noodles are cooked (*al dente*, little less cooked) drain the water with a strainer. Run the noodles under cold water and keep the noodles in the strainer till water from noodles drains out completely.
3. Keep aside the noodles but in between shuffle the boiled noodles with a fork till they completely cool down.
4. Heat oil in a medium wok and add all the finely sliced vegetables – peppers, carrots, beans, cabbage, onions (if using). Stir fry the vegetables on high heat for few minutes and then add salt.
5. Now add boiled noodles, chilli sauce, soy sauce, vinegar and black pepper.
6. Toss and cook on medium-high heat for another 2-3 minutes.
7. Garnish with spring onions and serve warm.

Chutneys, Pickles and Condiments

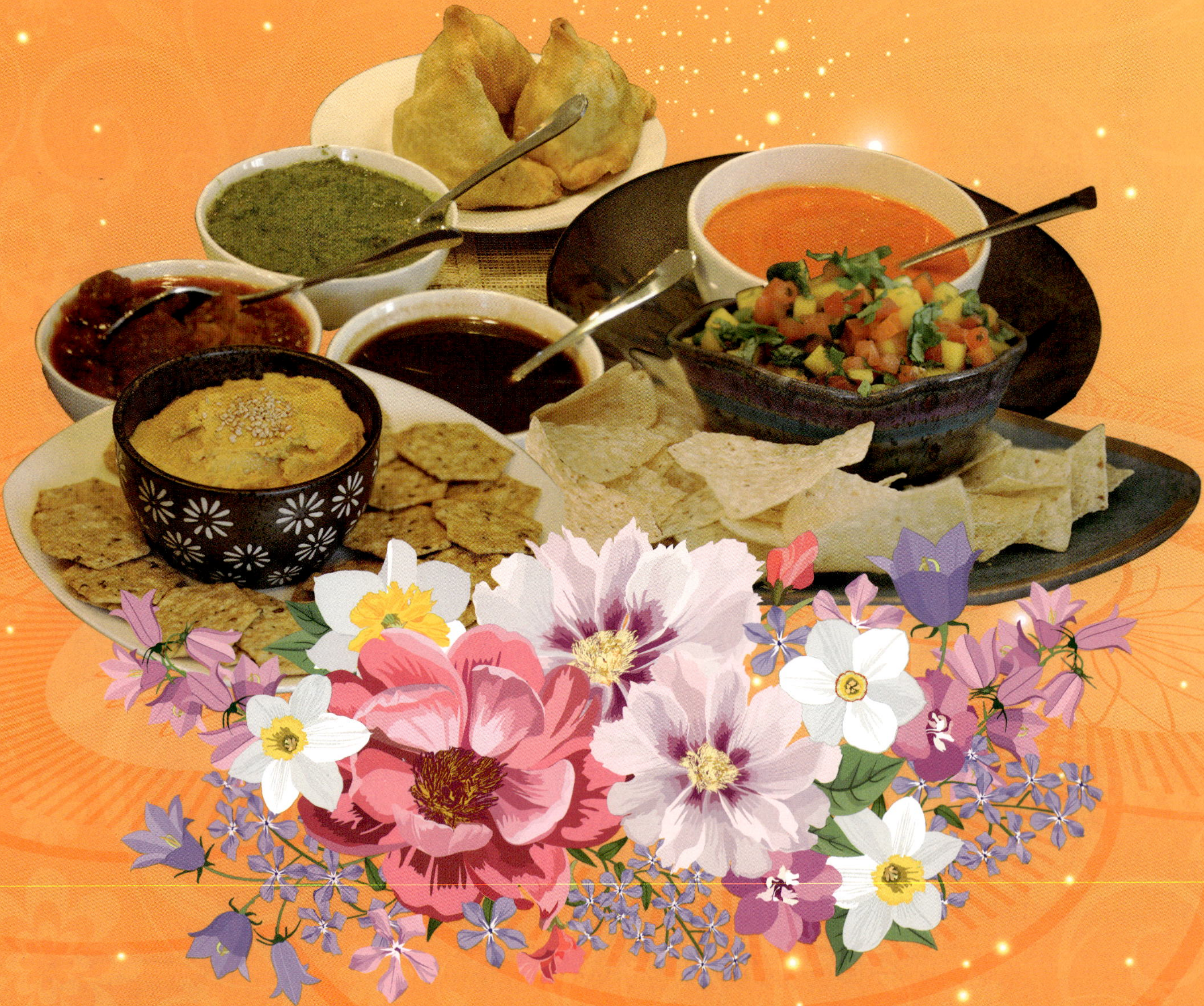

Chutneys, pickles and condiments with their spicier, tangier, sweet and sour tastes add the final 'zing' to many Indian dishes. We have attempted to include here a basic selection. They are the final accompaniments to any Indian meal/ snack.

Apple cilantro mint, tamarind date and apple butter chutney are best served with *chaats*, savory, fried or other snacks or even layered in sandwiches. *Almond, coconut, tomato* are the basic accompaniments to South Indian meals. *Hummus* of Mediterranean origin and *mango salsa* of Mexican are best served with pita bread and chips or even used in sandwiches. *Pickles* are served with meals or paranthas. Lastly the *vegetable raita* – spiced yogurt with vegetables tones down the heat of some Indian dishes.

1. Apple Cilantro Mint Chutney
2. Tamarind Date Chutney
3. Apple Butter Chutney
4. Almond Chutney
5. Coconut Chutney
6. Tomato Chutney
7. Hummus
8. Mango Salsa
9. Instant Lemon Pickle
10. Carrot and Green Chilli Pickle
11. Mango Pickle
12. Vegetable Raita

Apple Cilantro Mint Chutney

A sweet twist to a traditional evergreen recipe

Total time: 15 *minutes*

Yield: 8 *oz. bowl*

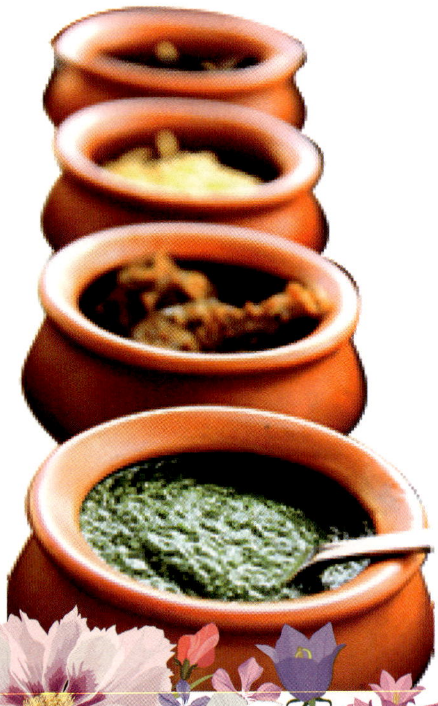

Ingredients

- 1 bunch cilantro leaves, chopped
- 1 small golden apple, cut in big slices
- 1-inch ginger
- 10 to 12 leaves of fresh mint
- 1-2 green chillies
- 1 teaspoon cumin seed
- 1 teaspoon peanuts (optional)
- 1 teaspoon lemon juice (preserves the green color of the chutney)
- salt to taste

Process

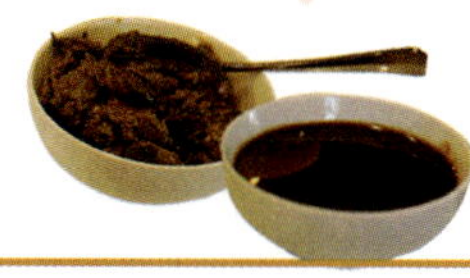

1. In a blender add coarsely chopped cilantro, apple, ginger, mint and green chilli.
2. Blend together with remaining ingredients – cumin, peanuts, lemon juice, salt and very little water to form a smooth paste.
3. Chutney can be refrigerated for about a week.

Optional tip: Peanuts are optional to add. If used, they act as a binding agent for various greens and create a smooth textured chutney.

Tamarind Date Chutney

A khathi–meethi (sweet and tangy) chutney to serve with savory snacks

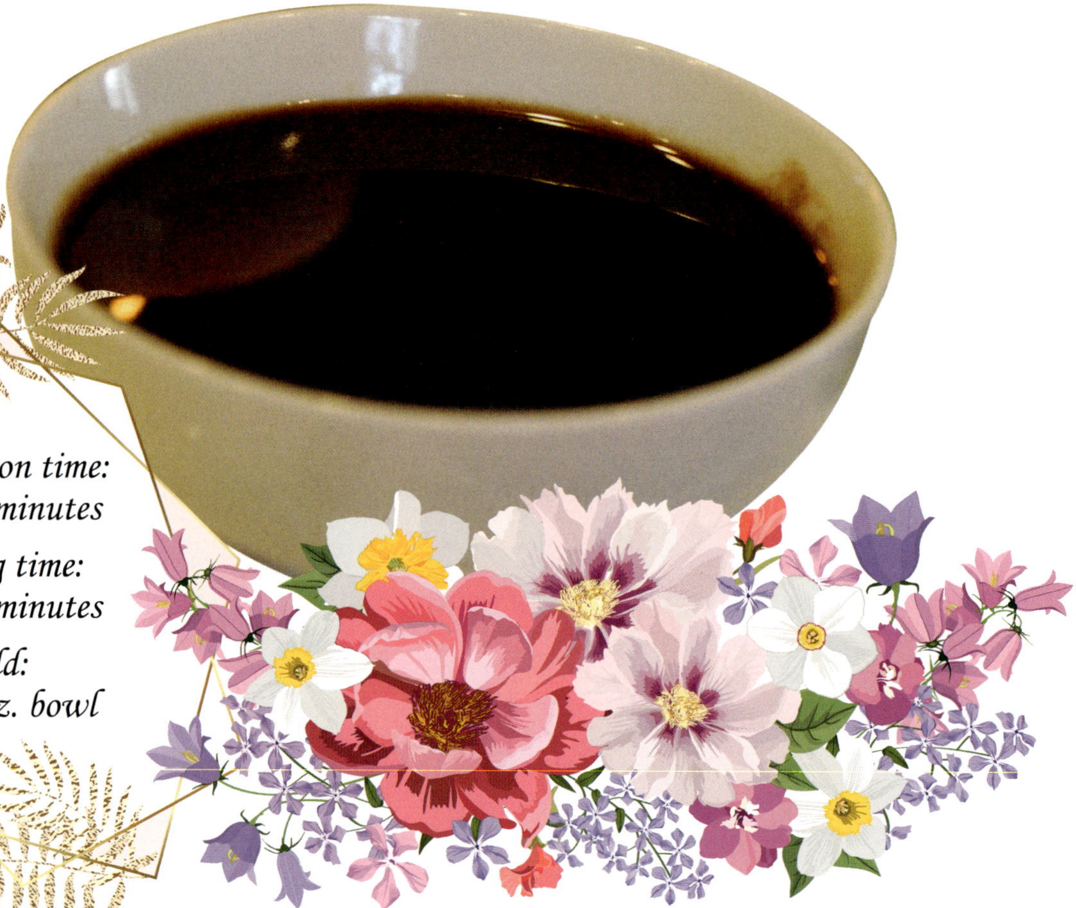

Preparation time:
10 *minutes*

Cooking time:
40 *minutes*

Yield:
8 *oz. bowl*

Ingredients

- ½ cup tamarind pulp
- 1 cup pitted dates, chopped
- ½ cup jaggery, chopped
- 2 teaspoons roasted cumin powder
- 1 teaspoon coriander powder (dhania powder)
- 2 teaspoons red chilli powder
- 4 cups water
- 2 teaspoons oil
- 1 teaspoon black salt (kala namak)
- 1 teaspoon salt

Process

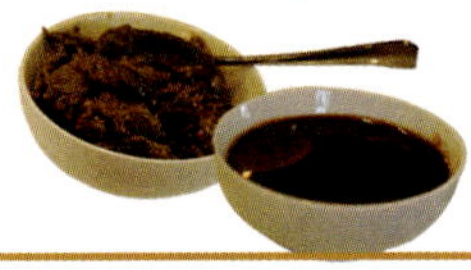

1. In a deep pan add water, tamarind pulp, dates and jaggery. Cook them all together for 10 minutes, checking that the dates get tender.
2. Cool the entire chutney mixture. Then, pour it in a blender jar and add roasted cumin powder, coriander powder, red chilli powder, salt and black salt.
3. Grind the entire mixture to a smooth liquid consistency.
4. Heat the oil in a small tempering pan and once oil heats up add cumin powder, roast for few seconds and add it to the date chutney. Mix it well.
5. If the chutney is thick then plain water may be added to get the desired consistency.
6. Serve with chaat or pakoras.

Apple Butter Chutney

A quick and easy chutney with healthy ingredients! A great substitute for tamarind chutney

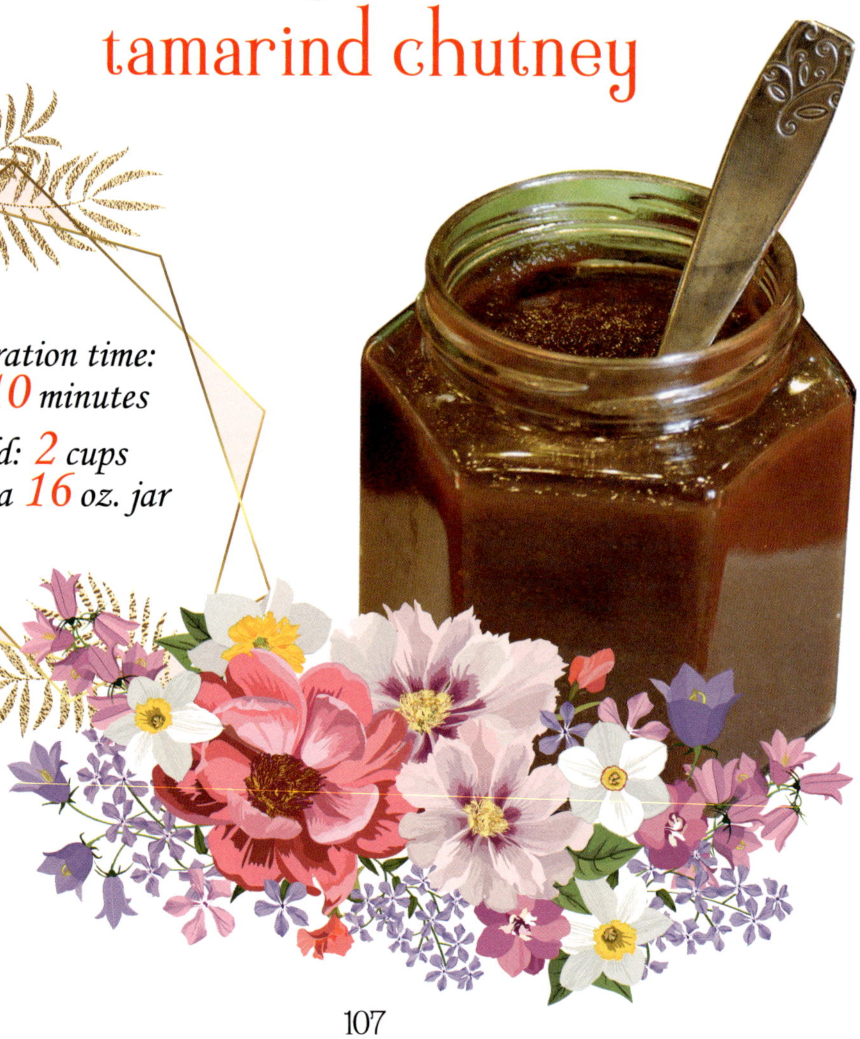

Preparation time: 10 *minutes*

Yield: 2 *cups or a* 16 *oz. jar*

Ingredients

- 16 oz. apple butter jar
- 2 teaspoons roasted cumin powder
- 1 teaspoon red chilli powder
- 4 tablespoons lemon juice (prefer bottled, as the preservative helps keep the chutney fresh longer)
- 1 teaspoon salt

Process

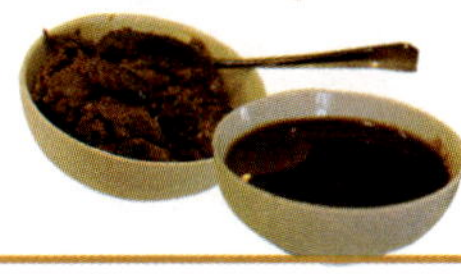

1. Pour apple butter into a mixing bowl.
2. Add cumin, chilli, lemon juice, salt and mix well with the apple butter. The chutney is now ready to serve.
3. Chutney may be refrigerated for up to 1 week.
4. It can be served with appetizers like dhokla and pakoras.

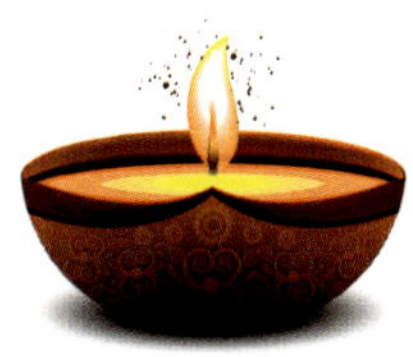

Almond Chutney

This chutney packs all the health benefits of almonds and tastes great too!

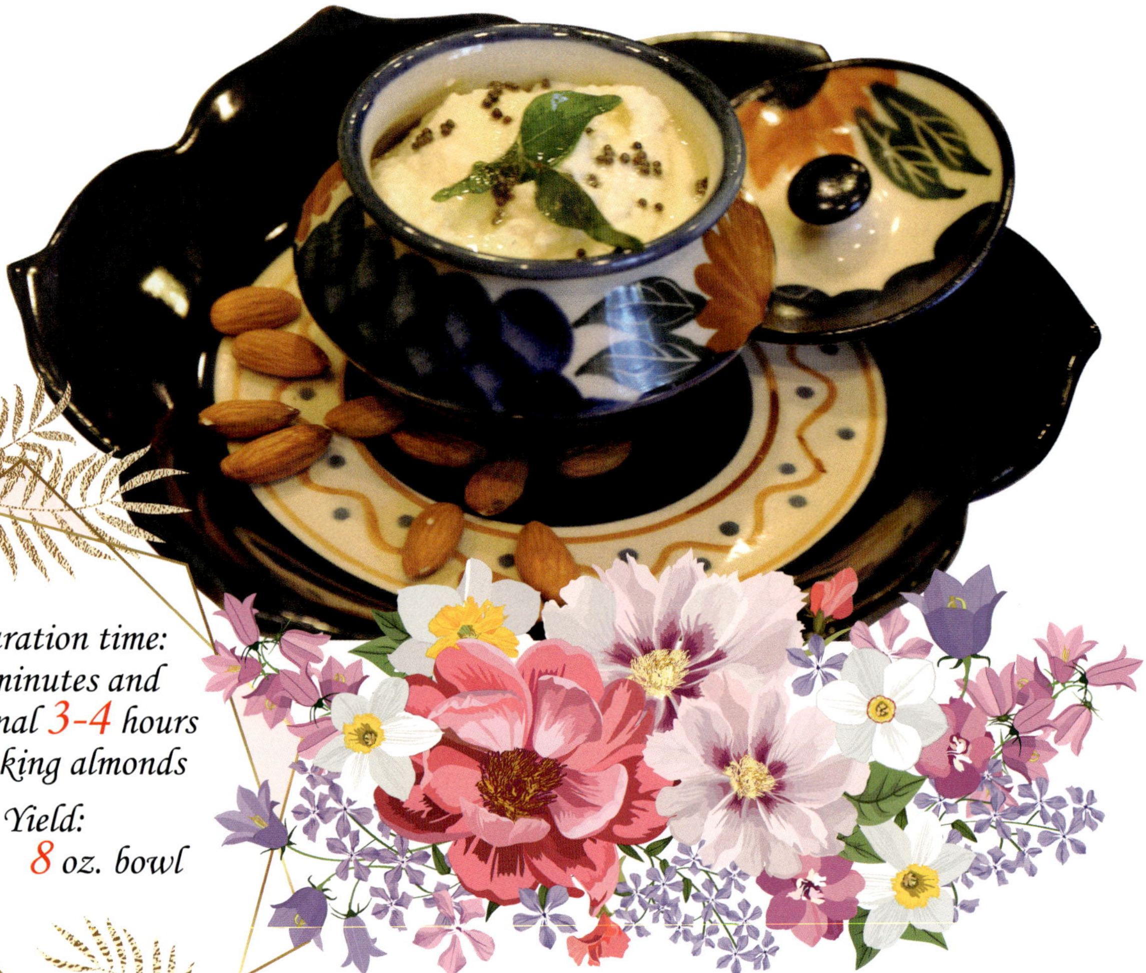

Preparation time:
10 minutes and additional 3-4 hours for soaking almonds

Yield:
8 oz. bowl

Ingredients

- ½ cup almonds, soaked
- 1 shallot onion (optional)
- ¼ inch piece ginger
- 2-3 green chillies
- 1 teaspoon salt or to taste

For tempering

- ⅛ teaspoon mustard seeds
- ⅛ teaspoon urad dal
- pinch asafoetida
- 3-4 curry leaves
- 1 teaspoon oil

Process

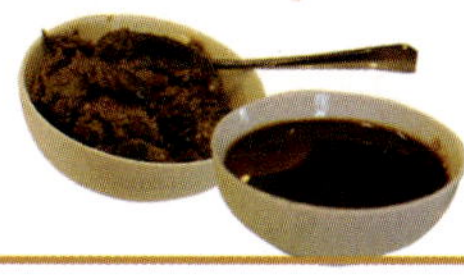

1. Soak the almonds in warm water for 3 to 4 hours. Drain the water and remove the skin of the almonds.
2. Grind the almonds, green chillies, ginger, onion (if using) and salt in a blender to a smooth paste with a little water.
3. For the tempering, heat oil in a pan and add mustard seeds, urad dal, asafoetida and curry leaves.
4. Pour this tempering on the chutney and serve.

Coconut Chutney

A popular earthy chutney served with South Indian meals

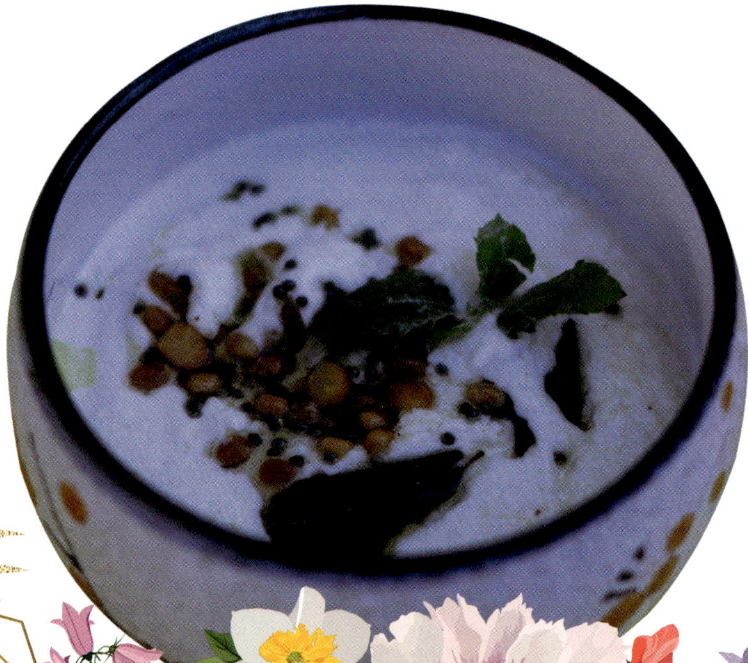

Preparation time:
10 *minutes*

Cooking time:
5 *minutes*

Yield:
8 *oz. bowl*

Ingredients

For chutney

- ½ cup chopped or grated coconut (fresh or frozen), defrost if using frozen
- 1 tablespoon roasted chana dal (dalia or fried gram)
- 1 tablespoon roasted peanuts (optional)
- 1 teaspoon tamarind paste
- ½ inch piece ginger
- 4-5 curry leaves (curry patta)
- 1 large green chilli or to taste
- ¼ cup water
- salt to taste

For tempering

- ½ teaspoon mustard seeds
- ¼ teaspoon urad dal
- ⅛ teaspoon asafoetida
- 1 tablespoon coconut oil

Process

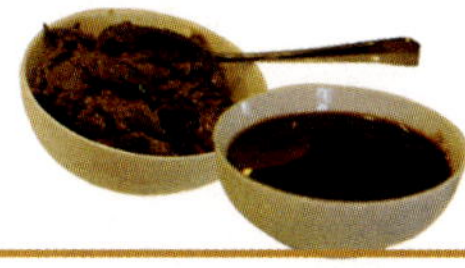

1. Blend all the chutney ingredients (coconut, chana dal, peanuts, green chilli, curry leaves, ginger and tamarind paste) with water to make a smooth paste. Adding water first makes it easier to grind. Transfer to a serving bowl.
2. In a small pan, heat the coconut oil on medium heat. Once oil is heated add mustard seeds and let them sputter.
3. Quickly add asafoetida and urad dal and roast the dal to a light brown color. Take it off heat immediately to prevent the dal from burning and pour this tempering over the prepared chutney paste.
4. Mix the tempering to the paste and the chutney is ready to be served.
5. Chutney stays good for 3-5 days if refigerated.

Tomato Chutney

A tangy delicious chutney can be served with appetizers or South Indian dishes

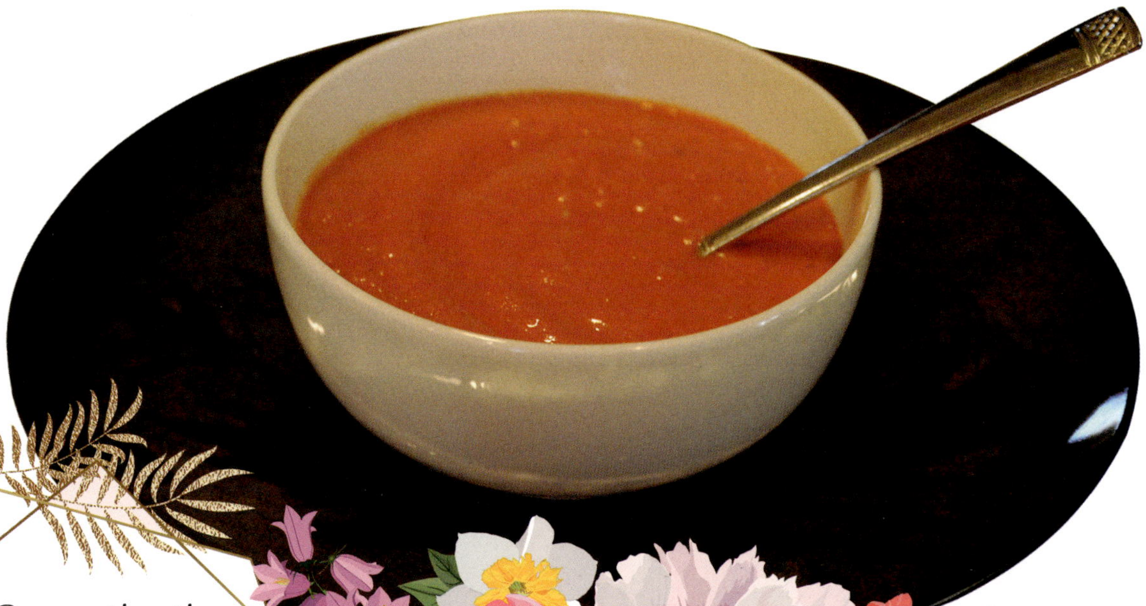

Preparation time:
10 minutes

Cooking time:
20 minutes

Yield:
1.5 to 2 cups

Ingredients

- 2 medium tomatoes, chopped
- 1 small onion, chopped (optional)
- 1 teaspoon tamarind paste
- 1-inch piece ginger, grated
- 1 green chilli, finely chopped
- handful of cilantro, finely chopped
- 5 curry leaves
- 1 teaspoon cumin seeds
- 1 teaspoon mustard seeds
- 1 teaspoon of fenugreek seeds
- 1 teaspoon turmeric
- 1 dry red chilli
- 1 teaspoon oil
- salt to taste

Process

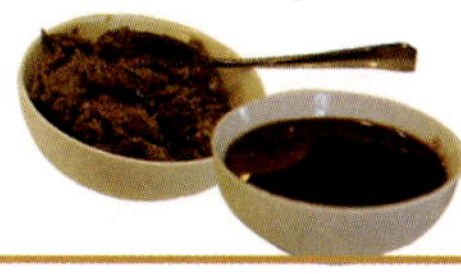

1. Heat oil in a medium pan and sauté the onions (if using) and then add the tomatoes.
2. Add all the spices (cumin seeds, mustard seeds, fenugreek seeds, turmeric, red chilli, salt) and cook for a few minutes until the ingredients are soft.
3. Add cilantro, green chillies, curry leaves, ginger, tamarind paste.
4. Remove from heat and bring to room temperature.
5. Let it cool. Use a blender, to make a smooth chutney that is now ready to serve.

Hummus

A protein rich spread made from chickpeas, garlic, tahini and olive oil

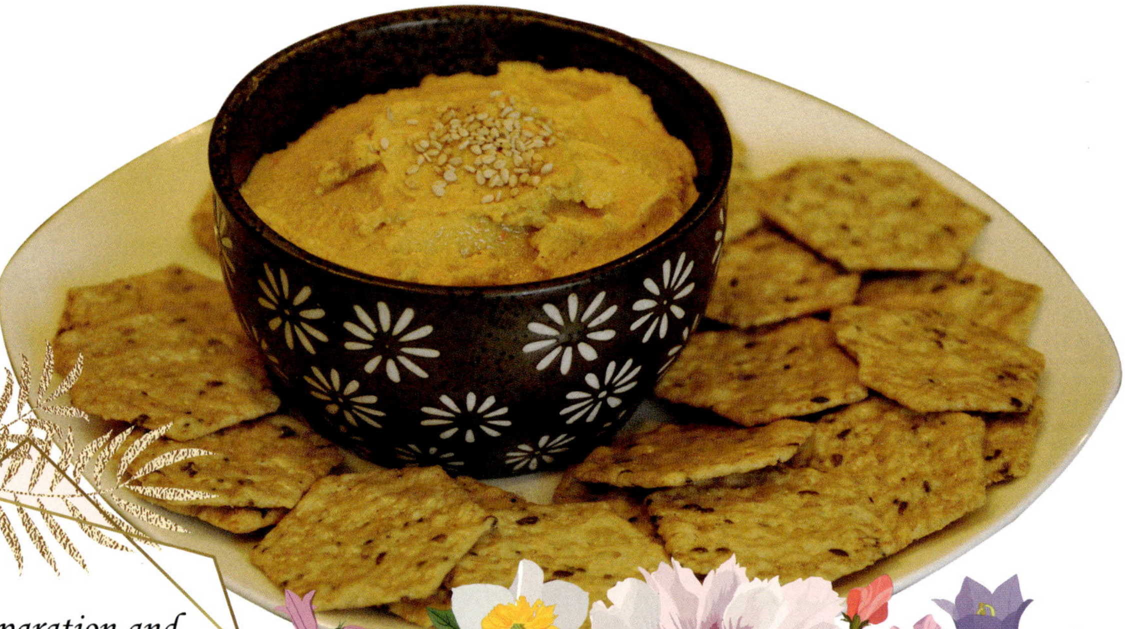

Preparation and assembling time:
15 *minutes or additional* 6-8 *hours soaking and cooking time for chickpeas if using uncooked ones*

Yield:
2 *cups*

Ingredients

- 15 oz. can rinsed chick peas or 1 ½ cups soaked and cooked chickpeas
- 1 small clove of garlic (optional)
- ¼ cup well stirred tahini or use ½ cup sesame seed ground in a paste
- 2 tablespoons extra-virgin olive oil
- ½ teaspoon ground cumin
- ½ cup red pepper
- dash of paprika for serving
- juice of one big lemon
- water - may need to add 2-3 tablespoons to get to right consistency
- salt and black pepper to taste

Process

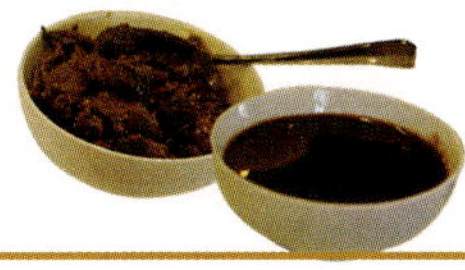

1. Blend the chickpeas, garlic, tahini, oil, lemon juice, cumin, peppers and salt together until smooth paste.
2. Keep adding a little bit of water and olive oil at a time while blending to get desired texture.
3. Sprinkle paprika and serve with tortilla chips or enjoy as a spread in sandwiches.

Substituting option: In case tahini is not available, roast ½ cup sesame seeds, and then grind them. Add some oil to these and they are ready to be used in place of tahini in the above recipe.

Mango Salsa

A sweet and spicy salsa with mango and jalapeños

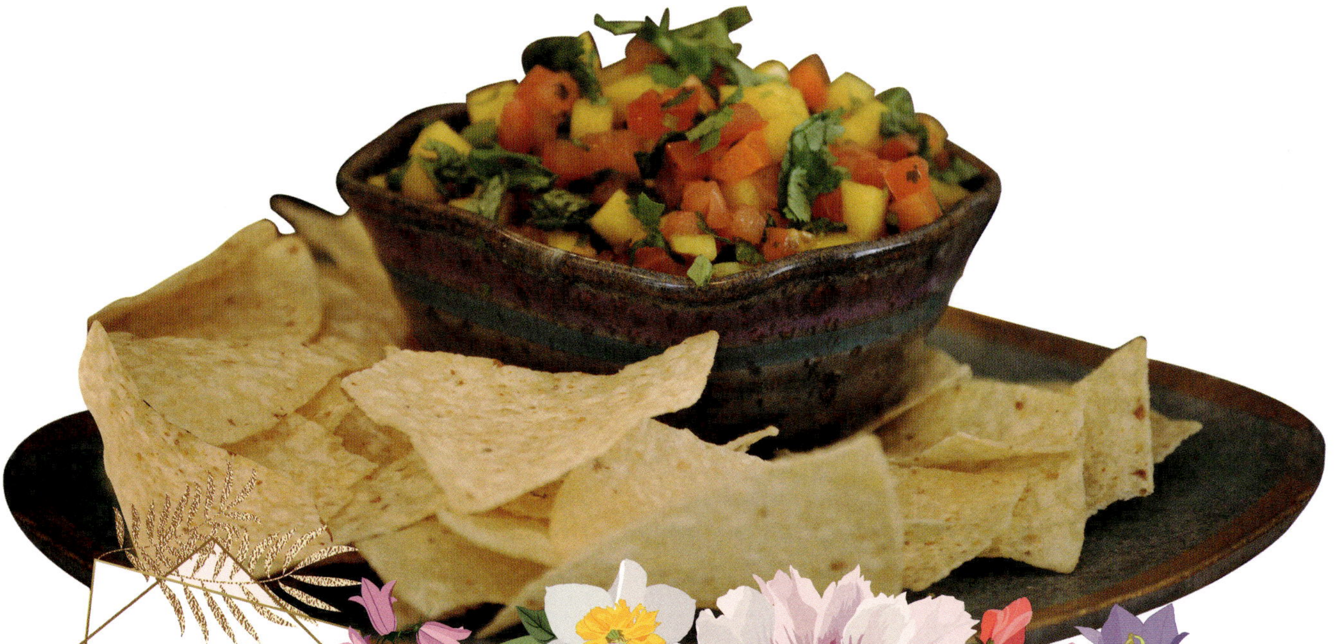

Preparation time: **10** *minutes*

Yield: **1.5** *cup*

Ingredients

- 1 cup ripe mango, cubed
- ½ cup red bell pepper, diced
- ¼ cup onion, finely chopped (optional)
- 1 jalapeño or to taste, finely chopped
- 1 bunch cilantro, finely chopped
- few mint leaves, finely chopped
- ½ teaspoon roasted and powdered cumin seeds
- lime or lemon juice to taste
- salt to taste

Process

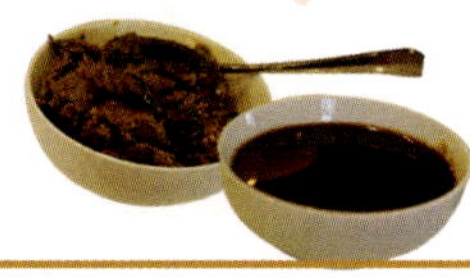

1. In a bowl, mix the mangoes, bell pepper, onion, jalapeños, cilantro and mint leaves. Add in salt, cumin powder and lemon or lime juice.
2. Toss and chill for 25-30 minutes.
3. Serve with tortilla chips, tacos, salad or as a side with grilled food.

Instant Lemon Pickle

A sweet and sour, hot spicy lemon pickle

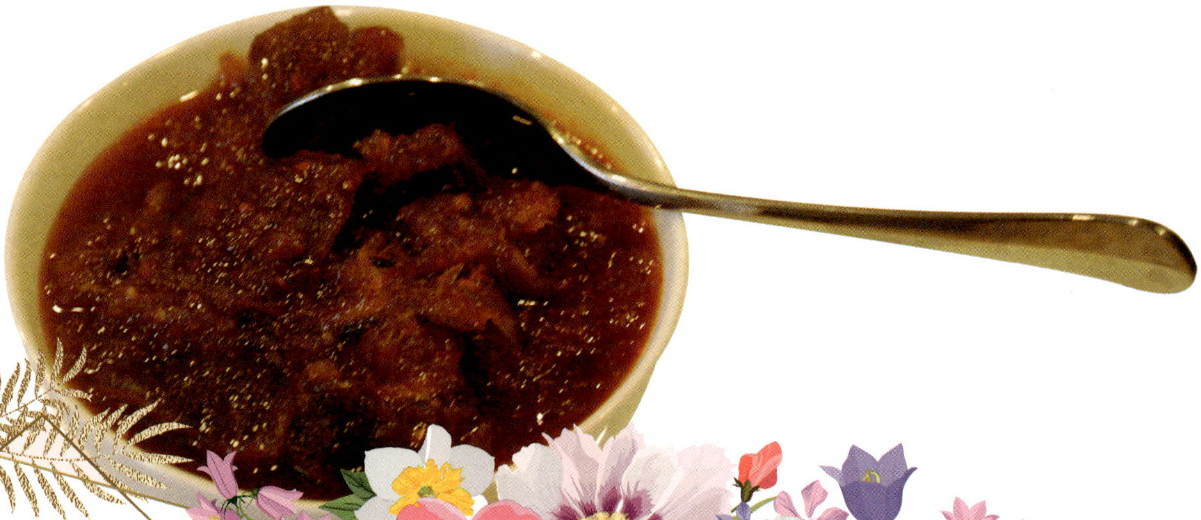

Preparation time: 15 *minutes*

Cooking time: 30 *minutes*

Yield: 12-16 *oz. jar*

Ingredients

- 5 lemons (4 lemons cut in quarters and juice of 1 lemon)
- ¼ cup red chilli powder
- 1 teaspoon turmeric powder
- pinch of asafoetida
- 1 teaspoon cumin powder
- 1 teaspoon dry coriander powder
- 1 teaspoon fenugreek seeds, roast and ground (optional)
- 1 cup sugar
- 1 tablespoon oil
- 3 teaspoons salt

Process

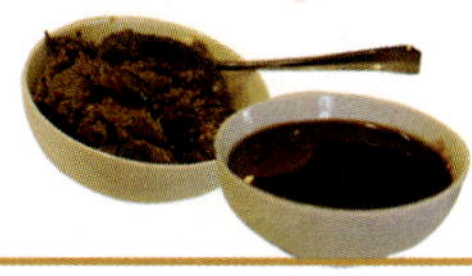

1. Cut 4 lemons into quarters and steam them for 15 minutes in a steamer.
2. Drain and set aside to cool.
3. Transfer the lemons to a mixing bowl. Mix in lemon juice, chilli powder, turmeric powder, asafoetida, cumin powder, coriander powder, fenugreek seeds, sugar, salt, and oil.
4. Mix all the ingredients well till the sugar is completely dissolved.
5. This pickle stays good for up to 3 months if stored in an airtight container.

Carrot and Green Chilli Pickle

An easy to prepare spicy vegetable pickle

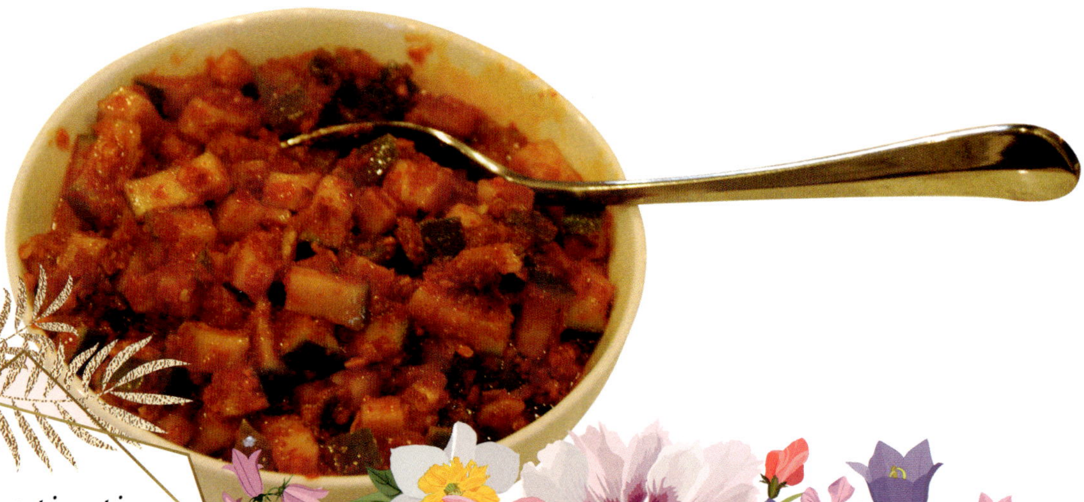

Preparation time:
45 *minutes*
(additional 18 *hours for overnight soaking and refrigeration)*

Yield:
16 *oz. jar*

Ingredients

- 2 big carrots, julienned on the thicker side
- 4 green jalapeño chillies, cut lengthwise and across the center to make one-inch julienne pieces
- 3 teaspoons ground mustard seeds
- 3 teaspoons ground fenugreek seeds
- ¼ teaspoon asafoetida
- 1 teaspoon red chilli powder
- 2 tablespoons white vinegar
- ¼ cup mustard oil
- 3 teaspoons salt, or to taste (used twice, 1 teaspoon for draining excess liquid from vegetables and 2 teaspoons in pickle masala)

Process

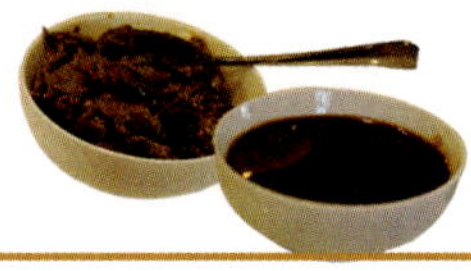

1. In a large mixing bowl, add carrots, green chillies, vinegar and only 1 teaspoon salt. Mix them well and keep aside for about 12 hours or overnight. Mix them again in between.
2. Transfer carrots/chillies to a colander to remove excess salt and vinegar, draining off all the liquid.
3. Now spread the carrot and chillies on paper towels for drying them and removing excess water.
4. In a separate mixing bowl add oil, mustard, fenugreek, chilli powders, asafoetida and salt. Whisk these until mixture is emulsified.
5. To the oil mixture add in the dried carrots and chillies. Mix well. Transfer to a glass/ceramic jar.
6. Cover and keep aside for 3-4 hours, shaking the jar several times.
7. The pickle is now ready to use and may be refrigerated for 15 days.

Mango Pickle

A delectable mango pickle that is quick and easy to make

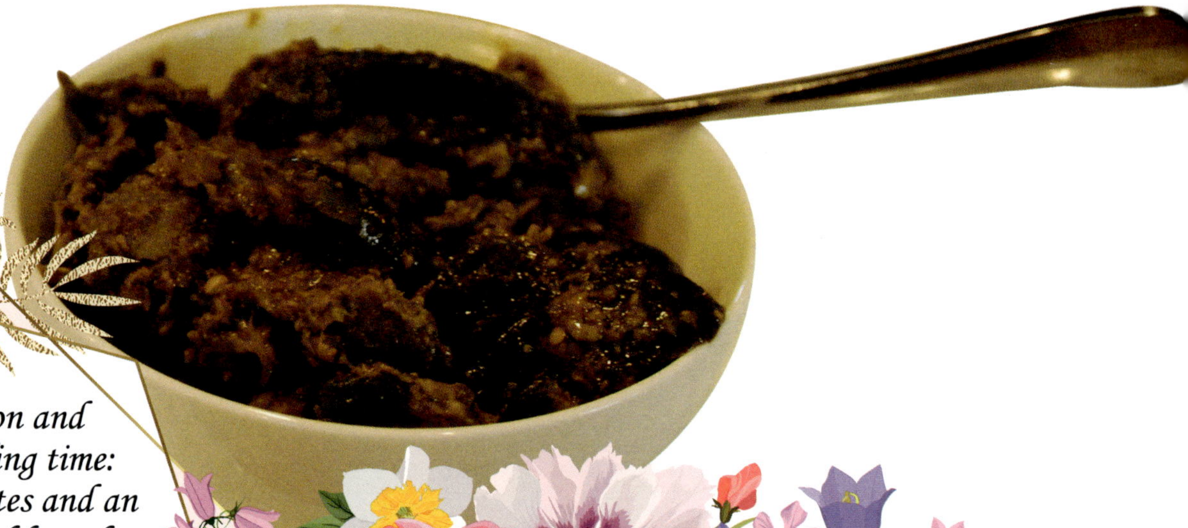

Preparation and assembling time:
60 *minutes and an additional hour for salting and setting aside mangoes*

Yield:
8 *oz. jar approx.*

Ingredients

- 2 cups raw green mangoes, peeled and cut in square pieces
- ½ teaspoon asafoetida
- ½ teaspoon turmeric powder
- 2 teaspoons roasted fennel seeds
- 2 teaspoons mustard powder
- 2 teaspoons chilli powder
- 2 teaspoons fenugreek powder
- 4 tablespoons mustard oil
- 1 tablespoon vinegar
- 3 teaspoons salt

Process

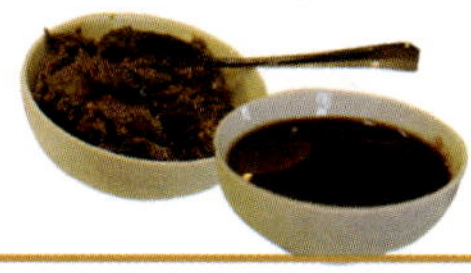

1. Add salt to the cut mangoes and mix well. Set aside for an hour.
2. Drain excess water from the mango pieces. Using paper towels, dry the mango pieces.
3. Combine the mango pieces, asafoetida, turmeric powder, fennel seeds, mustard powder, chilli powder, fenugreek powder, vinegar and mustard oil. Mix well.
4. The pickle may be used immediately or stored in the refrigerator for a few weeks.

Vegetable Raita

A spiced and whisked yogurt with a medley of vegetables, a perfect complement to the Indian meal

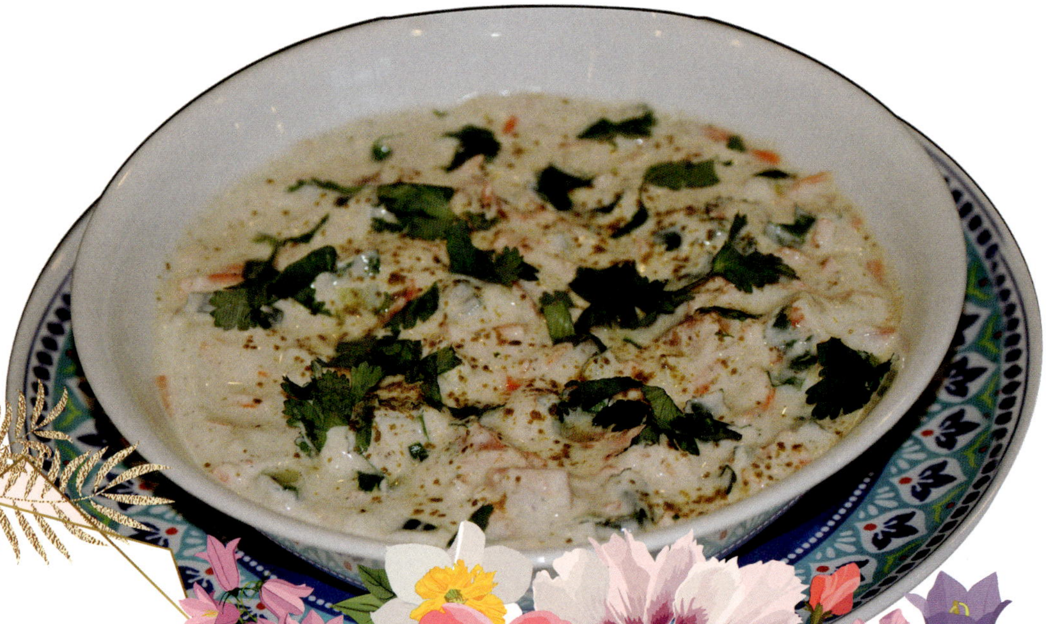

Total time: 15 *minutes*

Servings: 6 *small bowls*

Ingredients

- 2 cups fresh yogurt (not sour)
- 1 small cucumber, chopped
- 1 small tomato, chopped
- 1 small onion, chopped (optional)
- ½ cup carrot, shredded
- 1 small green chilli, chopped
- 1 tablespoon cilantro, chopped
- 2 teaspoons crushed roasted cumin seeds
- 1 teaspoon crushed black pepper
- ¼ teaspoon rock salt
- 1 teaspoon salt

Process

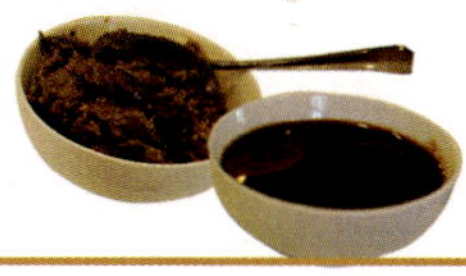

1. In a deep medium bowl add yogurt, roasted cumin, pepper, salt and rock salt and whisk them together.
2. Then add and mix in cucumber, tomato, onion (if using), carrot and green chilli.
3. Garnish with fresh chopped cilantro and serve with a typical Indian meal.

Alternate options: Other types of raita can be made in the same manner simply by replacing the vegetables with either boondi (fried tiny besan balls) or grated boiled lauki, boiled potatoes, fruits etc.

Sabzis, Dals and Curries

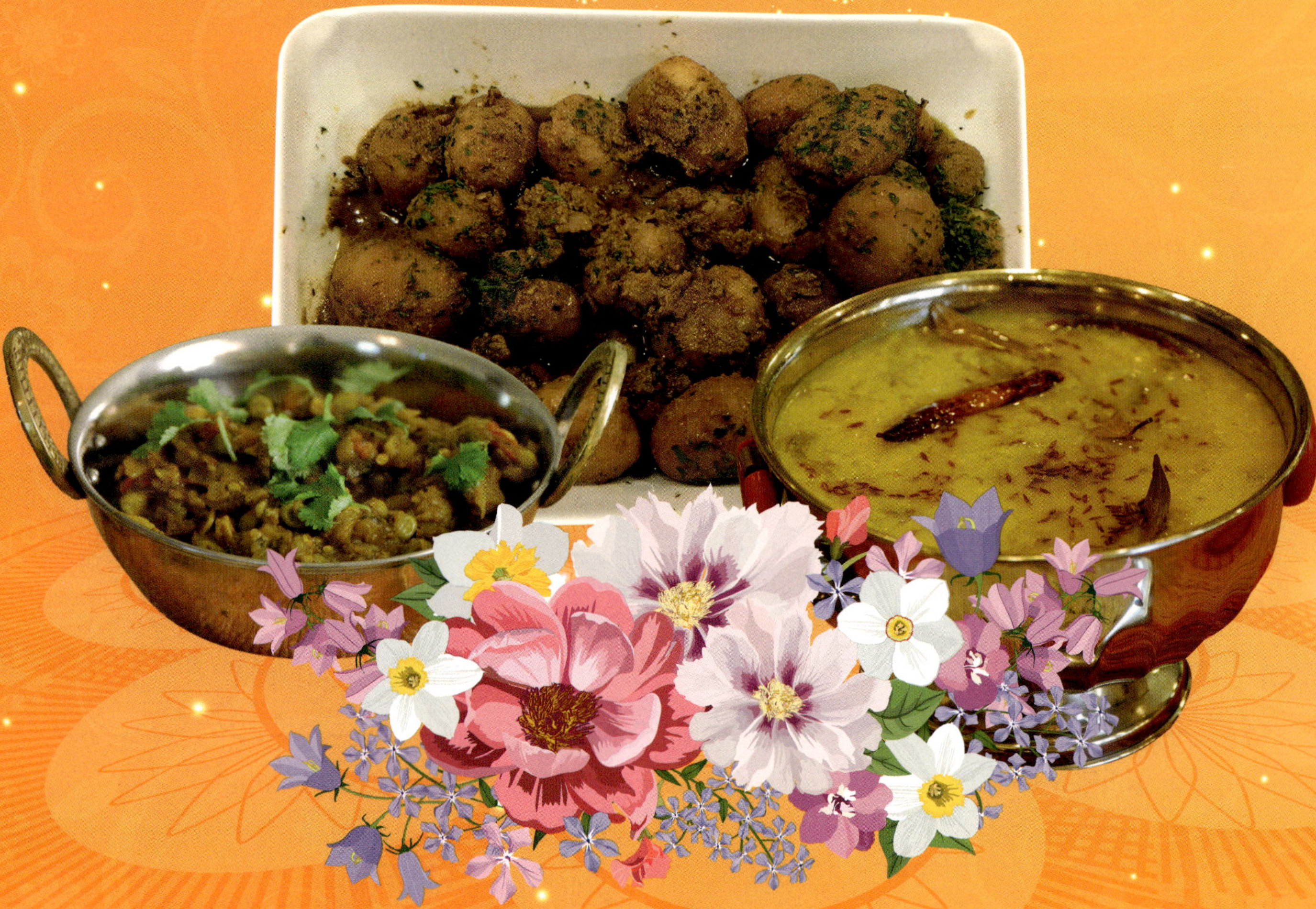

This chapter offers a wide selection of entrées that anchor the Indian meal - sabzis, dals and curries. These may be served with rotis, paranthas or rice preparations.

There is a range of vegetables used in these recipes from the greens-spinach, fenugreek, kale, to other commonly available vegetables like green and colored peppers, eggplants, okra (bhindi), lauki (bottle gourd), karela (bitter gourd), cabbage, cauliflower, mixed vegetables and potatoes.

Each of the dals has a different style and flavor – either by combining with vegetables as in the *karela dal* or *lauki chana dal*; or by tweaking the taste as the sweet and sour tastes in the *pineapple and Gujarati dal*, and the popular creamy taste of Punjabi *dal makhani*. Tempering with spices in the end further enhances the flavors.

Some vegetables and lentils are cooked together as curries such as the *mixed vegetable curry* and *cabbage and chana dal curry*. Popular dishes like *paneer makhani, Punjabi kadhi, chole* and *sambar* have also been included here to round up the selection.

All these preparations employ various cooking methods – sautéing, stir frying, steaming and boiling in the pressure cooker, cooking in the crock pot/slow cooker or in the instant pot.

1. Almond Sagu
2. Palak Paneer
3. Paneer Makhani
4. Cabbage and Red Pepper Flax Seeds Vegetable
5. Bharwaan Baingan with Aloo
6. Baingan Bharta
7. Kurkuri Bhindi
8. Gatte ki Sabzi
9. Kale and Peppers Sabzi
10. Aloo Gobi Masala
11. Kashmiri Mini Dum Aloo
12. Lauki Chana Dal
13. Pineapple Dal
14. Karela Dal
15. Gujarati Dal
16. Dal Makhani
17. Cabbage and Chana Dal Curry
18. Mixed Vegetable Curry
19. Punjabi Kadhi
20. Chole
21. Sambar

Almond Sagu

Mixed vegetables and potatoes cooked in rich almond gravy

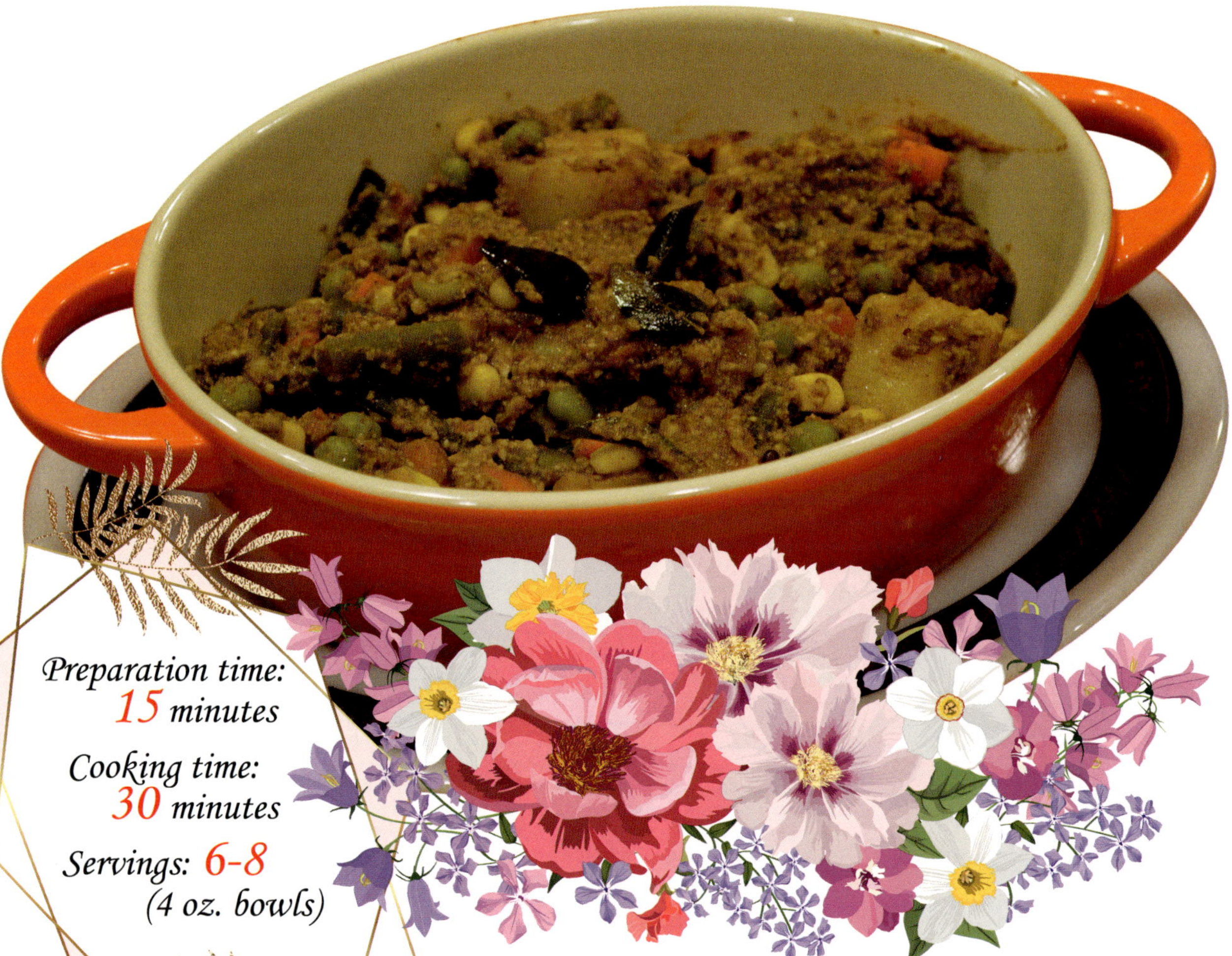

Preparation time: 15 *minutes*

Cooking time: 30 *minutes*

Servings: 6-8 *(4 oz. bowls)*

Ingredients

- 2 cups mixed vegetables (frozen mixed vegetables, with peas, corn, carrots, beans, steamed in the microwave for 2 minutes)
- 1 medium potato, cubed (microwave the cubes for 5 minutes approx.)
- 1 medium tomato, chopped
- 1 medium onion, chopped (optional)
- 1 teaspoon cumin seeds
- 1 teaspoon mustard seeds
- 1 tablespoon lemon juice
- 1 tablespoon vegetable oil
- 1½ teaspoons salt or to taste

To grind (for gravy)

- ¼ cup almonds (presoaking almonds in water for 15 minutes, microwaving them with water for 2 minutes, soften the almonds to make them easier to grind)
- ¼ cup onion, cut into big pieces (optional)
- ½ inch piece ginger
- 1 green chilli
- ½ cup cilantro, chopped
- 1-inch small piece of cinnamon (or 1 teaspoon of cinnamon powder)
- ¼ teaspoon or pinch of powdered cloves
- ¼ teaspoon of cardamom powder

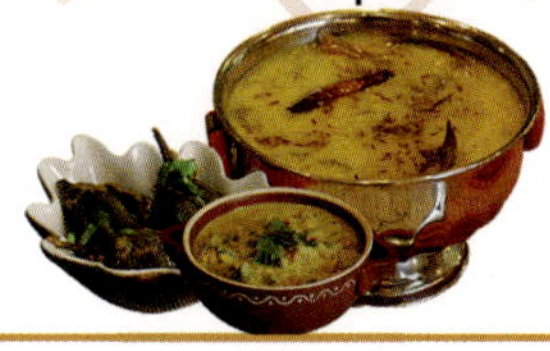

Process

1. Grind softened almonds (removing their skin), onion, ginger, green chilli, cilantro and the dry spices – cinnamon, cloves, and cardamom in a blender with approximately 2 cups water to make a purée for the gravy.
2. Steam the mixed vegetables and microwave the cubed potatoes. Keep aside.
3. Heat oil in a medium pan and add cumin seeds, mustard seeds, and curry leaves. When they start to pop, add the chopped onions (if using) and sauté until brown.
4. Now, add the chopped tomato, cook for a few more minutes. Then add the blended purée from step 1 above. Let it simmer for 15-20 minutes.
5. Once gravy seems thick, add cooked vegetables and potatoes. Add salt, and lemon juice and cook for a few more minutes.
6. Serve hot with rice or roti.

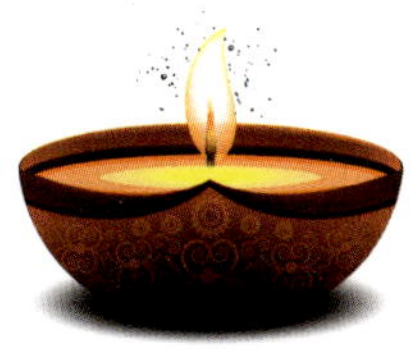

Palak Paneer

An evergreen healthy Punjabi staple served traditionally with makki ki roti, or just rotis

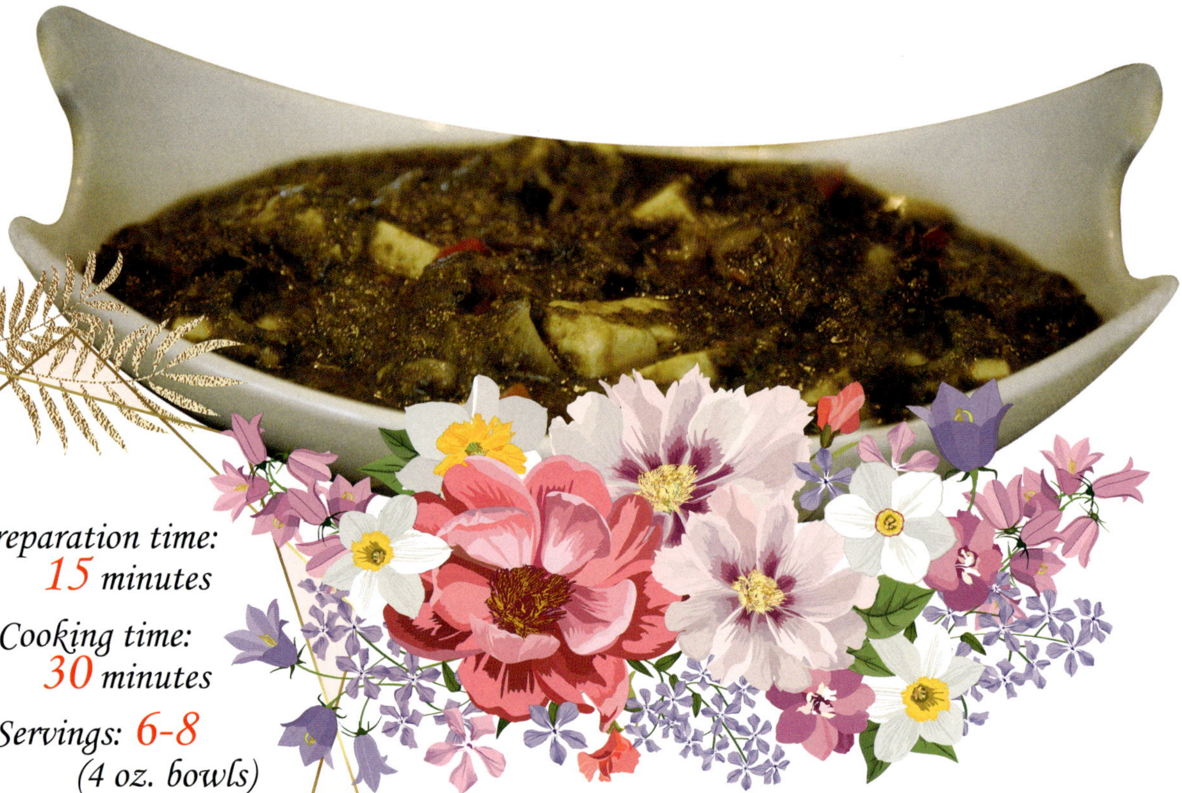

Preparation time: 15 *minutes*

Cooking time: 30 *minutes*

Servings: 6-8 *(4 oz. bowls)*

Ingredients

- 2 packets 24 oz. spinach, puréed
- 1 pack of 16 oz. paneer (cottage cheese), cubed and lightly fried
- 1 large tomato, chopped
- 1 small onion, coarsely chopped (optional)
- 1-inch ginger, finely chopped
- 2 teaspoons garlic, finely chopped (optional)
- 1 green chilli
- 1 teaspoon cumin seeds
- 1 bay leaf
- 2 teaspoons coriander powder
- ½ teaspoon garam masala powder
- ½ teaspoon red chilli powder
- 6 tablespoons oil
- salt to taste

Process

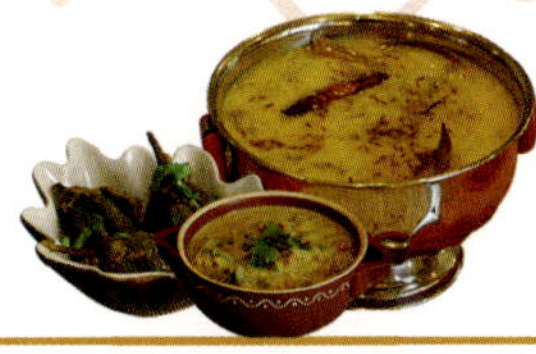

1. Heat 3 tablespoons of oil and sauté onion, garlic, ginger, green chilli in a small pan until light brown. Grind these ingredients in a blender/grinder.
2. Now in a bigger pan/kadai, heat 3 tablespoons of oil and add cumin seeds. When they splutter, add bay leaf and the onion mixture and cook well until the oil comes out.
3. Then, add tomatoes and cook over medium heat.
4. Once the tomatoes are well cooked, add garam masala, coriander powder, red chilli powder and salt. Stir them in until well mixed.
5. Then, add puréed spinach and cook for 10-15 minutes until the raw smell of the spinach goes away. Last, add the paneer cubes and cook for another 10 minutes.
6. Stir gently to not break the paneer cubes. Serve hot with rotis or makki ki roti.

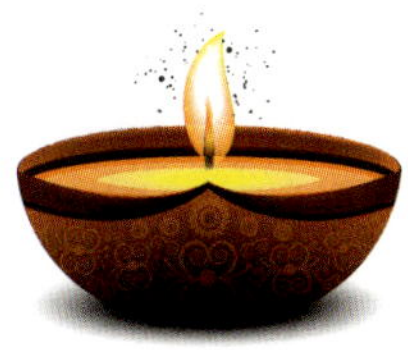

Paneer Makhani

An all-time favorite paneer dish made with a cashew-tomato-onion based gravy

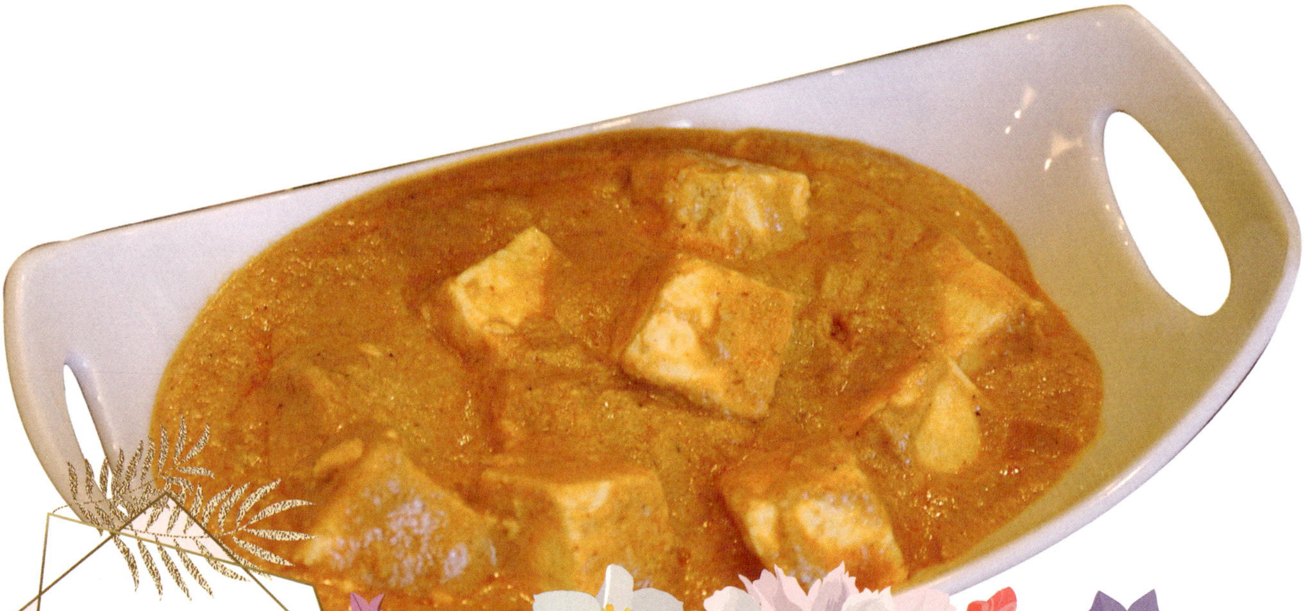

Preparation time: 10 *minutes*

Cooking time: 25 *minutes*

Servings: 8-10 *(4 oz. bowls)*

Ingredients

- 2 cups cubed paneer (If store bought can presoak paneer cubes to soften them)
- 4 medium tomatoes
- 1 medium onion (optional)
- 1-inch ginger
- ½ cup raw cashews
- ¼ teaspoon turmeric powder
- ¾ teaspoon red chilli powder
- 1 teaspoon coriander powder
- 1 teaspoon garam masala powder
- pinch of cardamom powder
- cilantro for garnishing
- ½ cup milk
- 3 tablespoons butter
- salt to taste

Process

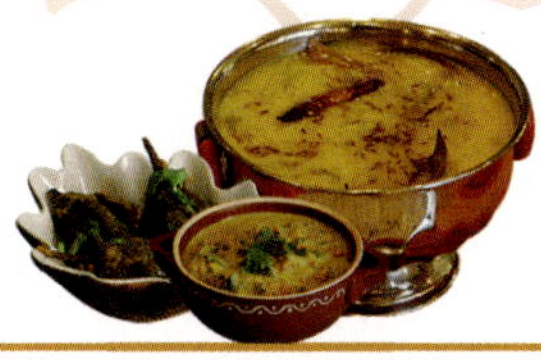

1. Cut paneer into cubes and soak them in hot water for 5 minutes to soften the cubes to better absorb the gravy.
2. In a blender, make a fine paste of onion, tomatoes, ginger and cashews.
3. Heat butter in a bigger pan/kadai. Add the above paste and sauté until oil appears on the sides of the pan.
4. Add all the dry spices – turmeric, red chilli, coriander powder, garam masala and cardamom powder to this masala and cook for about 5 minutes.
5. Now, add salt and a half cup of milk to this masala.
6. Then add the paneer cubes to the hot gravy and cook for about 5 minutes so that the paneer cubes are infused with gravy flavors.
7. Garnish the paneer makhani with cilantro and enjoy with roti or rice.

Alternate option: Instead of cashews, cream can be used as a base for a richer smoother taste.

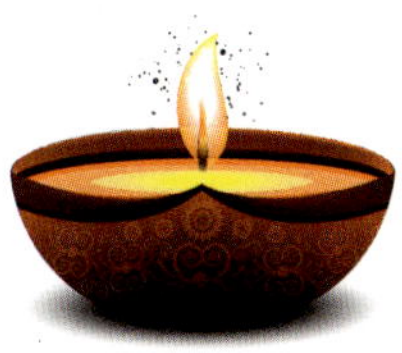

Cabbage & Red Pepper Sabzi with Flax Seeds

Crunchy cabbage dish with a healthy sprinkling of flax meal

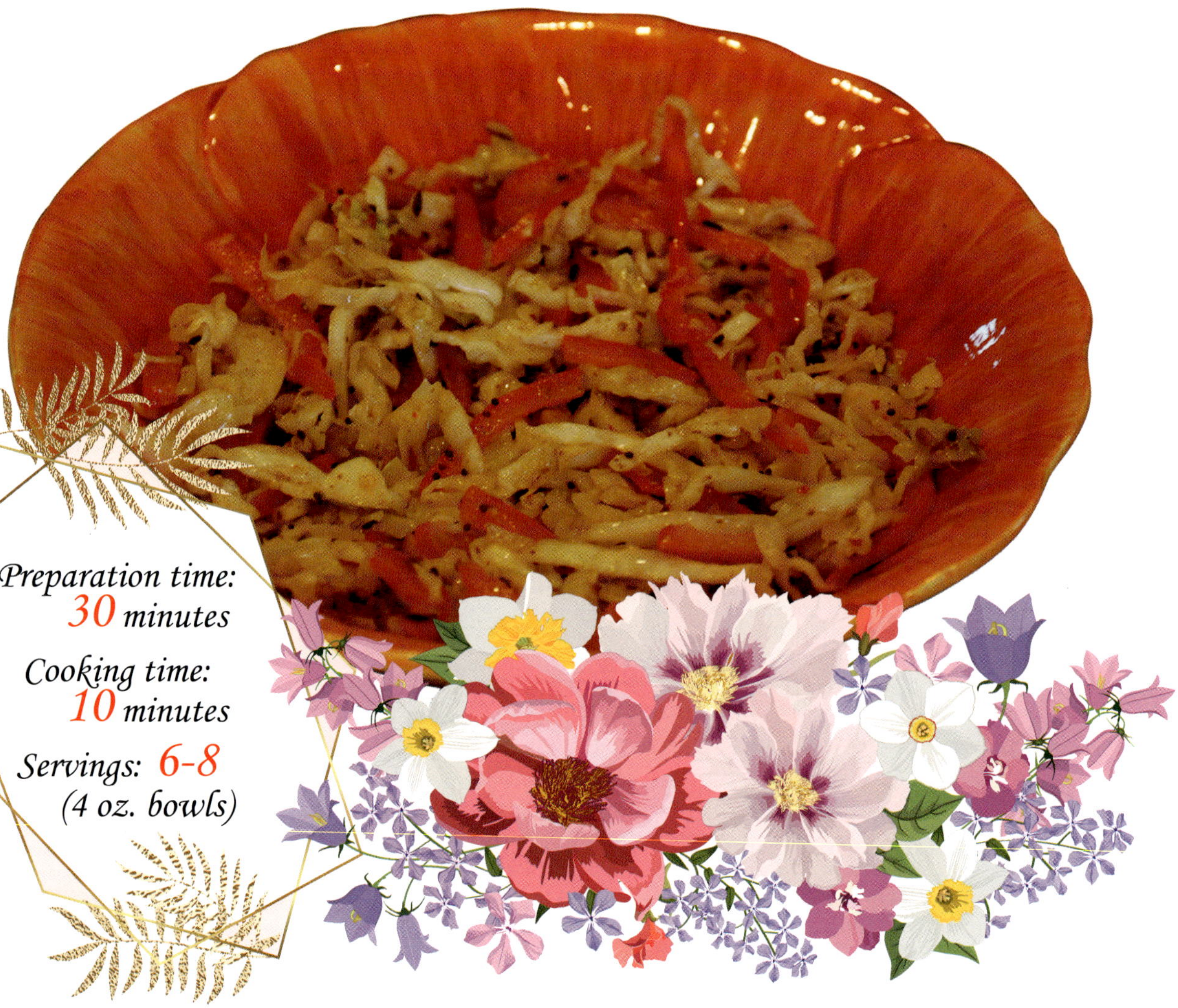

Preparation time: 30 *minutes*

Cooking time: 10 *minutes*

Servings: 6-8 *(4 oz. bowls)*

Ingredients

- ½ head cabbage, julienned
- 1 red bell pepper, julienned
- 4 teaspoons flax seed powder (flax meal)
- 1 teaspoon mustard seeds
- ½ teaspoon dried red chilli, coarsely ground
- ¼ teaspoon asafoetida
- 1 tablespoon urad and chana dal mix
- 6-7 curry leaves
- 1 tablespoon canola oil
- 1 ½ teaspoons salt or to taste (split in two)

Process

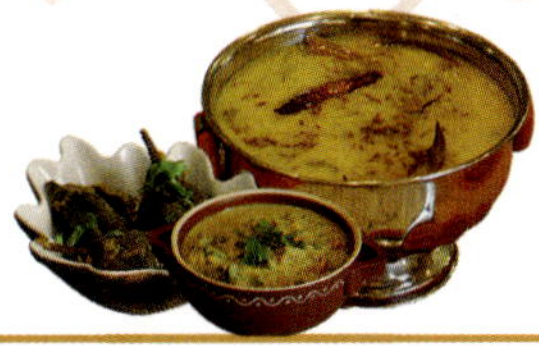

1. Place wok/pan on high heat and add 1 tablespoon of cooking oil.
2. Once oil is hot, add mustard seeds. When they start popping add curry leaves, dried red chilli flakes, asafoetida and urad-chana dal mix. Keep stirring for 10-15 seconds, until fragrant.
3. Now add cabbage and red bell pepper. Add 1 teaspoon salt and stir to mix in with the vegetables.
4. Reduce heat to medium and cover the wok/pan with a lid. After 4 minutes remove cover and toss vegetables. Cover again and let cook for another 3 minutes.
5. Remove lid and increase heat to high. Stir vegetables and cook for another minute or so. Vegetables should remain crunchy.
6. Then add remaining ½ teaspoon salt, flax seed powder and mix these well with the vegetables. Serve warm with roti.

Bharwaan Baingan with Aloo

Small eggplants stuffed with a medley of spices and tomatoes giving a unique flavor

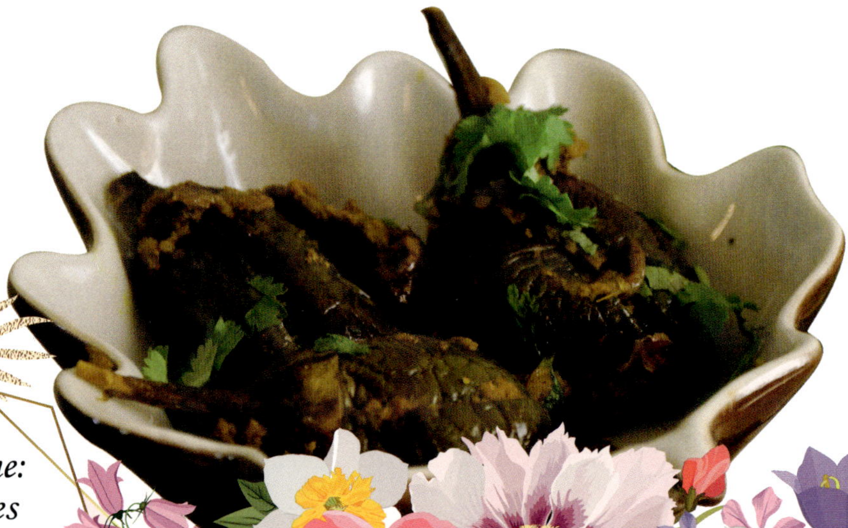

Preparation time: 40 *minutes*

Cooking time: 20 *minutes*

Servings: 8 *(4 oz. bowls)*

Ingredients

- 7-8 small eggplants
- 4-5 small red potatoes, peeled and quartered
- 1 tablespoon ginger, finely chopped
- 1 teaspoon green chillies, finely chopped
- 1 teaspoon red chilli powder
- 1 teaspoon cumin seeds
- 1 tablespoon cilantro for garnishing
- ⅓ cup canola oil
- ⅓ cup water

For the stuffing

- 2 cups tomatoes, finely chopped
- 1 cup cilantro, finely chopped
- ½ cup dry unsalted peanuts, powdered
- 3 teaspoons coriander powder
- 1 teaspoon turmeric powder
- 1 teaspoon mango (amchur) powder
- 1 teaspoon garam masala powder
- salt to taste

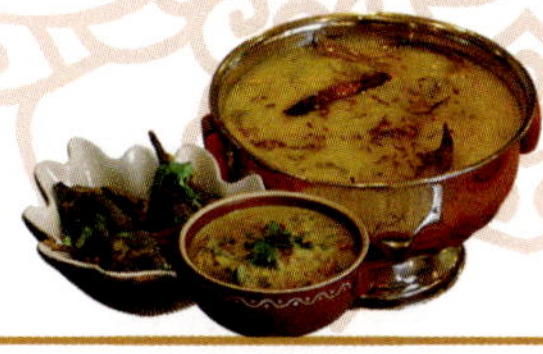

Process

1. Prepare the stuffing mixture by mixing together the chopped tomatoes, cilantro (reserving a tablespoon for garnish), powdered peanuts and dry spices (turmeric, coriander, amchur, garam masala powders and salt).
2. Wash and pat dry the eggplants. Remove the stems and make two slits to quarter them, about 1 cm from the base so that the pieces are joined together.
3. Stuff the eggplants very generously with the stuffing mixture, ensuring that the stuffing is tightly packed. Reserve the remaining mixture.
4. In a shallow large pan, heat ⅓ cup oil on medium high heat and add cumin seeds. When the seeds splutter, add chopped ginger and green chillies, until the ginger begins to turn light brown in color.
5. Then, add the quartered potatoes and fry potatoes for 3-4 minutes until very light brown.
6. Now, add the remaining tomato mixture and eggplants and stir gently and turn off stove.
7. Transfer contents of the pan into a pressure cooker carefully and add ⅓ cup water.
8. Pressure cook on high heat till one whistle.
9. When the pressure cooker has cooled, open the lid and very gently transfer the contents with a spoon into the serving dish.
10. Garnish with cilantro and serve hot with rotis.

Baingan Bharta

A traditional roasted eggplant recipe with a smoky flavor

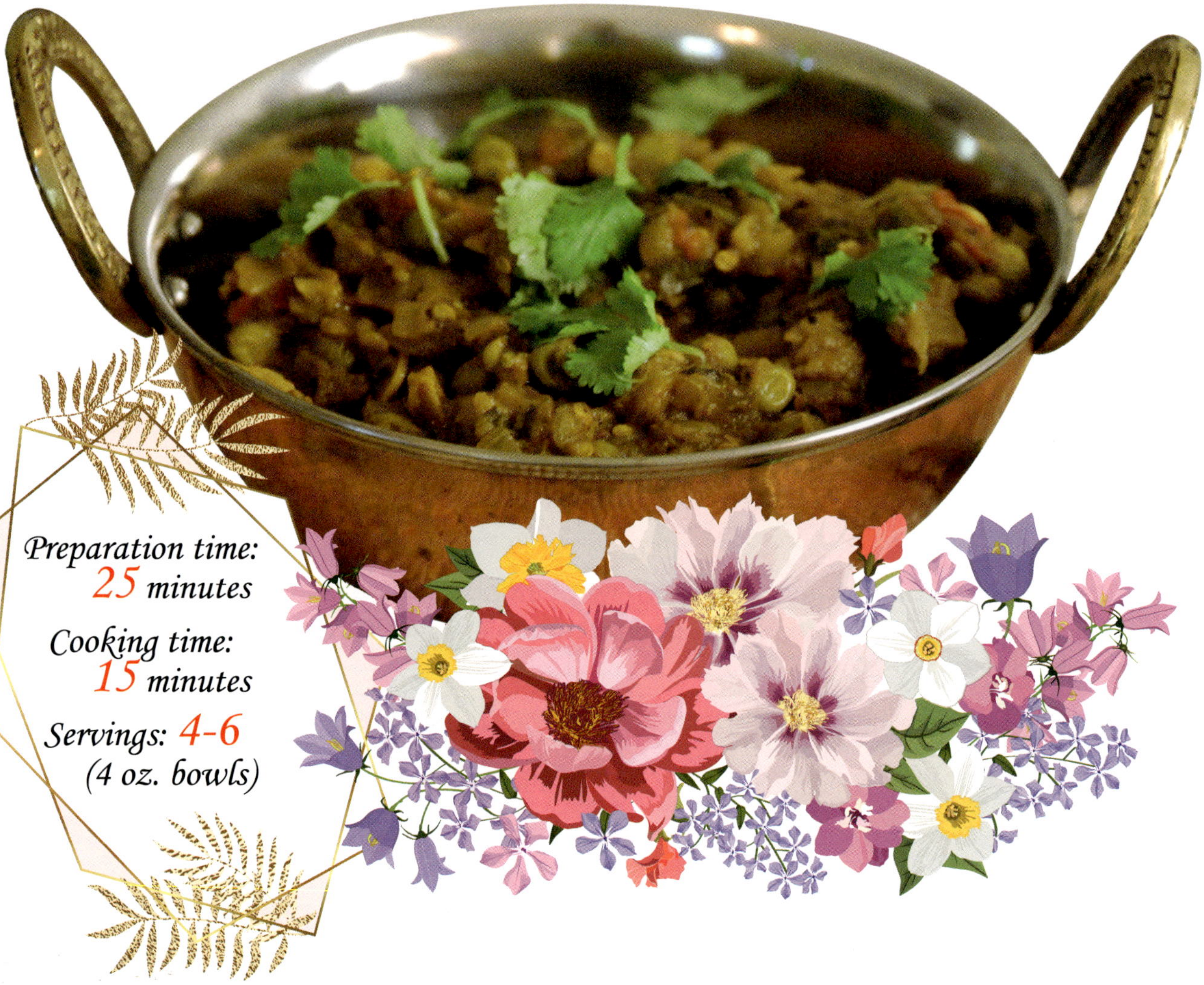

Preparation time: 25 *minutes*

Cooking time: 15 *minutes*

Servings: 4-6 *(4 oz. bowls)*

Ingredients

- 1 large eggplant
- 1 tomato, finely chopped
- 1 medium-sized onion, chopped (optional)
- 2 green chillies
- ½ teaspoon turmeric powder
- 1 tablespoon coriander powder
- 1 teaspoon red chilli powder
- ½ cup cilantro, chopped for garnishing
- 2 tablespoons vegetable oil or sesame oil
- salt to taste

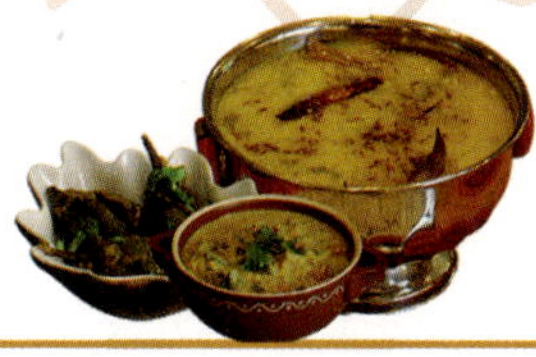

Process

1. Wash and pat dry the eggplant with a napkin. Apply little oil all over the eggplant and roast it on the open flame/stove or in the oven. If you are roasting the eggplant on an open flame, turn the eggplant every two minutes so that it gets evenly cooked.
2. Once completely roasted, rinse eggplant with water so that the roasted skin comes off easily. Now smash roasted eggplant using a fork. Keep aside.
3. Heat oil in a separate pan/kadai and add chopped onions (if using), and tomatoes. Sauté onions and tomatoes for 5 minutes.
4. Add the smashed eggplant and turmeric, coriander and red chilli powder, green chillies and salt. Cook on low flame for 10-15 minutes with the lid uncovered.
5. Garnish with cilantro and serve hot with naan, roti or parantha.

Optional: Green peas may be added to the bharta, as in the photo.

Kurkuri Bhindi

Crispy twist to a traditional vegetable

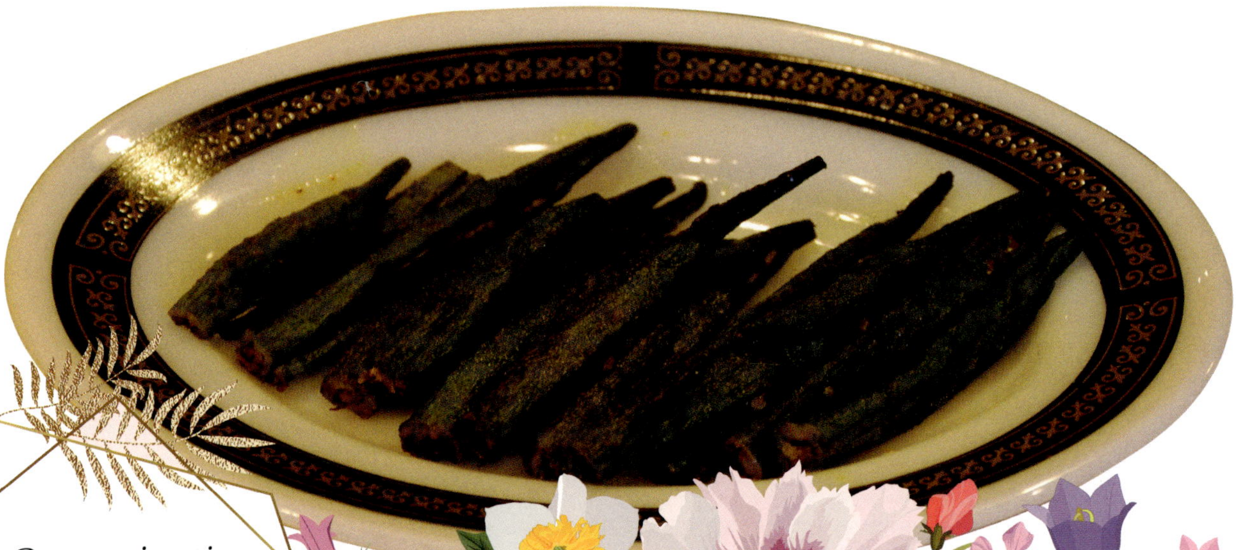

Preparation time: 20 *minutes*

Cooking time: 15 *minutes*

Servings: 3-4

Ingredients

- 15-20 pieces of bhindi (okra)
- 1 teaspoon gram flour (besan)
- ½ teaspoon rice flour
- ½ teaspoon turmeric powder
- 1 teaspoon red chilli powder
- ¼ teaspoon cumin powder
- ½ teaspoon mango (amchur) powder
- ¼ teaspoon chaat masala powder
- oil for frying
- salt to taste

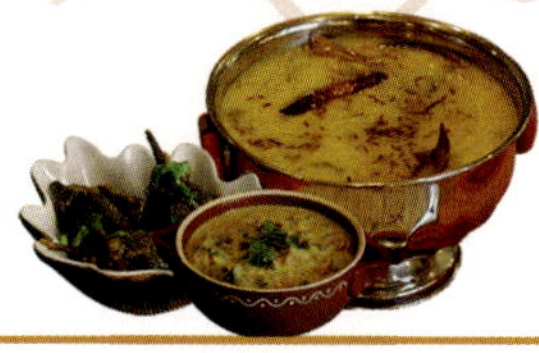

Process

1. Wash and dry bhindi.
2. In a mixing bowl, cut the bhindi lengthwise and deseed them.
3. Add all the masala ingredients–besan and rice flour, turmeric, red chilli, cumin and amchur powders, to the bowl and mix well.
4. Add some salt to taste in the end just before frying.
5. In a pan/kadai heat oil for frying.
6. Deep fry the bhindi till it turns crisp in hot oil.
7. Remove excess oil from the bhindi by placing it on paper towels.
8. Sprinkle some chaat masala on top before serving with rotis or paranthas.

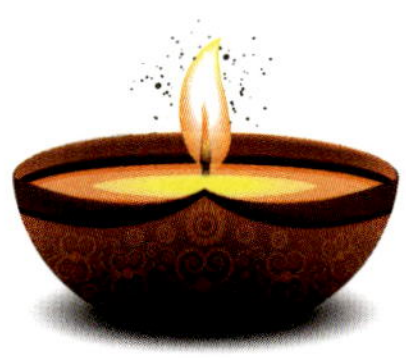

Gatte ki Sabzi

A typical Rajasthani dish made with boiled gram flour dumplings in spicy curd gravy

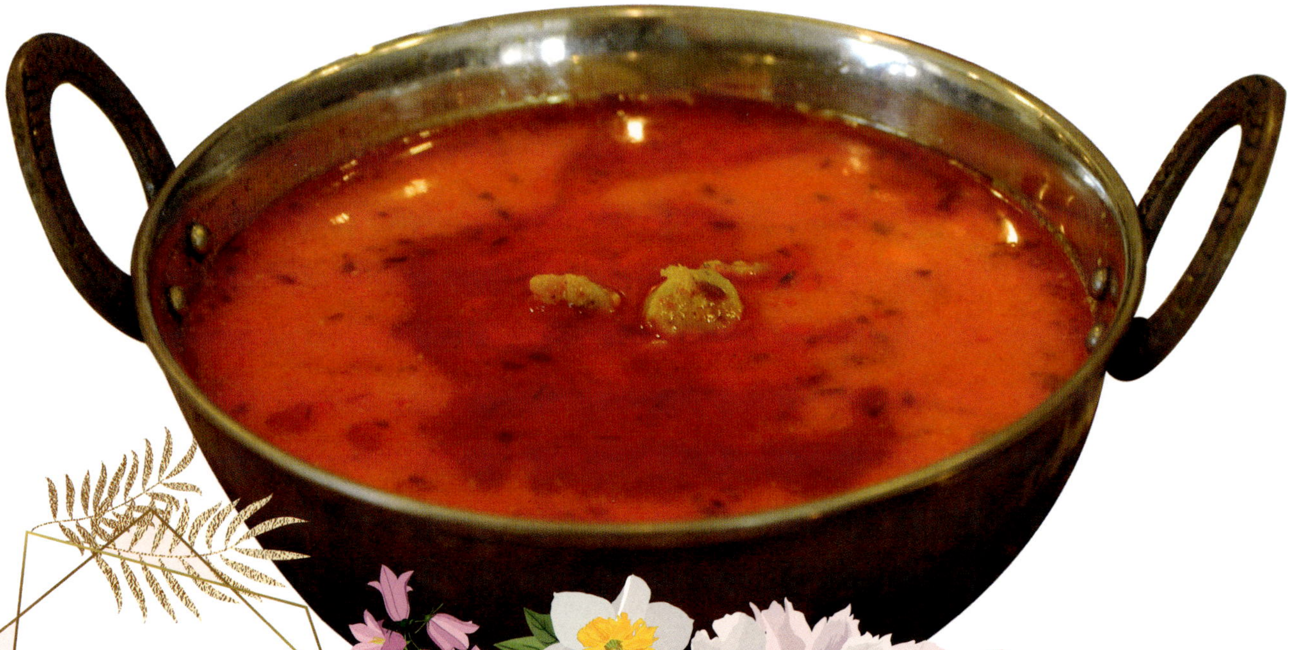

Preparation time: 1 *hour*

Cooking time: 30 *minutes*

Servings: 8-10 *(4 oz. bowls)*

Ingredients

For the gatte

- 2 cups gram flour (besan)
- 1 tablespoon fennel seeds (saunf)
- 2 teaspoons red chilli powder
- 2 tablespoons oil
- 2 teaspoons salt
- water for kneading (add gradually to make a semi-hard dough)

For the gravy

- 1-inch ginger, minced
- 2-3 green chillies, finely minced
- 1 teaspoon cumin seeds
- 2 teaspoons asafoetida
- 1 teaspoon turmeric powder
- 1 teaspoon red chilli powder
- 1 cup yogurt at room temperature
- 3 tablespoons ghee
- salt to taste

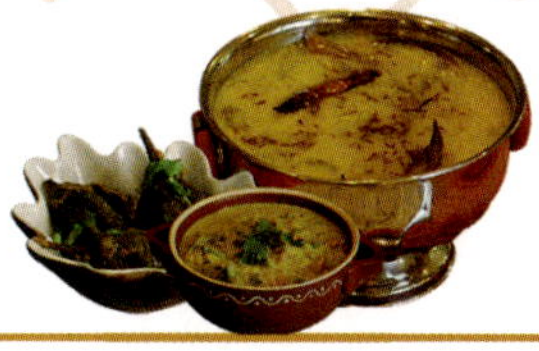

Process

For the gatta

1. Mix fennel seeds, red chilli powder and salt to the gram flour.
2. Using water and oil now knead the gram flour with the mixed spices to a dough like consistency.
3. Boil water with a few drops of oil in a deep pan.
4. Make long rolls of gatta (7-10 inches) and submerge them in water that is on a rolling boil. Boil for 20 minutes.
5. Take gatta rolls out and slice them into discs.
6. Reserve the liquid.

For the gravy

7. Make a paste of ginger and green chillies.
8. Heat oil, then add cumin seeds, asafoetida, red chilli powder and ginger-green chilli paste in the order mentioned. Cook till fragrant.
9. Then add the reserved liquid and more water if so desired (the liquid tends to thicken over time).
10. Add salt and turmeric powder.
11. Let it come to a boil, then add gatte discs and boil for another 5 minutes.
12. Now reduce the heat and add the yogurt. Keep stirring in the yogurt till the sabzi comes to a boil.
13. Reduce heat and cook for approximately 10 minutes on medium heat.
14. Serve with rice or puris.

Additional tips: Asafoetida is the key flavor so add liberally. Once you add the yogurt, cook only on reduced heat. High heat will make the yogurt curdle. Also, to add an extra zing, temper in the end with ghee, asafoetida, red chilli powder and a spoonful of water.

Kale and Bell Pepper Sabzi

Packed with healthy ingredients and great flavor

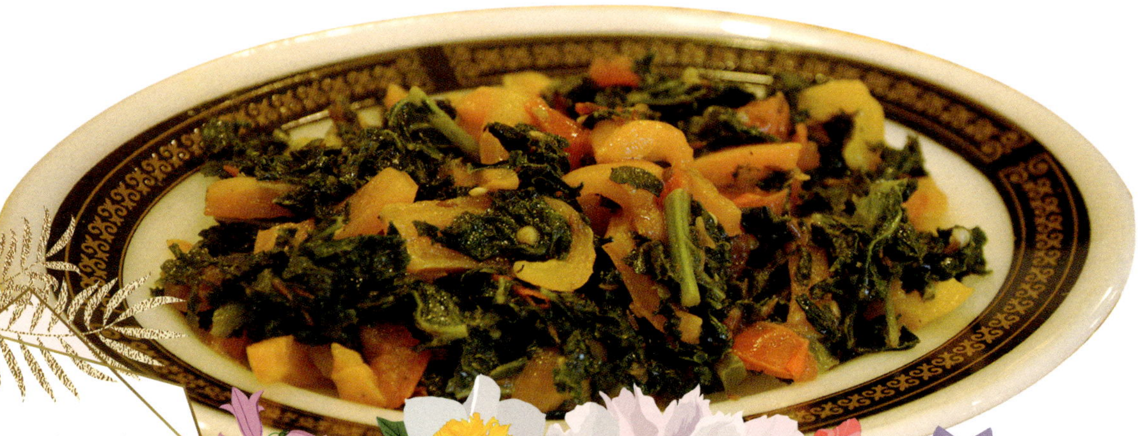

Preparation time: 20 *minutes*

Cooking time: 20 *minutes*

Serves 4-6 *(4 oz. bowls)*

Ingredients

- 6-7 oz. or 1 bunch kale
- 1 cup fresh spinach leaves
- 1 red bell pepper, sliced
- 1 medium tomato, chopped
- 2 Thai green chillies, finely diced
- pinch asafoetida (hing)
- 1 teaspoon cumin seeds
- ½ teaspoon black pepper powder
- 1 tablespoon ghee
- salt to taste

Process

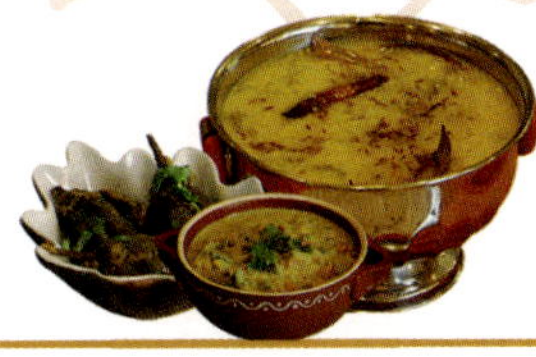

1. Roughly pluck kale leaves by hand from the stem.
2. Warm ghee and add cumin seeds and once they start sputtering, add green chilli and asafoetida.
3. Sauté bell pepper for 3-4 minutes.
4. Then add kale and salt.
5. Once kale reduces in volume, add spinach.
6. Add black pepper. Cover and cook for 5-6 minutes.
7. Then add the tomatoes and cook uncovered for another 2-3 minutes. Check on salt.
8. Enjoy with rotis.

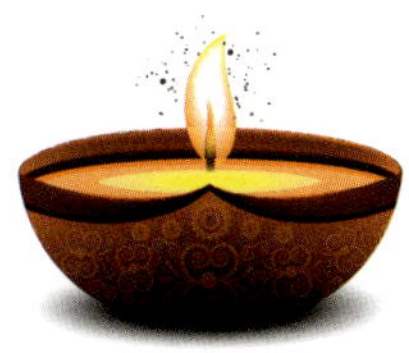

Aloo Gobi Masala

Another all-time favorite sabzi cooked in tomatoes and spices

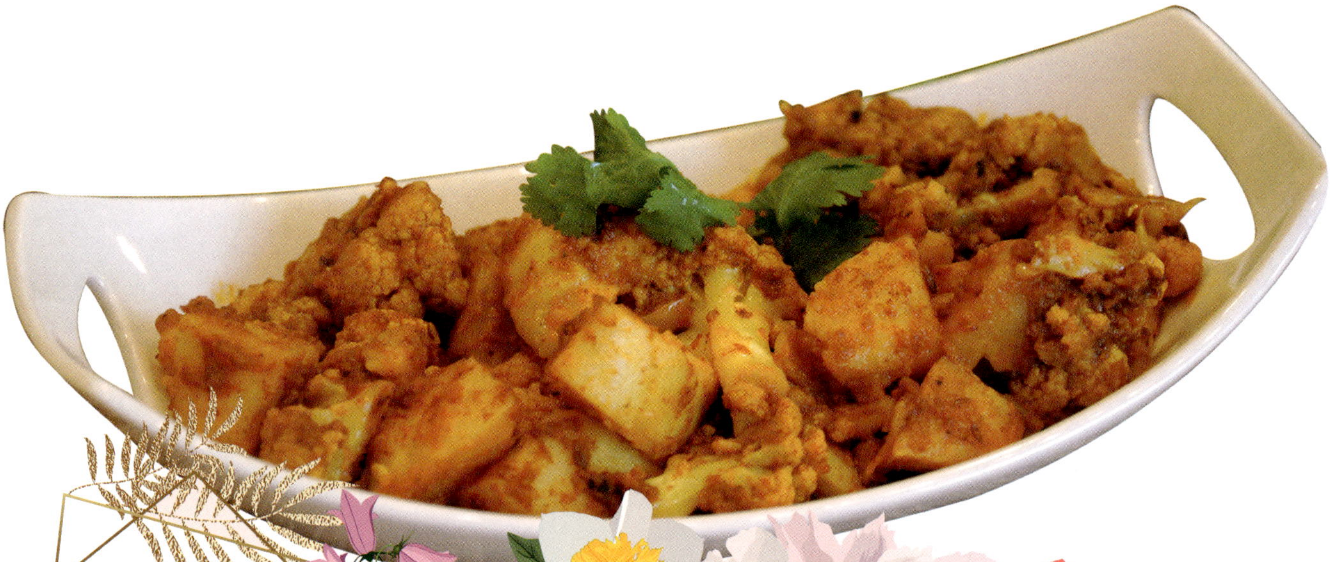

Preparation time: 20 *minutes*

Cooking time: 20 *minutes*

Servings: 10-15 *(4 oz. bowls)*

Ingredients

- 1 large sized cauliflower (gobi), cut in medium size florets
- 5 to 6 medium size potatoes, boiled and cubed
- 2 medium size tomatoes, chopped
- 2-inches ginger, chopped
- 1 teaspoon cumin seeds
- 1 bay leaf
- 1 teaspoon turmeric powder
- 1 teaspoon red chilli powder
- 2 teaspoons coriander powder
- ½ teaspoon garam masala powder
- cilantro leaves for garnish
- 4 tablespoons oil or ghee
- salt to taste

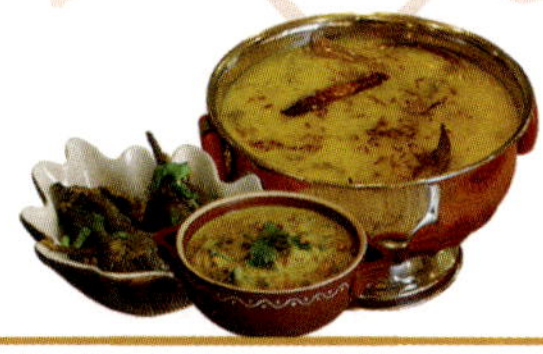

Process

1. Cut cauliflower in medium florets. Rinse the florets well in water.
2. Spread them on a plate and cover with wet paper towel. Microwave for 4 minutes until they are tender.
3. Boil potatoes for approximately 10 minutes or until they are cooked. Once cool chop in cubes.
4. In a thick bottomed pan, heat oil or ghee. Add cumin seeds and when they sputter add the chopped ginger, tomatoes and spices and salt except for garam masala to the pan. Cook for 3-4 minutes, until tomatoes are soft.
5. Lower the flame and add the cauliflower and potatoes and cook for 5-7 minutes. Add garam masala.
6. Garnish with cilantro, serve warm with roti or parantha.

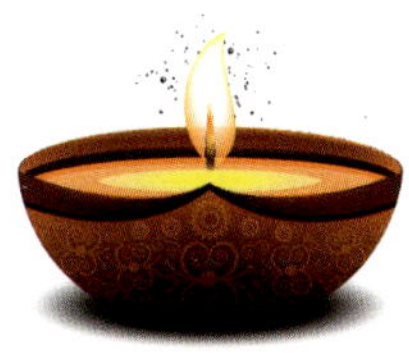

Kashmiri Mini Dum Aloo

A delightful blend of potatoes cooked in yogurt and spices in this popular dish

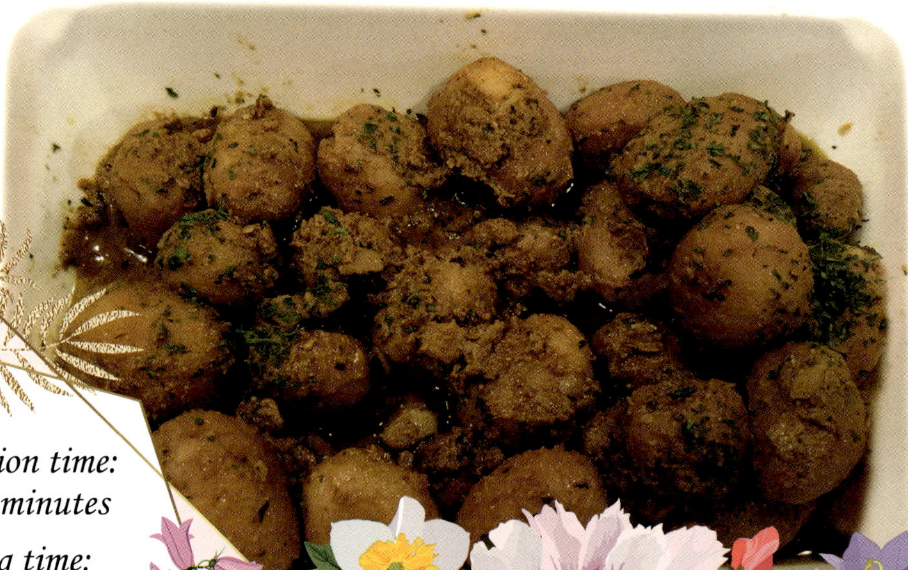

Preparation time: 20 *minutes*

Cooking time: 40 *minutes*

Servings: 10-12 *(4 oz. bowls)*

Ingredients

- 20 small potatoes
- 2 cups whole milk yogurt
- 2 tablespoons fennel powder
- ½ tablespoon cumin powder
- ½ tablespoon coriander powder
- ½ tablespoon red chilli powder
- ½ teaspoon green cardamom powder
- 2 big (black) cardamoms, the pods cracked open
- 1 tablespoon cumin seeds
- 2-3 cloves
- 2-3 cinnamon, small pieces
- a pinch asafoetida
- salt to taste

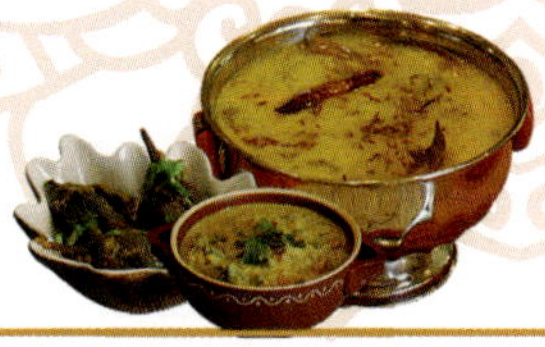

Process

1. Boil potatoes in a microwave till they are soft but not mushy (probably 10-15 minutes). Peel the potatoes and prick them slightly with fork.
2. Heat oil in a wok/pan and fry the potatoes till evenly golden brown. Prick potatoes one more time and keep them aside.
3. In a bigger pan, heat oil and add cumin seeds, cloves, black cardamoms, asafoetida powder and cinnamon sticks. Stir for few seconds till fragrant. Now, add the fried potatoes to this oil.
4. In a bowl whisk yogurt with cumin, coriander, green cardamom, red chilli and fennel powders, and salt. Pour this yogurt mixture on to the potatoes with some water.
5. Allow potatoes to cook in the gravy for 30 minutes on low heat, with the lid covered, checking in between ensuring that the masala does not stick to the bottom of the pan.
6. Before serving, garnish with coriander leaves and serve hot with steamed rice.

Cooking note: The dum aloo's are first pricked with a fork and later cooked on low heat with monitoring so that the spices and flavors of the masala seep deep inside the potatoes to give them their unique taste.

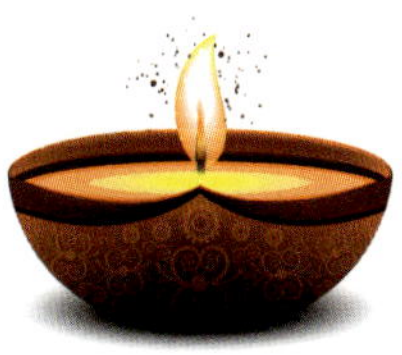

Lauki Chana Dal

A great way to incorporate lauki with the nutrition packed chana dal

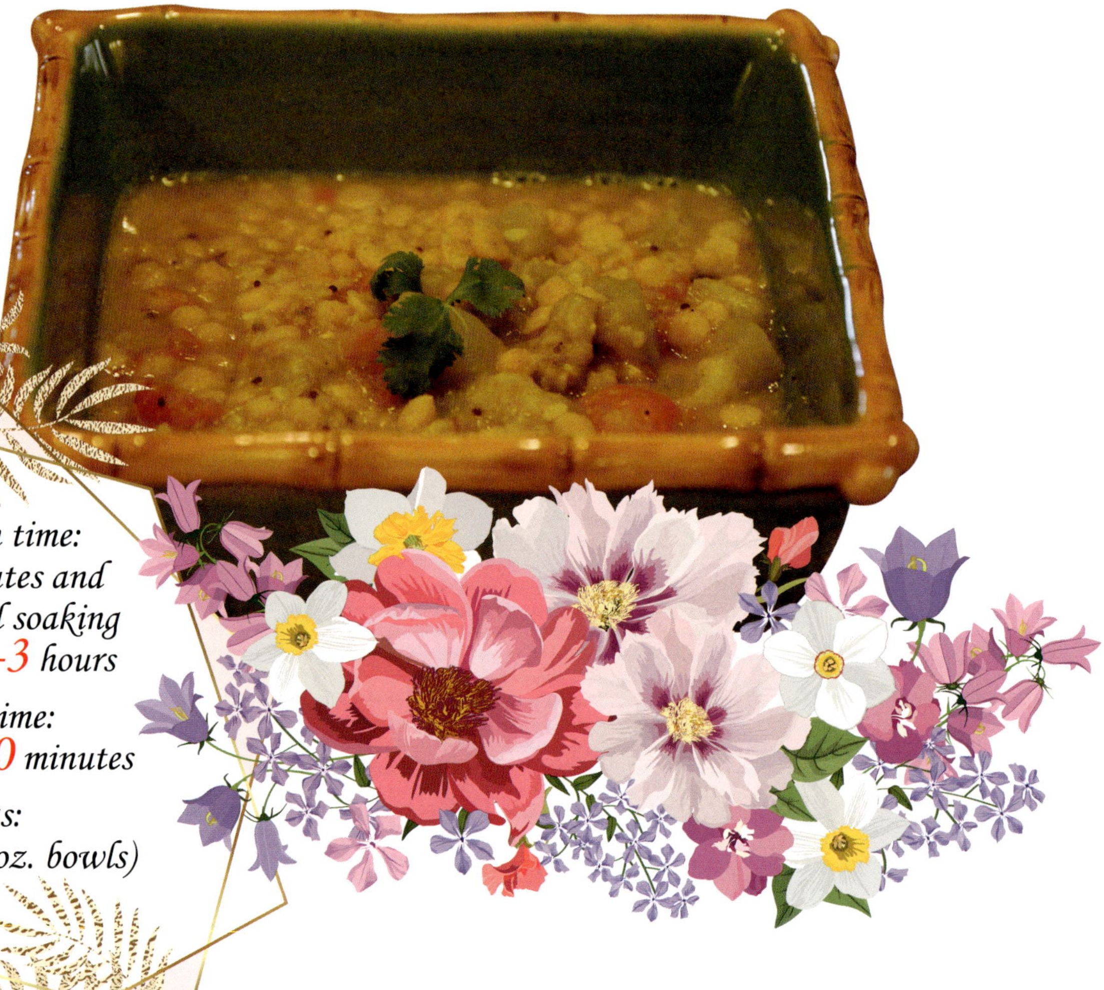

Preparation time:
10 minutes and additional soaking dal for 2-3 hours

Cooking time:
40 minutes

Servings:
8 (6 oz. bowls)

Ingredients

- 1 lauki (bottle gourd), thin long one, or about 3 cups chopped in cubes
- 1 cup chana dal, soaked in water for 2-3 hours
- ½ teaspoon mustard seeds
- ½ teaspoon cumin seeds
- 1 teaspoon turmeric powder
- 1 teaspoon coriander powder
- 2-count dry red chillies
- 1 pinch asafoetida
- 1 tomato, finely chopped
- 1 teaspoon ginger paste
- 1 teaspoon green chillies paste
- ½ tablespoon lemon juice
- 1 teaspoon jaggery
- 1 ½ cup water
- 1 tablespoon olive oil
- salt to taste

Process

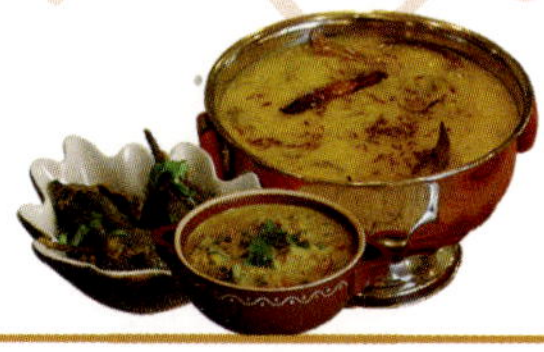

1. Heat oil in a pressure cooker and add mustard seeds and cumin seeds. Once they start spluttering add asafoetida and tomatoes. Cook for a minute.
2. Now add chana dal and lauki. Then add coriander powder, ginger and green chilli paste, turmeric powder, lemon juice, jaggery and salt.
3. Add water and mix everything well. Pressure cook for about 1 whistle.
4. Cool completely then open the lid. Check for dal consistency and add more water if needed at this point and boil for a few more minutes.
5. Serve hot with rice or roti.

Pineapple Dal

Delicious sweet and sour dal served best with rice

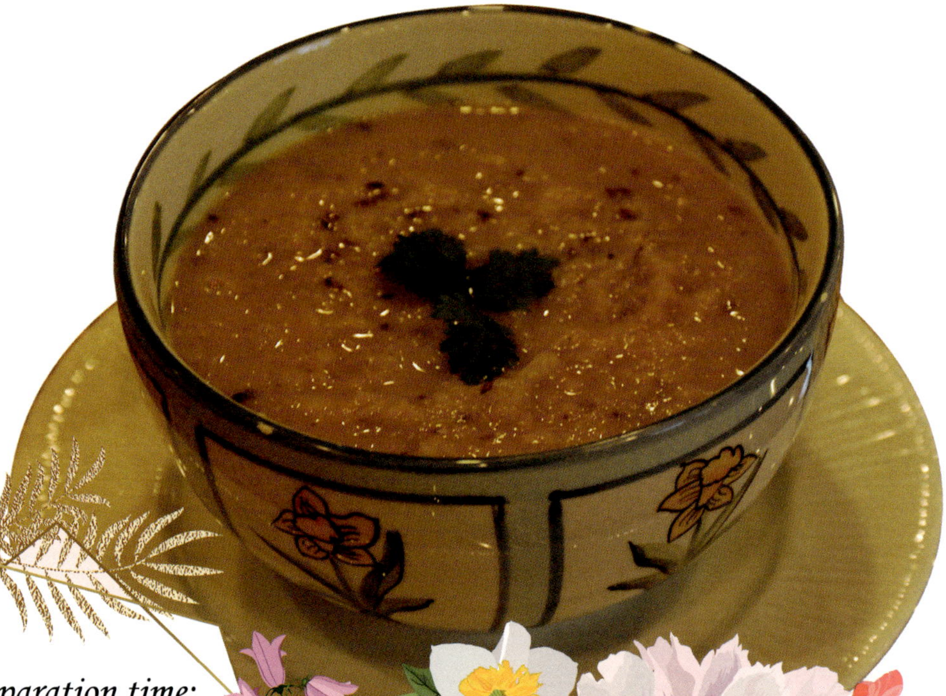

Preparation time: 10 *minutes*

Cooking time: 30 *minutes*

Servings: 8-10 *(4 oz. bowls)*

Ingredients

- 1 cup masoor dal (husked)
- 1-inch ginger, grated
- 1 green chilli, or to taste
- 1 stalk curry leaves
- 20 oz. can pineapple tidbits in 100% pineapple juice
- ¼ teaspoon turmeric
- ½ teaspoon mustard seeds
- ½ teaspoon cumin seeds
- few pinches asafoetida
- 4 cups water
- ¼ cup of coriander for garnishing
- 4 tablespoons vegetable oil
- salt to taste

Process

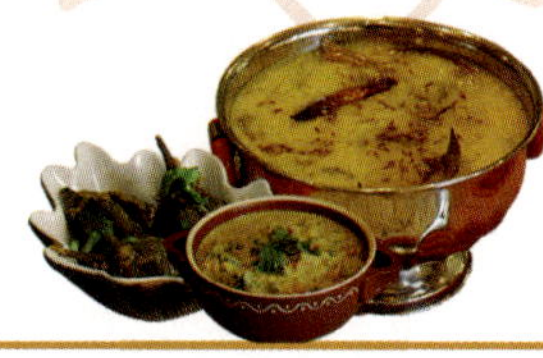

1. In a big pot add mustard and cumin seeds to heated oil. When they start to pop, add green chilli, curry patta, ginger and asafoetida.
2. Then add washed masoor dal. Stir it for 2-3 minutes until there is a nice aroma.
3. Now, add salt, turmeric and pineapple tidbits including the juice. Let all this cook together for another minute.
4. Add 4 cups of water. Cover the pot with a lid and cook until the dal breaks down. Because this dal cooks fast, it can be done on the stovetop without using a pressure cooker. When cooked, you can mash the dal well with a ladle.
5. Garnish with coriander leaves and serve hot with rice.

Karela Dal

An innovative recipe to incorporate the bitter tasting karelas in family meals

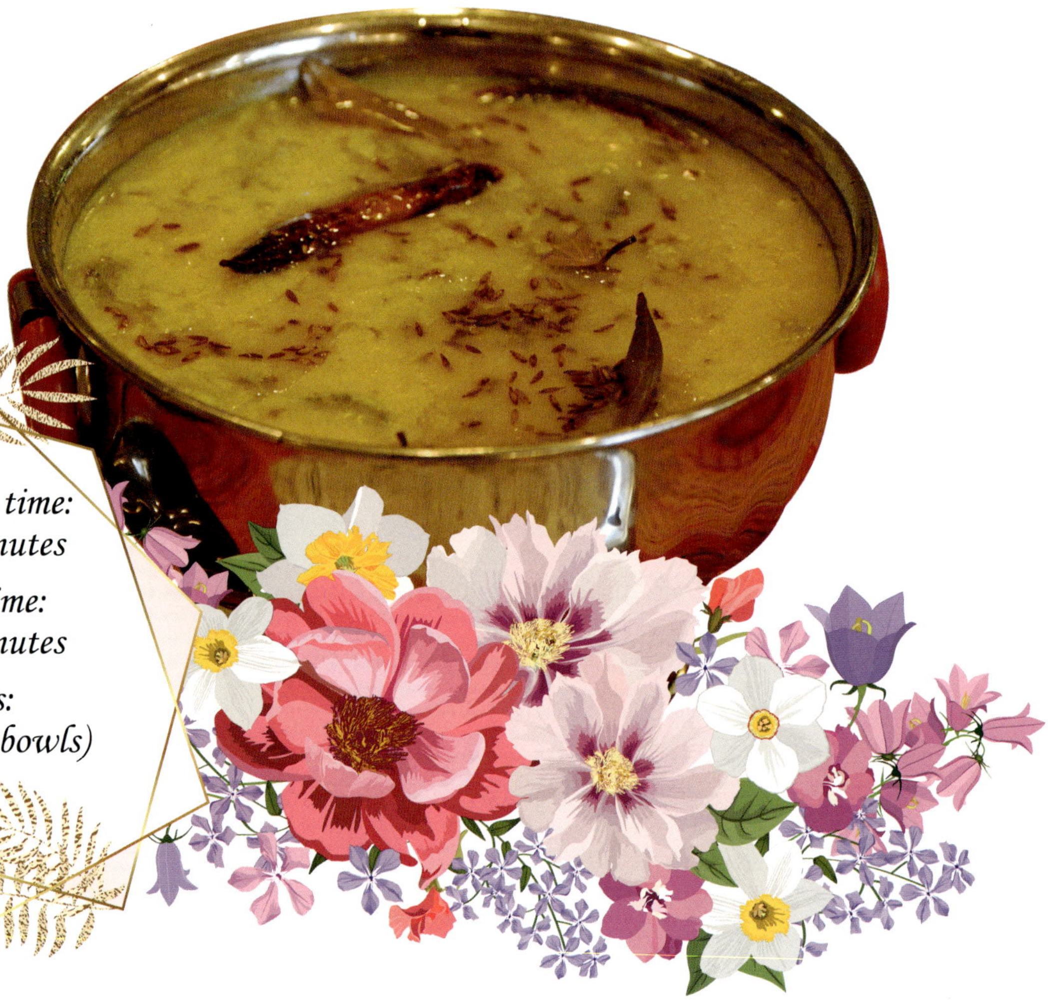

Preparation time:
15 *minutes*

Cooking time:
30 *minutes*

Servings:
8 *(4 oz. bowls)*

Ingredients

- 1 cup whole moong dal
- 3 medium sized karelas
- 1 teaspoon turmeric powder
- 1 teaspoon cumin seeds
- 2-3 red chillies
- 2-3 bay leaves
- 1 teaspoon sugar
- 3 cups water
- 2 tablespoons ghee
- 1 tablespoon oil
- salt to taste

Process

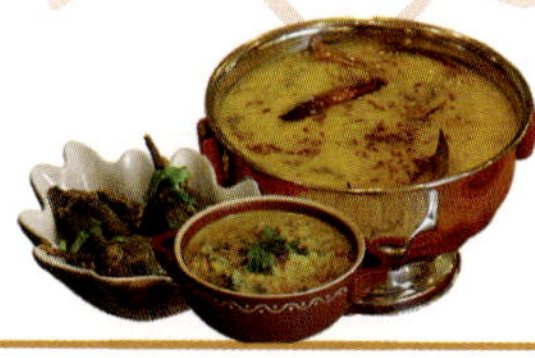

1. Wash the dal and pressure cook with 3 cups of water for 2-3 whistles.
2. Wash the karelas and lightly scrape the outer skin. Slice them in round discs. In a bowl, add salt and ¼ teaspoon turmeric powder to these and mix them well. Let them sit for 5 minutes.
3. Heat oil in a thick-bottom pan. Fry the salted karela pieces for about 5 minutes.
4. Once the karela pieces are soft, add the cooked moong dal to the pan. Also add remaining turmeric powder, salt and sugar. Cook for another 5 minutes.
5. In another small pan prepare the tempering with ghee. Add bay leaves, cumin seeds and red chillies to the heated ghee. Once it crackles, pour the tempering over the dal.
6. Serve hot with rice.

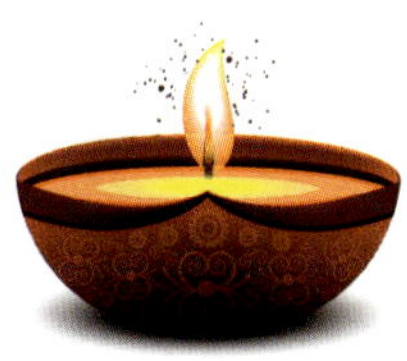

Gujarati Dal

A Gujarati staple – sweet and sour dal made with a variety of spices and peanuts

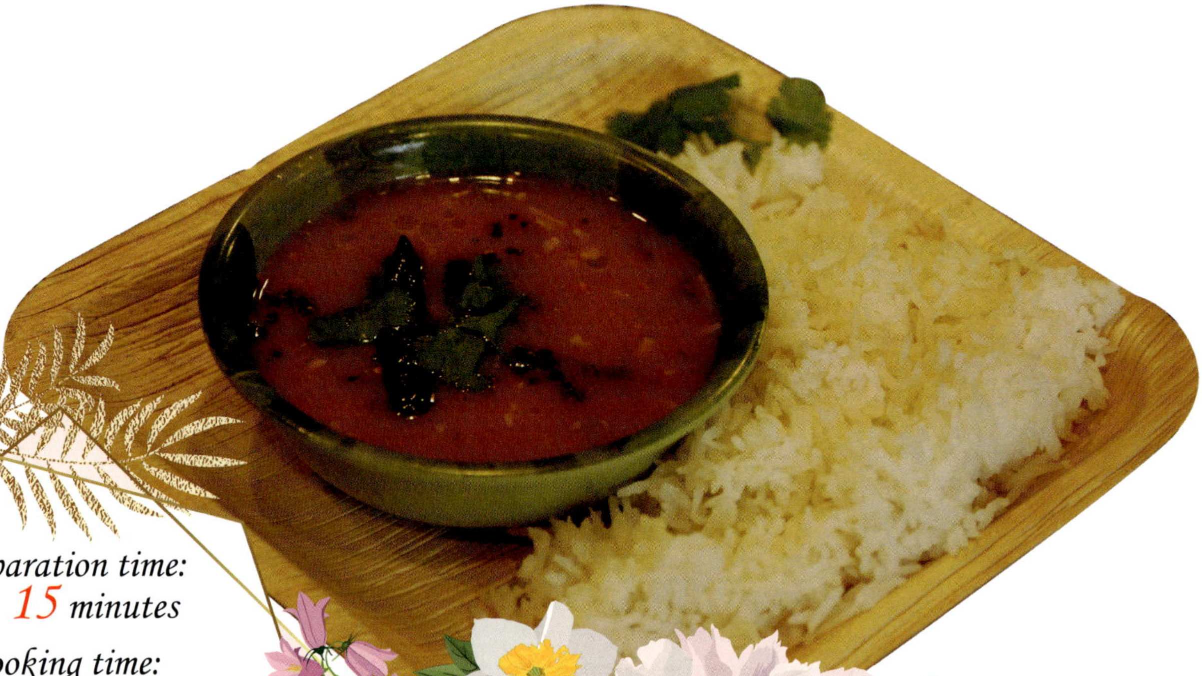

Preparation time: 15 *minutes*

Cooking time: 45 *minutes (in a slow cooker, it takes* 4-6 *hours to cook)*

Servings: 10-12 *(4 oz. bowls)*

Ingredients

- 1 cup toor dal
- 2 tablespoons peanuts
- 1 teaspoon lemon juice
- 5 count kokum
- 2 tablespoons grated jaggery or to taste
- 1 tablespoon dry coriander powder
- ½ teaspoon turmeric powder
- 1 teaspoon red chilli powder
- 2 cups water to cook dal
- cilantro for garnishing
- salt to taste

For Tempering

- 1 tablespoon oil
- 1 tablespoon ghee
- 1 large tomato, chopped
- 1-2 green chillies, slit
- 1-inch ginger, grated
- 5 curry leaves
- 3 cloves
- 1 cinnamon stick
- 1 teaspoon mustard seeds
- 1 teaspoon fenugreek seeds
- 2 dry red chillies
- 1 teaspoon asafoetida

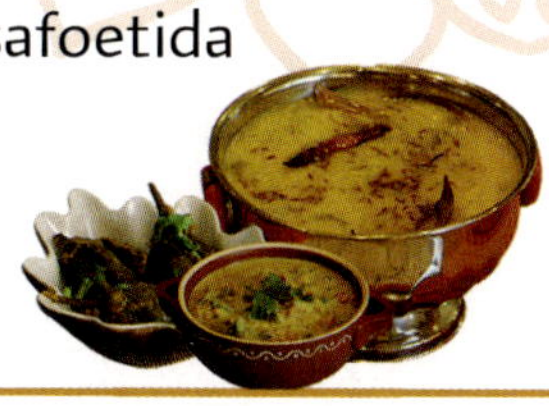

Process

1. Wash the toor dal and cook in a pressure cooker by adding two cups water for 3 whistles or in a crock pot till it is cooked properly.
2. In a separate deep vessel add cooked dal, 2 cups water, chopped tomatoes, green chillies, ginger, peanuts, kokum and lemon juice and cook for 10 minutes till all masalas blend in well.
3. In a deep medium pan add oil and ghee. Once it melts add the mustard seeds, wait for few minutes for them to crackle then add fenugreek seeds, dry chillies, asafoetida, curry leaves, cinnamon stick and cloves. Cook for few seconds till fragrant.
4. Pour this tempering over the dal. Then add red chilli powder, turmeric powder, coriander powder, jaggery and salt to it. Bring it to boil and cook on high heat for 15-20 minutes.
5. Garnish with coriander and serve hot with rice or roti.

Note: If one prefers the dal to be of smooth texture then after pressure cooking the dal can be blended. Peanuts and other ingredients can be added after blending.

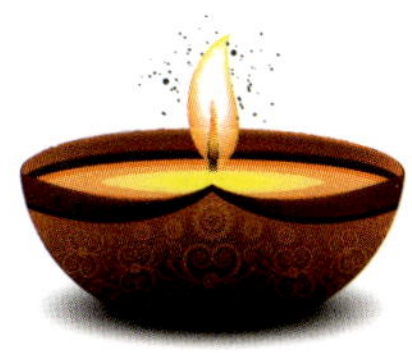

Dal Makhani

A rich creamy spicy north Indian lentil delight slow cooked in spices

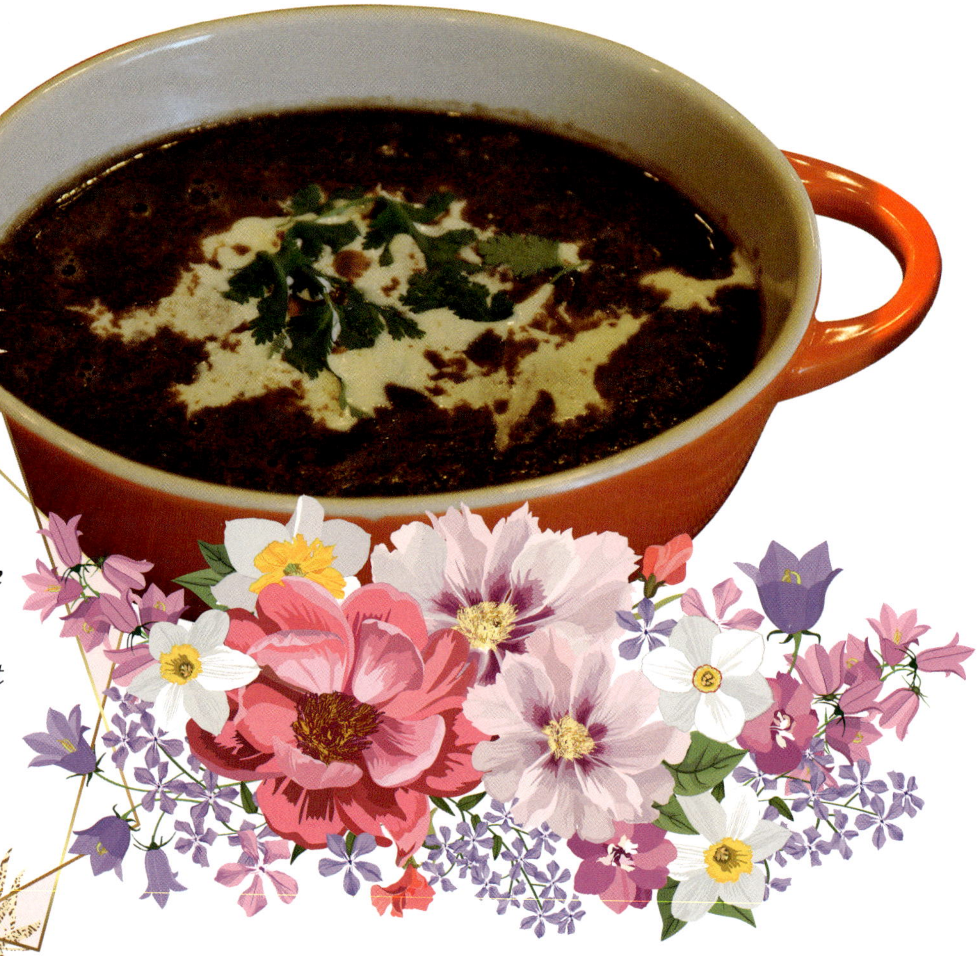

Preparation time:
10-15 minutes and additional 30 minutes soaking time

Cooking time:
overnight in crockpot

Servings: 25-30
(4 oz. bowls)

Ingredients

- 1 ½ cups whole urad dal (black matpe, black gram)
- ½ cup red kidney beans (rajmah)
- ½ cup chana dal (split Bengal gram)
- 2 big tomatoes, chopped
- 2-inch ginger, chopped
- 1 onion, chopped (optional)
- 8 garlic cloves, chopped (optional)
- 2 teaspoons garam masala powder
- 2 teaspoons red chilli powder or to taste
- 1 teaspoon turmeric
- ½ cup whipping cream
- 3 tablespoons butter
- salt to taste

Process

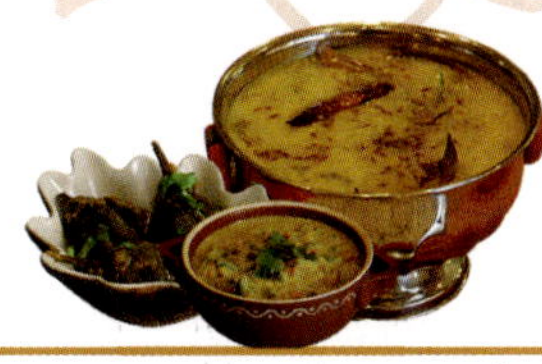

1. Soak whole black urad dal, red kidney beans and split Bengal gram in a big bowl in 3-4 cups of water. Rinse and wash all the lentils well after 30 minutes and put them in an 8-quart crockpot.
2. Add chopped onions, ginger, garlic, salt and turmeric to the crockpot.
3. Set the crockpot overnight (8-9 hours) with 10-11 cups of water on the low temperature setting.
4. Half hour before serving, heat butter in a thick-bottomed pan. Add tomatoes, red chilli powder and garam masala. Cook for 5-10 minutes until it is a thick paste.
5. Ensure that the dal is cooked (soft and mushy), then add the tomatoes to the boiled dal in crockpot.
6. Add whipping cream (save a little for garnish) and let it simmer on warm setting for 15-20 minutes.
7. Garnish with cilantro and a little cream and serve hot with a naan or rice.

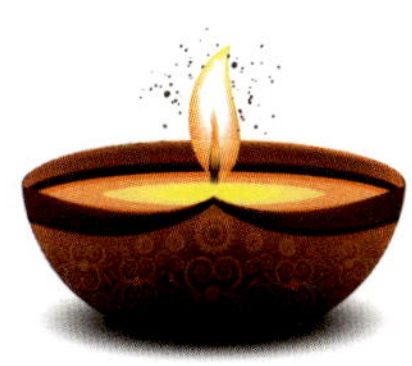

Cabbage and Chana Dal Curry

An easy to make delicious combination of cabbage and gram lentils

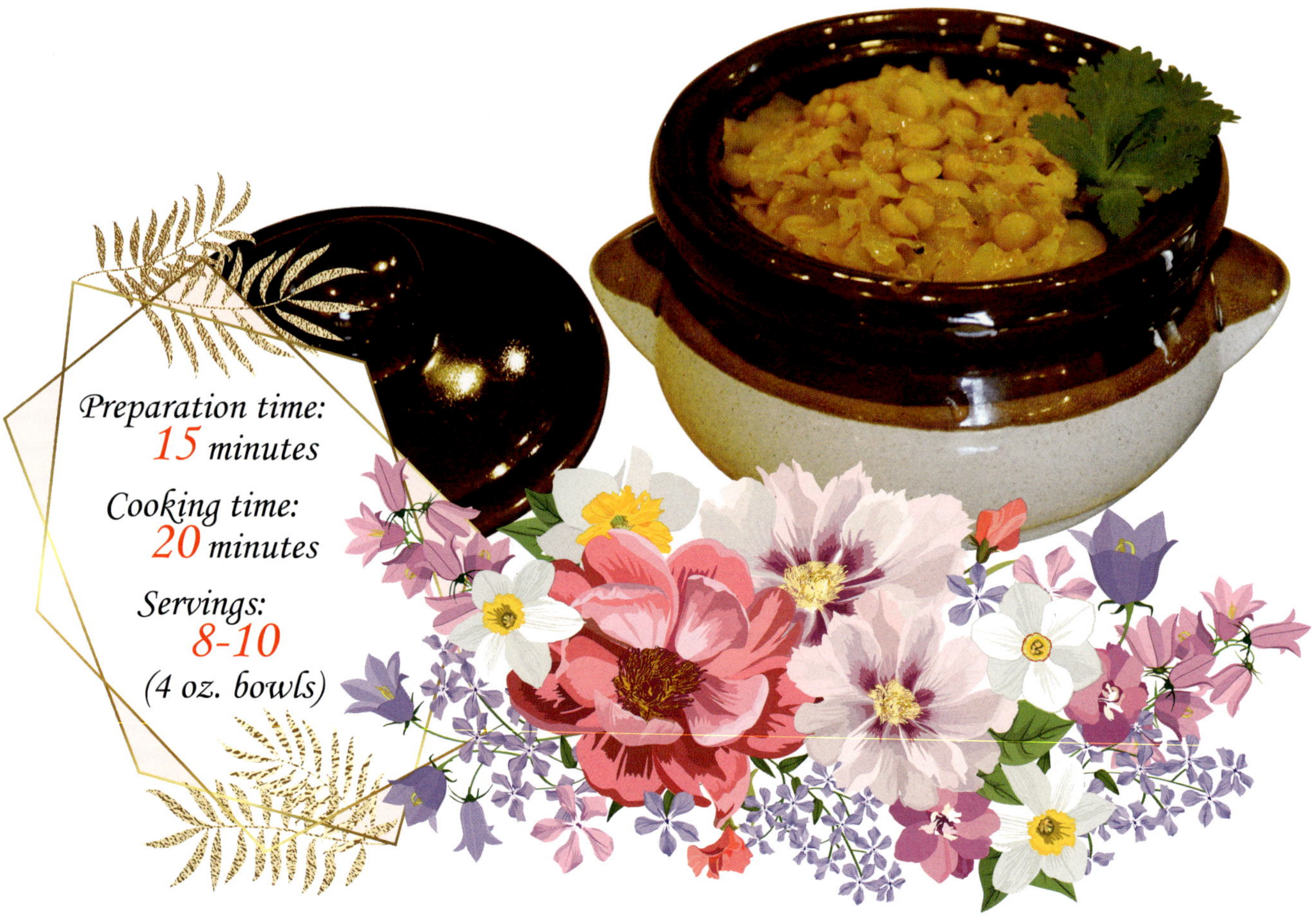

Preparation time: 15 *minutes*

Cooking time: 20 *minutes*

Servings: 8-10 *(4 oz. bowls)*

Ingredients

- 3 cups cabbage, chopped
- ¼ cup chana dal (gram dal)
- ¼ teaspoon mustard seeds
- ¼ teaspoon turmeric powder
- ½ teaspoon red chilli powder
- a pinch of asafoetida
- 3 tablespoons vegetable oil
- salt to taste

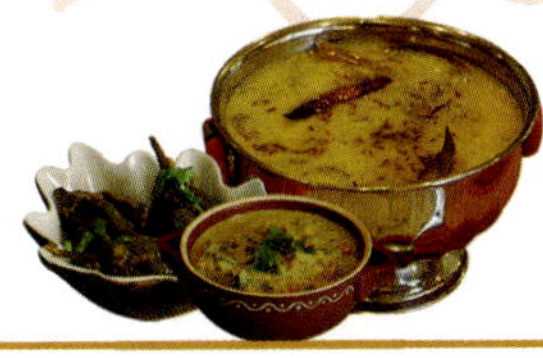

Process

1. Boil chana dal in a pan with little water for ten minutes until it becomes a little soft.
2. Heat oil in a non-stick pan and add mustard seeds. After they start popping, add cabbage, boiled chana dal and asafoetida.
3. Then add turmeric, red chilli powder and salt.
4. Cover the curry and cook for five minutes on medium heat.
5. Garnish with cilantro and serve the curry with roti or puri.

Mixed Vegetable Curry

A rich mixed vegetable sweet curry made with cashews and onion–ginger–garlic masala

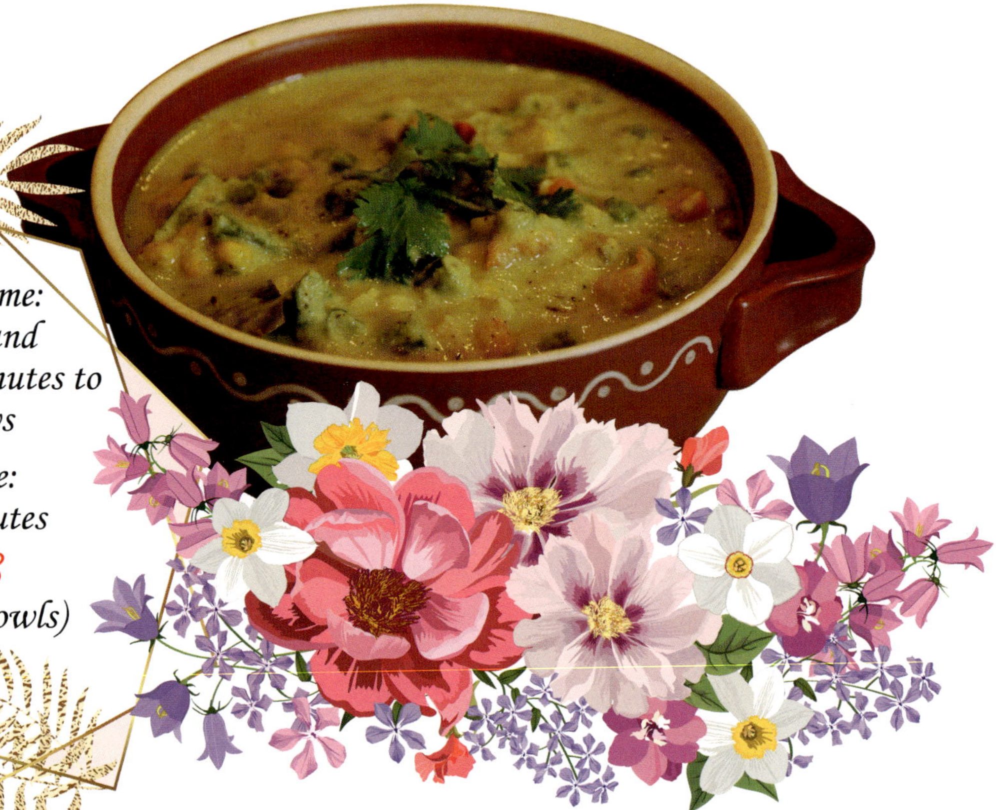

Preparation time:
20 minutes and additional 30 minutes to soak cashews

Cooking time:
20 minutes

Servings: 8
(4 oz. bowls)

Ingredients

- 2 cups of frozen mixed vegetables (corn, peas, beans, carrots)
- 1 big white onion (optional), cut in quarters
- 5-6 cashews soaked 30 minutes in water or 4 tablespoons cashew powder/water paste
- 1-inch ginger, minced (optional)
- 1 small clove garlic, minced (optional)
- 1-2 green chilli, slit
- cilantro for garnish
- 1 small piece cinnamon
- 2-3 small bay leaves
- 4-5 black peppercorns
- 2 cardamoms
- 1 teaspoon turmeric
- 1 tablespoon cumin seeds
- 1 teaspoon sugar
- 3-4 tablespoons oil
- salt to taste

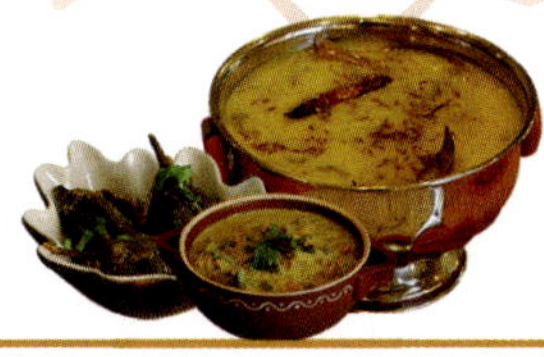

Process

1. Boil/steam mixed vegetables until soft, drain and set aside.
2. Boil onion, chillies, cinnamon, cardamom and black peppercorns in ½ cup of water. Grind into a paste.
3. Separately, make a paste of cashews or cashew powder-water paste and keep aside.
4. In a bigger pan heat oil on medium heat. Add cumin seeds, and bay leaves. Then add onion paste and minced ginger garlic (if using). Add turmeric and salt. Sauté this well (till oil leaves the sides of the pan) on medium heat.
5. Now add the cashew paste to it. Keep stirring. Add water to make a gravy type consistency.
6. Add the boiled vegetables. Add sugar. Cook for another 10 minutes until ingredients are blended in.
7. Garnish with cilantro and serve hot with rice, roti or parantha.

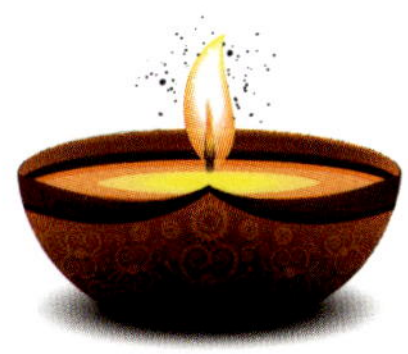

Punjabi Palak Kadhi

A favorite dish with pakodas added to besan and sour yogurt gravy

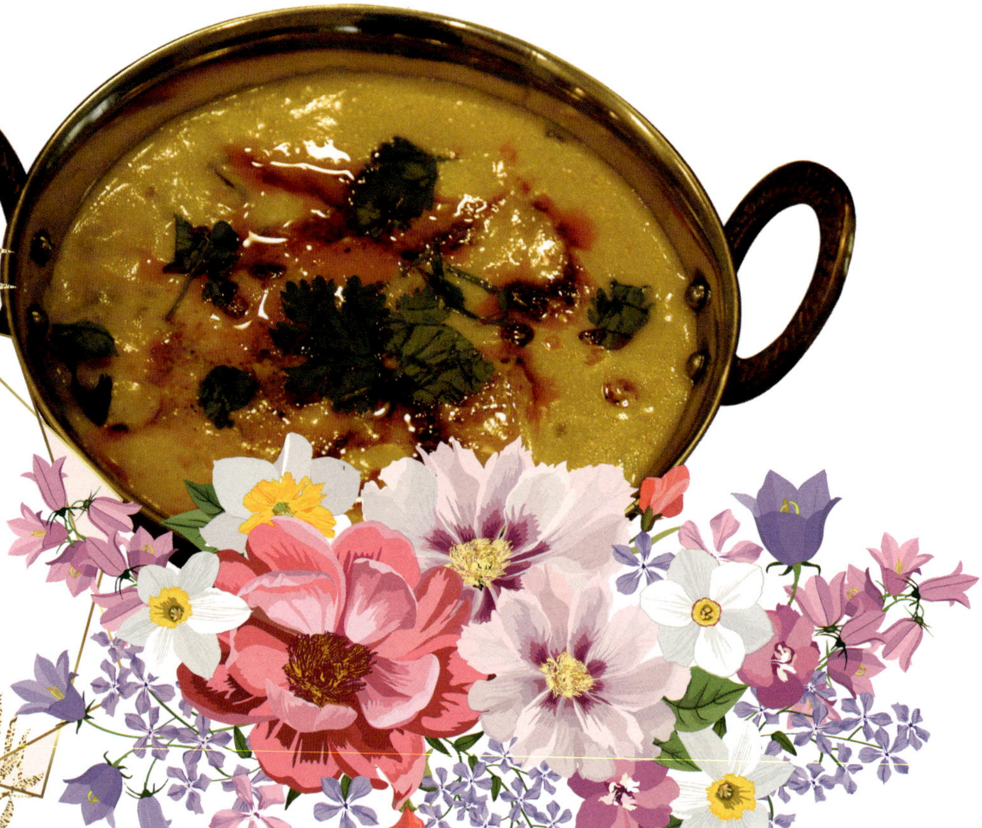

Preparation time: 20 *minutes*

Cooking time: 1 *hour or more*

Servings: 20 *medium bowls*

Ingredients

For kadhi

- 1 cup besan (gram flour)
- 3 cups sour yogurt
- 2 to 3 cups spinach, washed and finely chopped
- 1 teaspoon turmeric powder
- 2 teaspoons coriander powder
- ½ teaspoon red chilli powder
- 10 cups water
- 1 teaspoon ginger paste
- 3 teaspoons salt

For tempering

- 2 tablespoons ghee
- ¼ teaspoon cumin seeds
- 1 teaspoon fenugreek seeds
- 1 teaspoon coriander seeds
- 4 count dry red chillies
- 10 count curry leaves
- 1 teaspoon asafoetida
- 6 cloves

For pakodas

- 2 cups besan flour
- 1 onion, finely chopped (optional)
- 1 cup spinach (palak), washed and finely chopped
- 1 small potato, chopped
- 1 to 2 green chillies, finely chopped
- ¼ teaspoon asafoetida
- 1 ½ teaspoon salt or according to taste
- 4 cups corn oil for frying

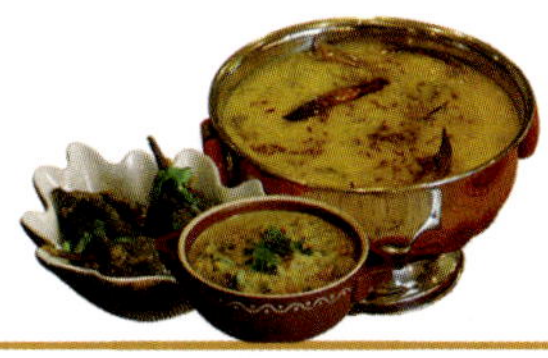

Process

For kadhi

1. In a big bowl mix besan, yogurt and spices–turmeric, chilli powder, coriander powder and salt until the besan lumps disappear. It is easier to do this in a blender.
2. In a big deep pot, heat the ghee for tempering. To this add chilli, cumin seeds, coriander seeds, fenugreek seeds, cloves, curry leaves and asafoetida. When fragrant add the ginger paste and cook for a minute.

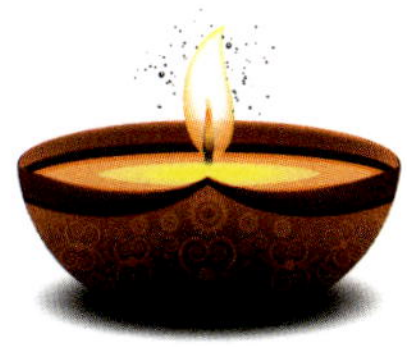

3. Now, add the besan-yogurt mix to this and add 10 cups or more of water and mix it in well. Bring it to a boil. The kadhi tends to froth and can spill over so reduce the heat and stir often so it does not stick to the bottom of the pot.
4. You can then add the spinach and let the curry simmer while you make the pakodas.

For pakodas

5. In a big bowl mix besan, onions, potatoes, spinach, chillies, asafoetida and salt with water to make a smooth batter. Batter should not be too thick or very watery.
6. Keep it aside for 5-10 minutes so that the ingredients blend in nicely.
7. In a kadai heat oil to fry the pakodas in batches. Once oil is hot, you can lower the heat to medium.
8. To fry the pakodas, using fingers or a spoon carefully drop batter in the oil. Turn them over when done and fry till they are medium brown, but not crispy.
9. Remove on paper towels to drain excess oil.
10. *Putting it together*: Then add pakoras to the kadhi. If one prefers them to be soft, then let them soak in the curry for a while. If the preference is for crispy pakoras, then soak for 5-10 minutes only.
11. Garnish with coriander and the palak kadhi is ready to serve with rice or rotis.

Chole

An all-time favorite dish cooked faster using the Instant Pot Pressure Cooker

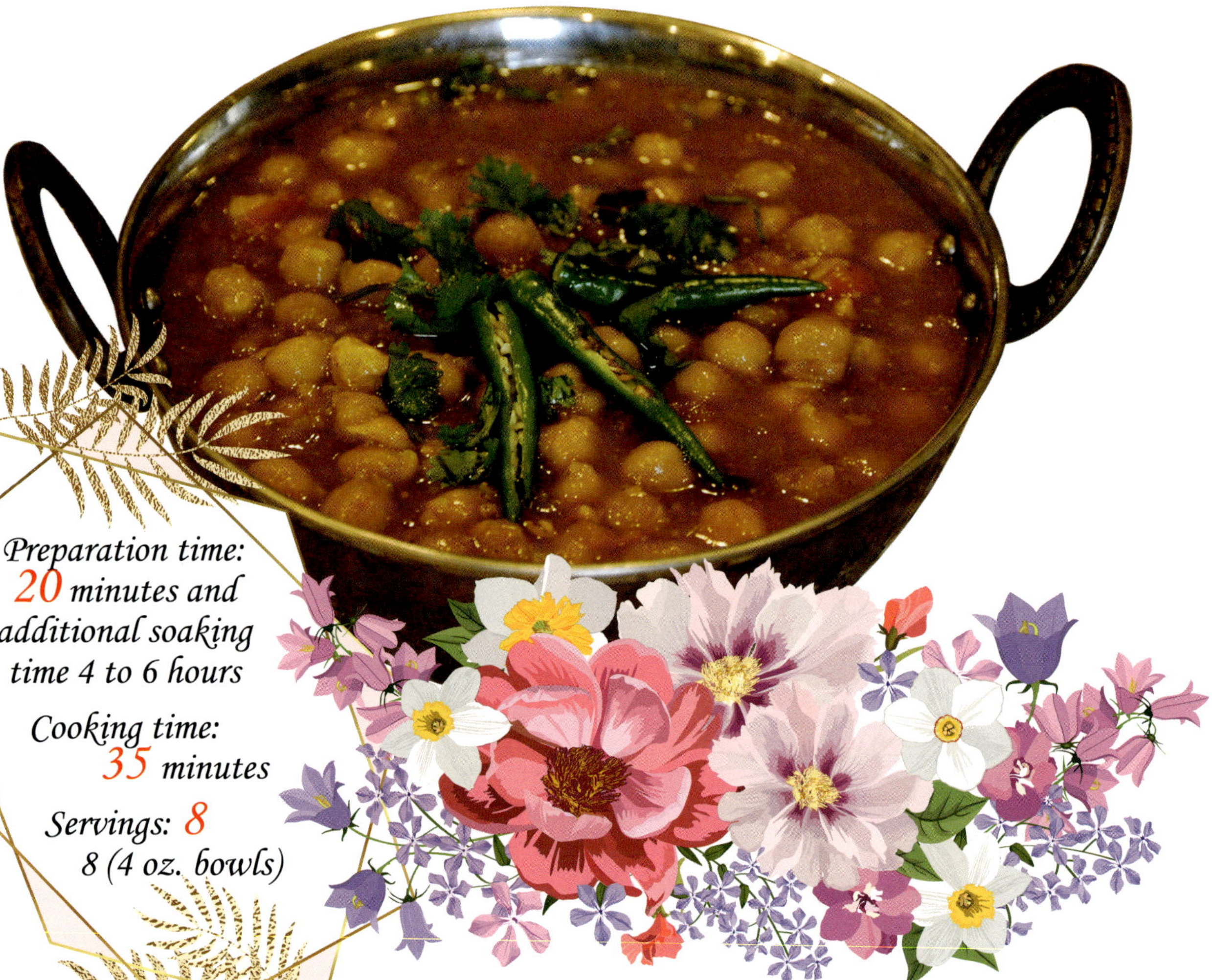

Preparation time:
20 minutes and additional soaking time 4 to 6 hours

Cooking time:
35 minutes

Servings: 8
8 (4 oz. bowls)

Ingredients

- 1 cup dry white Kabuli chanas
- 1 medium tomato, chopped
- 1 medium onion, coarsely chopped (optional)
- 1 tablespoon tomato paste, or can use an additional chopped tomato instead
- 1 tablespoon cilantro, chopped
- 1 tablespoon coriander powder (dhania powder)
- 1 tablespoon garam masala powder
- 1 tablespoon kasuri methi (dried fenugreek leaves)
- 2 teaspoon amchur (mango) powder
- 1 teaspoon turmeric (optional)
- 3 cups water for soaking
- 3 cups water for cooking
- 2 teaspoons salt, or to taste

For tempering

- 1 teaspoon cumin seeds
- ½ teaspoon asafoetida
- 1 stick cinnamon
- 2 small bay leaves
- 3 curry leaves
- 1 teaspoon ginger paste
- 1 tablespoon ghee

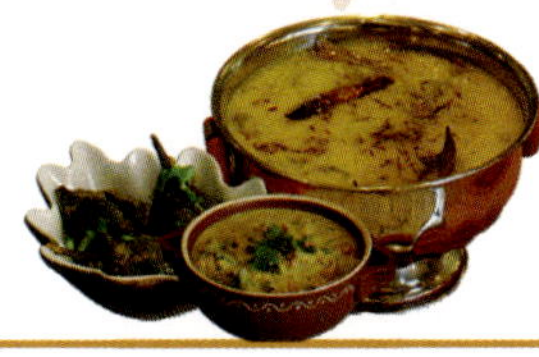

Process

1. Soak the chanas in 3 cups warm water for minimum 4 to 6 hours or more. Then drain the water and keep aside.
2. In a 6-quart instant pot turn on the sauté mode. To prepare tempering, heat ghee and add cumin, cinnamon, asafoetida, bay leaves and ginger paste.
3. When the above is fragrant, add chopped onions (if using) and salt and sauté until golden in color. Then add chopped tomatoes followed by tomato paste. Cook for few minutes and add coriander powder, garam masala, amchur and kasuri methi. Finally add the drained chanas and 3 cups of water.
4. Close the instant pot lid and keep the vent into sealing position. Change the mode of cooking into manual mode (high setting) for 25 minutes.
5. Once it is done let the instant pot release the pressure by itself. It would take another 10 minutes.

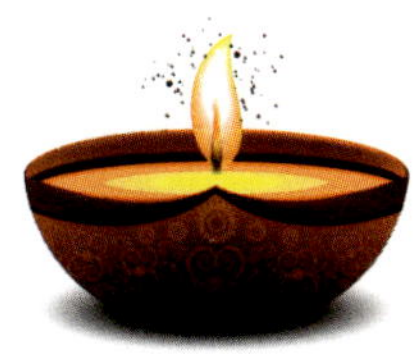

6. Open the pot and garnish with chopped coriander and serve with bhaturas, naan or rotis.

Time-saver option: Using chickpea cans/garbanzo beans can save substantial time required in soaking and cooking chanas and can be cooked without a pressure cooker too.

The same recipe can be made in the regular pressure cooker, simply adjusting the time settings. However, cooking in an Instant Pot is more efficient, time saving and does not need monitoring.

Sambar

Traditional sambar with vegetables and different spice blends

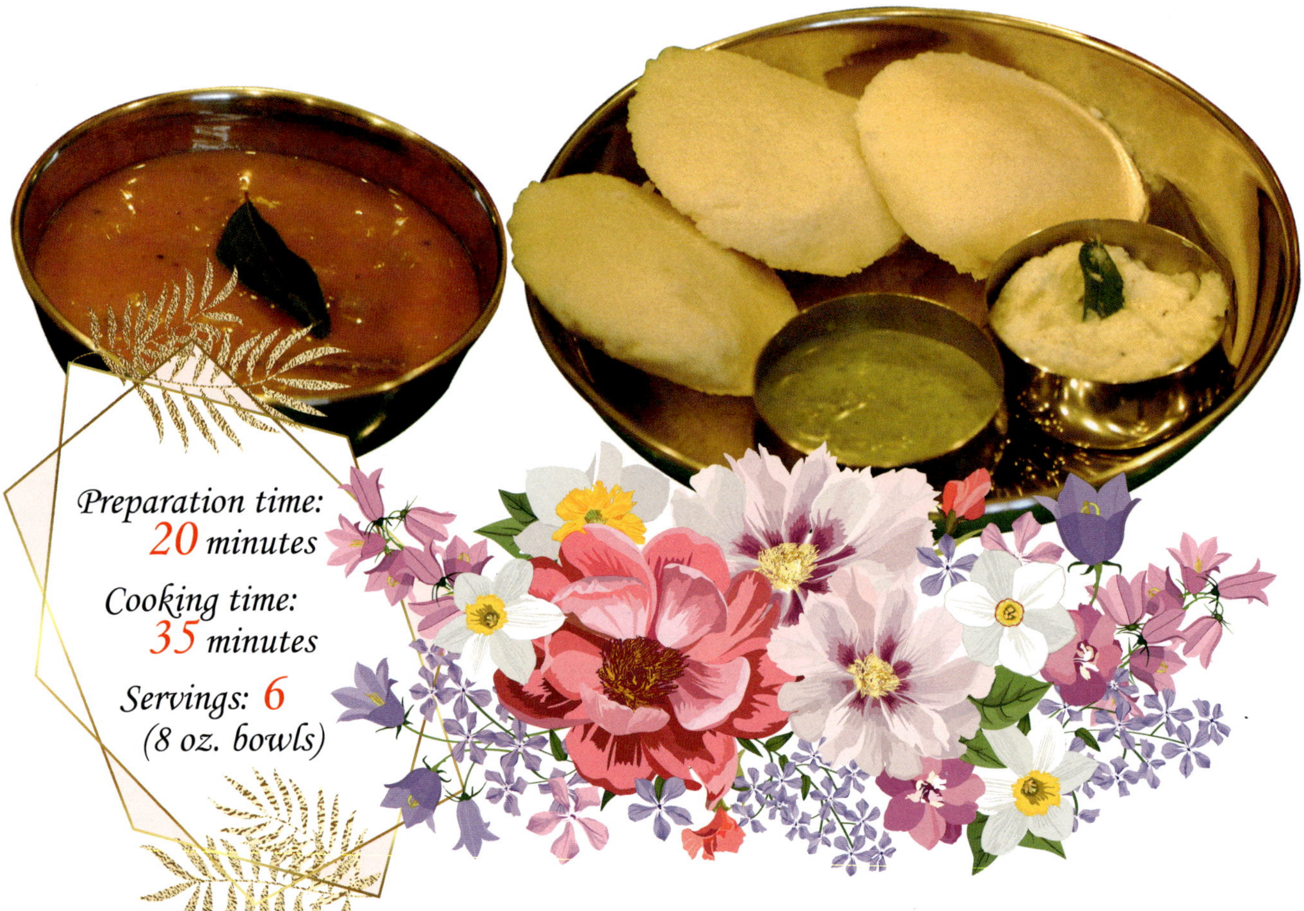

Preparation time: 20 *minutes*

Cooking time: 35 *minutes*

Servings: 6 *(8 oz. bowls)*

Ingredients

- 1 cup toor dal
- 1 cup lauki (bottle gourd), big cubes
- 1 cup potatoes, chopped in cubes
- 1 cup chopped onion, chopped big (optional)
- 3-4 drumsticks (2-3 inches in size)
- ½ cup Chinese eggplant, chopped in cubes
- ½ teaspoon turmeric powder
- ½ teaspoon mustard seeds
- ¼ teaspoon fenugreek (methi) seeds
- pinch asafoetida
- 10-15 curry leaves
- 1 cup fresh cilantro, chopped
- 3 cups water for dal, 2 cups for vegetables, or more
- 4 teaspoons oil, split two times
- 1 tablespoon jaggery or dark brown sugar
- 2 teaspoons salt, split twice for dal and vegetables, or to taste

For spice blend

- 1 tablespoon coriander seeds, heaped
- 1 teaspoon cumin seeds
- 2 Kashmiri chillies
- 1 New Mexico chilli
- 1 tablespoon store bought sambar powder (any brand)

For tamarind pulp

- 1 oz. or about 2 tablespoons tamarind
- 1 cup water, split two times

Process

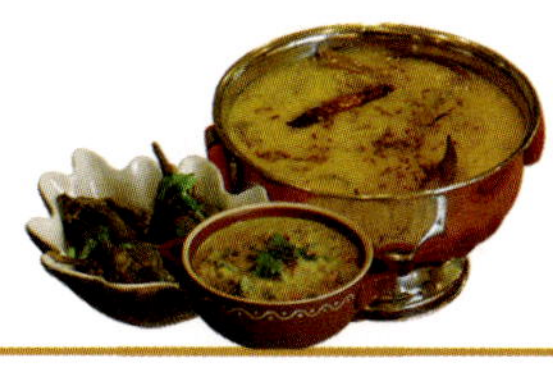

Preparing the dal

1. In a pressure cooker heat oil. Temper with mustard seeds. When popping sound calms down, add methi seeds, sauté for 20 seconds then add turmeric powder, asafoetida and curry leaves.
2. Cook 20 seconds then add toor dal, salt and 2 cups water. Once water starts to boil add 1 more cup water.
3. Cover the lid and cook until two whistles are blown. Turn off the stove.

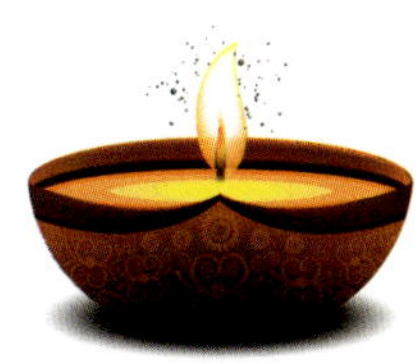

For spice blend

4. Gently roast coriander seeds and cumin seeds until aromatic. Let them cool.
5. Then grind to fine powder along with Kashmiri chillies and a New Mexico chilli. The New Mexico chilli adds a beautiful red hue to the sambar without adding any heat.
6. To this home ground spice blend, add 1 heaped tablespoon ready-made sambar powder and keep it aside.

Helpful tip: Mixing two brands of ready-made sambar powder enhances the taste of the sambar.

For tamarind extract

7. In a microwave safe bowl, add tamarind with half cup water. Cook for 2 ½ minutes without letting it overflow.
8. Once it cools down, mash and squeeze to extract pulp, add half cup more water. Use a tea strainer to get fine tamarind extract.

Helpful tip: To save time, use store bought tamarind pulp.

Preparing sambar vegetables

9. In a 4-quart thick bottom pot heat 2 teaspoons oil, sauté onions first (if using), followed by lauki, potatoes and drumsticks for 5-6 minutes on medium heat. Then add 2 cups water, tamarind pulp and salt and let this boil.
10. Cook covered for 5-6 minutes over medium heat. Add the spice blend mix (home ground and store-bought sambar powder). Stir and mix it in with vegetables

Adding cooked dal and vegetables

11. Then add prepared dal to the vegetables. Gently stir with wooden spoon. Add jaggery and ½ cup cilantro. Adjust sambar consistency by adding more water, if needed.
12. Now cover and cook for another 10-12 minutes over medium heat, gently stirring at intervals. Turn off heat, let it sit over stove for some time. Add remaining half cup chopped cilantro just before serving.

Optional tip: For more authentic sambar, vegetables such as chayote (kind of squash), or similar ones like dosa kai (yellow cucumber) and white winter melon (sufed kaddu/white pumpkin) can be used. Additionally, zucchini, carrots, green beans, radish, bell peppers, plantain and cucumber may also be added.

Rotis, Breads and Rice

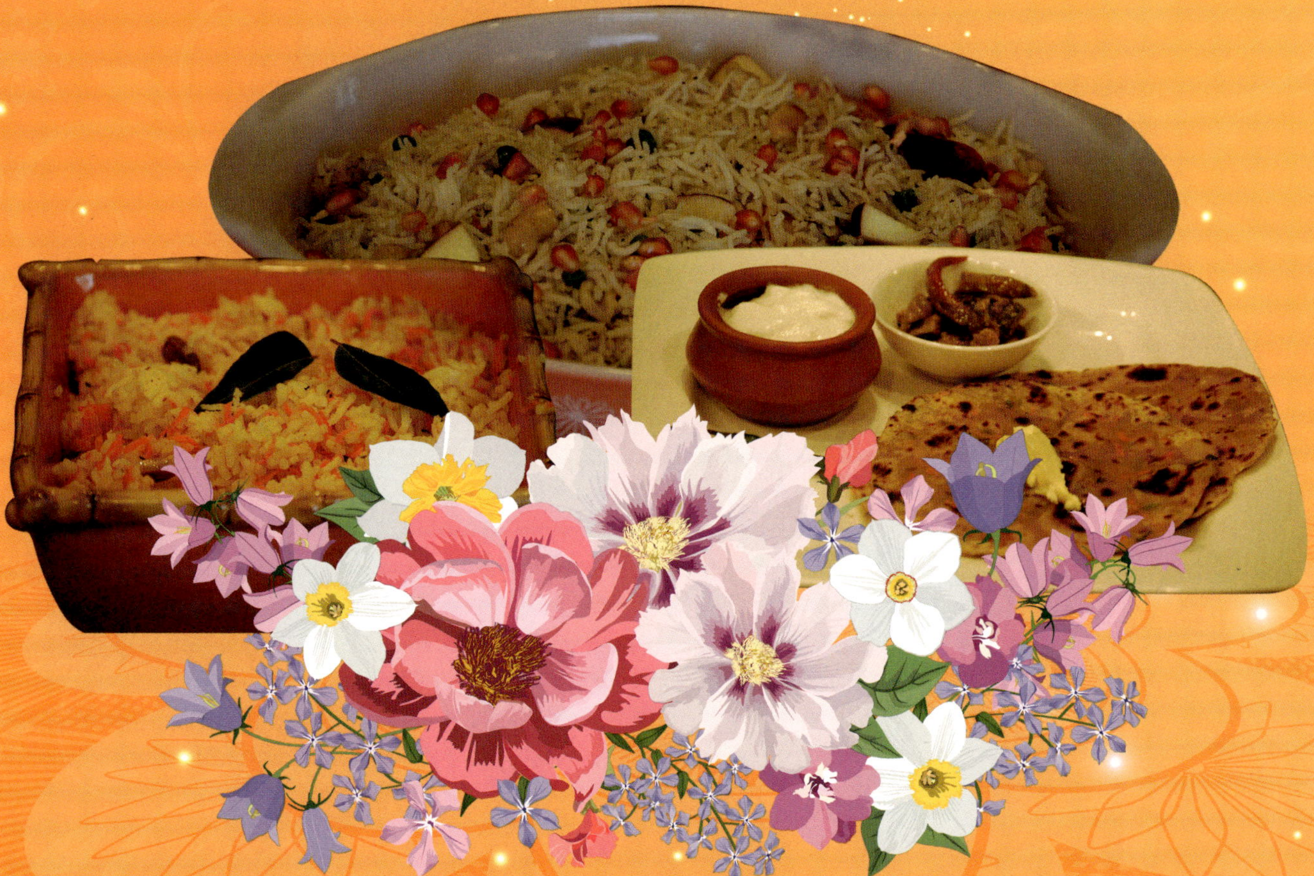

This chapter primarily includes rotis/paranthas, baked breads and several kinds of rice preparations.

The different flat breads presented here include the paranthas that are cooked with oil on a griddle as the last step. If one prefers a healthier version, the last step may be omitted to simply make rotis with the same dough that is kneaded with different vegetables, grains, cheese or mix of spices. *Thepla* the Gujarati staple is made using fenugreek leaves, *paneer parantha* has cottage cheese as the main ingredient, *kale and cheese parantha* provides an example of how greens can be easily blended in the dough itself. *Muli aloo parantha* is a great way to incorporate radish or other vegetables and *jowar methi parantha* and *mixed grain rotis* depict how different grains can be easily incorporated in our everyday diets.

Amongst the baked breads are the nutty *cranberry walnut bread,* the simple and wholesome *oatmeal whole wheat bread* and the popular Italian *Focaccia bread*. This small sampling of bread recipes is not only tasty but also nutritious. These easy to try recipes are a perfect replacement for store bought bread.

The rice dishes are also extremely easy to make and there is something to appeal to different tastes and palettes. The *spinach and corn rice* are packed with the goodness of spinach. The *Himachali pulao is* a unique preparation blending both dry (cashews, raisins) and fresh fruits (pomegranates, apples) in one dish. *Tamarind rice* and *carrot lemon rice* are popular South Indian preparations. *The bise bele bath* is a more involved recipe in which rice is simmered with vegetables and lentils to make a wholesome meal.

1. Thepla
2. Paneer Parantha
3. Kale and Cheese Parantha
4. Muli Aloo Parantha
5. Jowar Methi Parantha
6. Mixed Grain Roti
7. Cranberry Walnut Bread
8. Oatmeal Whole Wheat Bread
9. Focaccia Bread
10. Carrot Lemon Rice
11. Spinach and Corn Rice
12. Tamarind Rice
13. Bisi Bele Bath
14. Himachali Pulao

Thepla

A Gujarati staple, theplas are a flat bread made with whole wheat, besan and fenugreek leaves

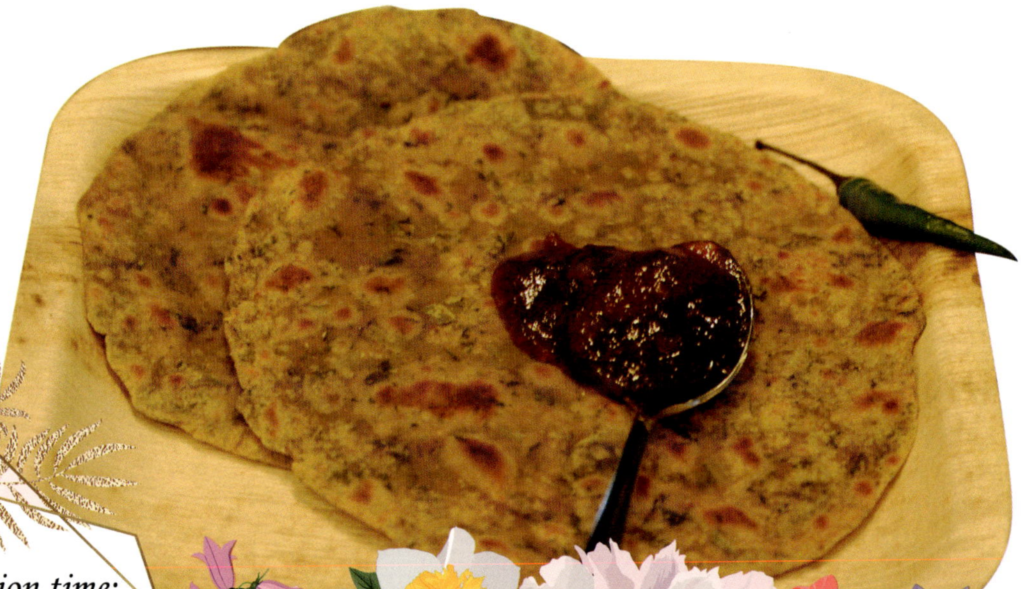

Preparation time:
30 minutes

Cooking time:
1 hour or more

Makes approx.
25 theplas

Ingredients

- 3 cups whole wheat flour and extra 1 cup flour for dusting
- ½ cup gram flour (besan)
- 1 cup fresh chopped fenugreek leaves (if using dried leaves, soak leaves in luke-warm water for 10 minutes prior to use)
- 1 cup yogurt or buttermilk
- 2 tablespoons oil for dough and 1 tablespoon oil per thepla
- 1 teaspoon cumin powder
- 1 teaspoon carom seeds
- 1 teaspoon turmeric powder
- 1 teaspoon red chilli powder
- 1 tablespoon garlic, minced (optional)
- ½ cup cilantro, chopped
- ¼ cup warm water
- 2 teaspoons salt or to taste

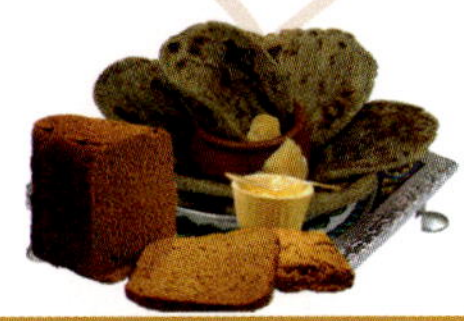

Process

1. In a big bowl, mix whole wheat flour, gram flour and 2 tablespoons oil. Mix well.
2. In a separate medium bowl, mix yogurt, cumin powder, carom seeds, turmeric powder, red chilli powder, chopped fenugreek leaves, garlic (if using), cilantro and salt.
3. Mix the yogurt mixture with the flours and gradually adding little water to form a smooth texture dough.
4. Smear a little oil on the dough, knead the dough again, cover and leave aside for 15-20 minutes.
5. Heat a flat skillet on medium flame to make the theplas.
6. Dusting with dry four, roll out a 2-inch dough ball into a 6-inch round. Cook this on both sides using little oil. Repeat for the rest of the dough.
7. Serve the theplas hot with yogurt, pickles or any vegetable dish.

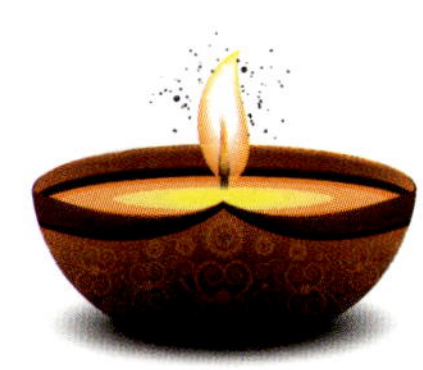

Paneer Parantha

A fried flat bread stuffed with grated cottage cheese and spices

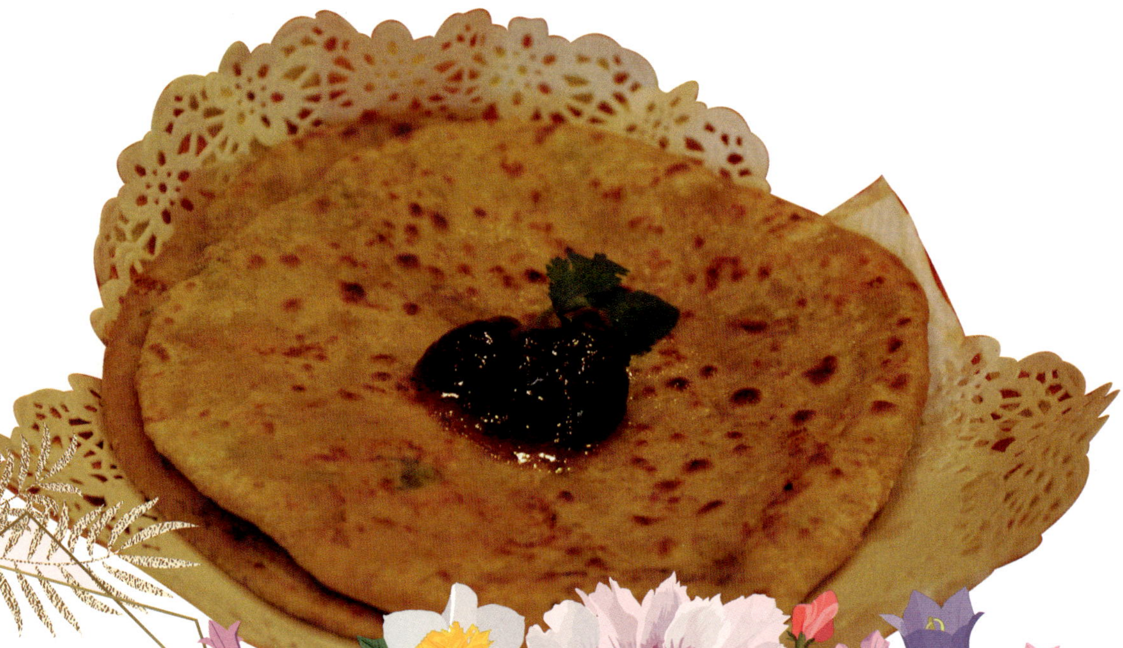

Preparation time: 15-20 *minutes*

Cooking time: 2-3 *minutes each*

Makes approx. 15 *paranthas*

Ingredients

- 1 cup whole wheat flour
- ½ cup all-purpose flour (maida)
- 2 tablespoons gram flour (besan)
- ½ block or 8 oz. paneer, grated
- 2 teaspoons garlic, finely chopped, or garlic paste (optional)
- 2 teaspoons green chillies, finely chopped
- 4 tablespoons cilantro, finely chopped
- ½ teaspoon garam masala powder
- ½ teaspoon chilli powder
- ½ teaspoon amchur powder
- whole wheat flour for rolling
- water to knead dough
- 2 teaspoons oil/ghee per parantha

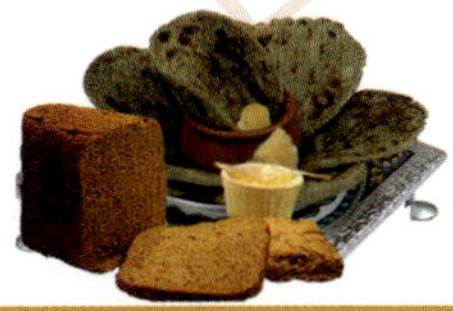

Process

1. Combine the three flours, grated paneer, cilantro, garlic (if using), green chillies, garam masala, chilli powder, amchur and salt and knead into a soft and smooth dough using enough water.
2. Keep aside for 30 minutes.
3. Divide the dough into equal portions, about 15.
4. Using a rolling pin roll the balls into approximately 5-inch rounds using dry flour.
5. Cook on a hot griddle, using a little ghee, till both sides are golden brown in color.
6. Repeat with the remaining dough to make more paranthas.
7. Serve warm with chutney, pickle or yogurt.

Kale and Cheese Parantha

A tasty way to savor the health benefits of kale

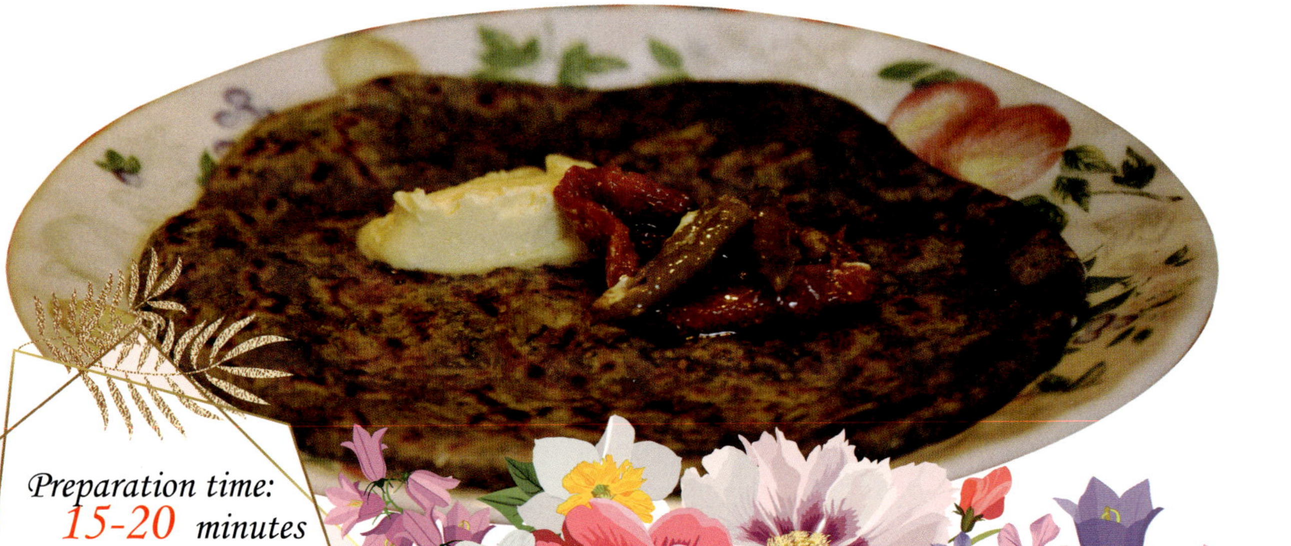

Preparation time:
15-20 *minutes*

Cooking time:
30-45 *minutes*

Makes approx.
15 *paranthas*

Ingredients

- 2 cups whole wheat flour
- 6-7 oz. or one bunch kale
- 2 cloves of garlic (optional)
- 8 oz. cheddar cheese for stuffing
- whole wheat flour for rolling
- water to knead the dough
- 2 teaspoons oil plus more for cooking each parantha
- 2 teaspoons salt or to taste

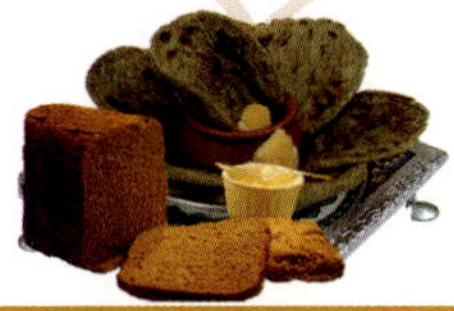

Process

1. Wash kale thoroughly and remove the stem or rib of kale. Chop it into thin and small pieces.
2. Heat 1 teaspoon oil, add garlic (if using). Add the kale leaves and let them cook for 3 minutes in a closed lid.
3. Remove the lid and stir the kale and add salt. Cook for another 2-3 minutes. When cool, grind into a paste with water.
4. Now add the kale paste to the flour and mix it well with 1 teaspoon oil and salt to make a smooth dough. Kale mixture should have enough water, if not add just enough to make a smooth dough which is not too soft. Keep it aside for 10 minutes.
5. Now divide the dough into equal parts and make them into golf-sized balls. Use grated cheese as a stuffing.
6. With a rolling pin, roll out the balls using whole wheat flour into approx. 5-inch circles.
7. Cook on a hot griddle, using a little oil, till both sides are golden brown in color.
8. Repeat with the remaining dough and stuffing to make more paranthas.
9. Serve warm with pickle and chutney.

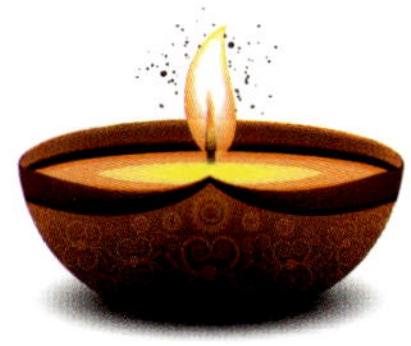

Muli Aloo Parantha

A popular North Indian breakfast choice

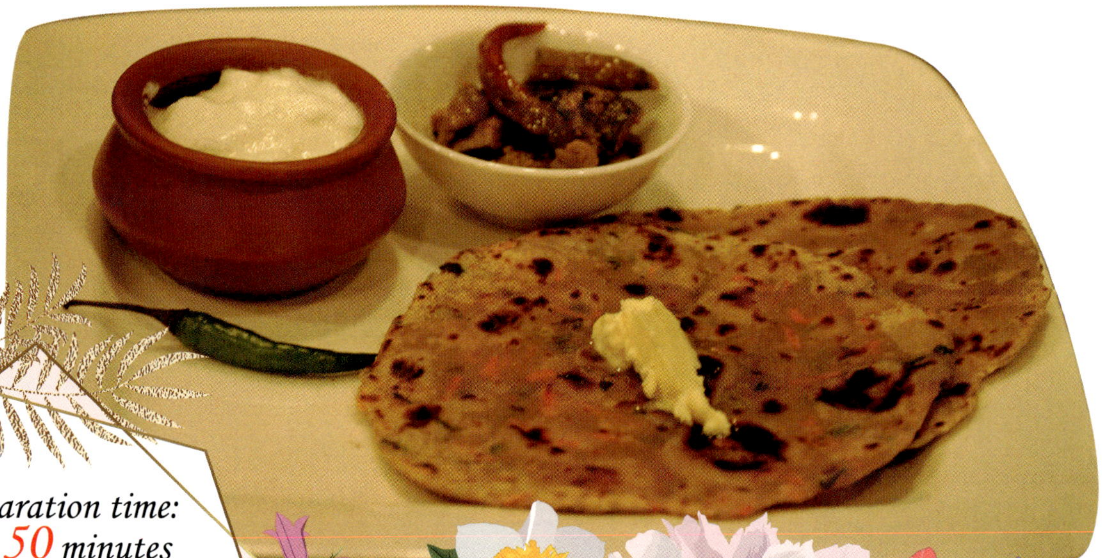

Preparation time: 50 *minutes*

Cooking time: 1 *hour or* 2-3 *minutes per parantha*

Makes about 20 *paranthas*

Ingredients

- 2 cups whole wheat flour and 1 cup extra flour for dusting
- ½ cup gram flour
- 1 large white radish (muli), peeled and shredded
- 2 small boiled potatoes, mashed
- 1 teaspoon turmeric powder (optional)
- ½ teaspoon carom seeds
- 1 teaspoon ginger, grated
- 1 teaspoon chillies, finely chopped
- ½ cup cilantro, finely chopped
- 1 tablespoon oil in the dough
- 1 teaspoon oil for each parantha for frying
- 1 teaspoon lemon juice
- salt to taste

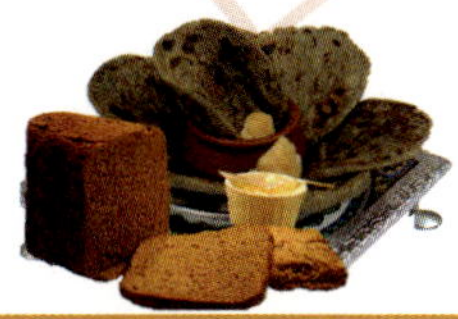

Process

1. Mix both the flours-whole wheat flour and gram flour with the dry ingredients-carom seeds, turmeric and salt. Add the radish, mashed potatoes, ginger, chillies, lemon juice, cilantro and oil in the flour. Knead the flour to form a soft dough. Note that water has not been added here as the water from the radish will help make the dough. A little additional water may be added if needed.
2. Make dough into equal portions of 1.5-inch diameter balls (size of golf balls).
3. Using a rolling pin and dusting with dry flour roll these out into 6-7-inch diameter circles/paranthas.
4. Cook these on a hot skillet using oil on one or both sides.
5. Serve paranthas hot with yogurt, butter or pickle.

Alternate tips: Similar paranthas may be made with shredded carrots or lauki (bottle gourd) as well. Lemon juice can be replaced with amchur powder or yogurt.

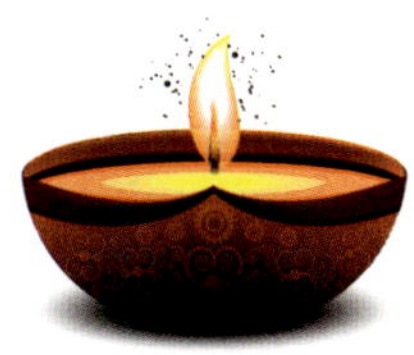

Jowar Methi Parantha

A tasty and healthy way to boost your hemoglobin levels

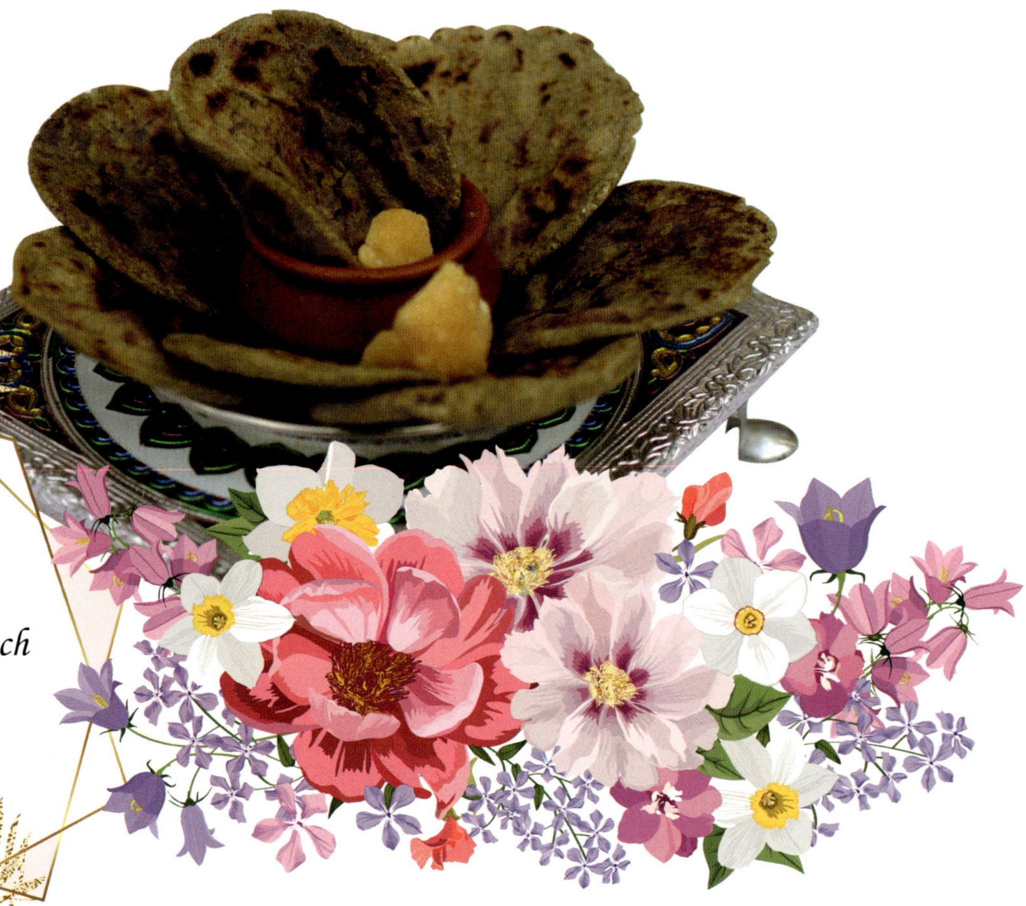

Preparation time:
10 minutes

Cooking time:
2-3 minutes each

Makes approx.
8 paranthas

Ingredients

- 1 cup jowar (white millet/sorghum) flour
- ½ cup whole wheat flour
- ¼ cup gram flour
- 1 teaspoon turmeric
- 1 cup fenugreek leaves, chopped
- ½ cup onion, chopped (optional)
- ¼ cup cilantro, chopped
- 1 teaspoon crushed ginger
- 1 teaspoon green chillies, finely chopped
- 1 teaspoon sesame seeds
- ½ cup yogurt
- 1 ½ teaspoon oil for cooking each parantha
- jowar (white millet/sorghum) flour for rolling
- salt to taste

Process

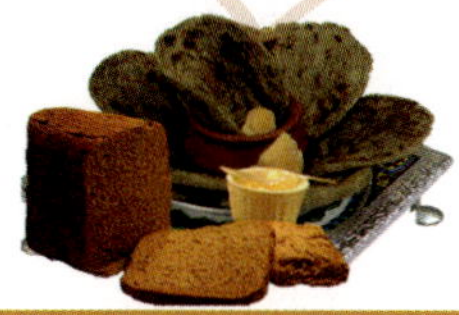

1. In a big bowl, combine all the ingredients–flours, turmeric, fenugreek, onion, cilantro, ginger, chillies, sesame seeds, yogurt, oil and salt and knead into a soft dough using enough warm water. Cover with a lid and keep aside for 10 minutes.
2. Make about 8 golf sized balls and using little jowar flour roll them out into circular shape.
3. Cook each parantha on a hot nonstick pan using a little oil until it turns golden brown on both sides.
4. Serve hot immediately with gud/jaggery.

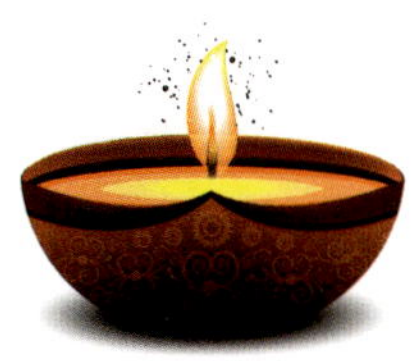

Mixed Grain Roti

The flours are a powerhouse of nutrition with superb flavor

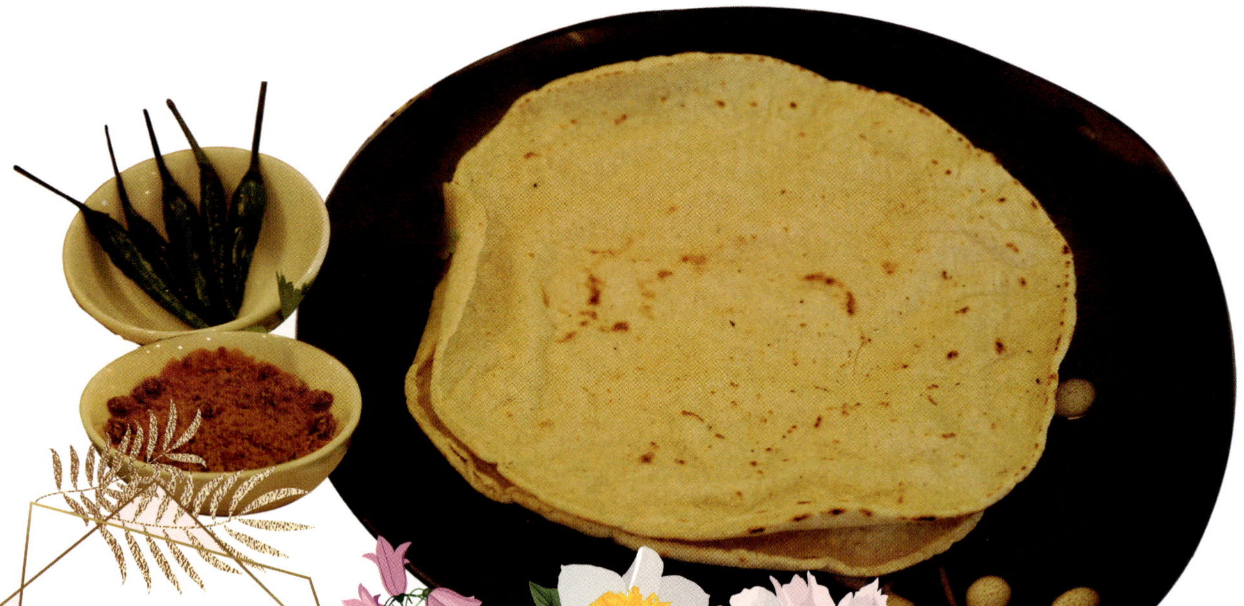

Preparation time: 15-20 *minutes*

Cooking time: 20 *minutes*

Makes approx. 15 *rotis*

Ingredients

- ½ cup barley flour
- ¼ cup soya flour
- ½ cup sorghum flour
- ½ cup gram flour
- water to make dough
- whole wheat flour for rolling
- salt to taste

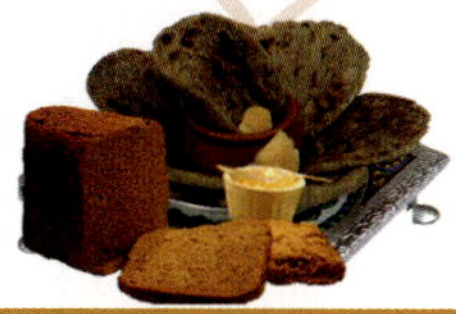

Process

1. Combine all the four flours-barley, soya, sorghum, gram and salt. Knead into a semi-soft dough using enough water. Keep aside for 10 to 15 minutes.
2. Make about 15 balls for the dough and roll them out into 8-9-inch diameter rounds/chapatis.
3. Cook these rotis on a griddle.
4. Serve hot with gud/jaggery, green chillies or as chapatis/rotis with the meal.

Cranberry Walnut Bread

A moist nutty bread with a hint of orange

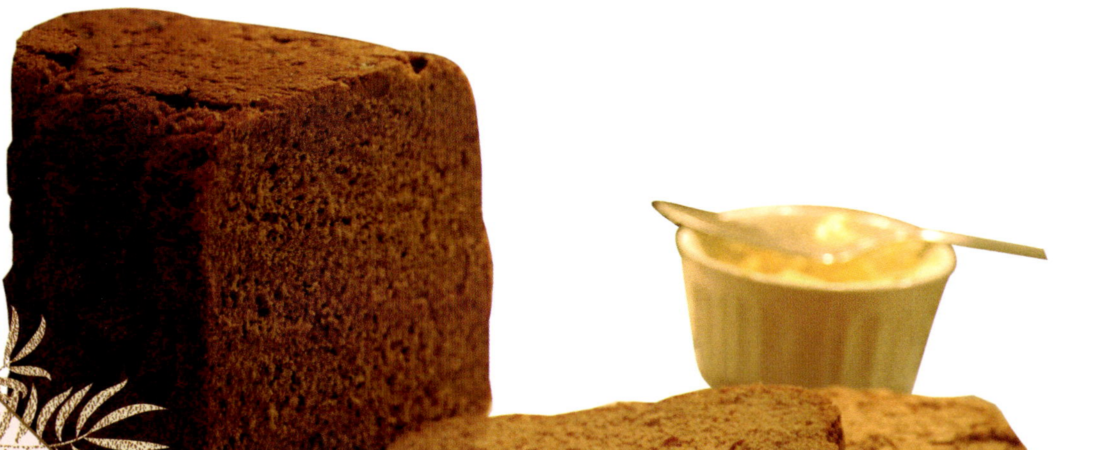

Preparation time:
20 *minutes and additional* 2 *hours rest time for dough*

Baking time:
40 *minutes*

Servings: 15 *slices*

Ingredients

- 3 ½ cups all-purpose flour (or 1 cup all-purpose flour and 2 ½ cups whole wheat flour)
- 1 cup yogurt or buttermilk
- 1 egg substitute (1 tablespoon flax seed powder plus 3 tablespoons warm water - mix well and keep aside for 7 to 8 minutes till it becomes gooey)
- ½ cup dried cranberries
- ½ cup chopped walnuts
- 1 teaspoon grated orange zest (optional)
- 1 teaspoon cinnamon powder
- 2 ½ teaspoons active dry yeast
- ¼ cup water, lukewarm (to activate the yeast)
- 1 teaspoon sugar, for the yeast
- ¼ teaspoon baking soda
- 1 ½ tablespoons butter
- 1 teaspoon kosher Salt

Process

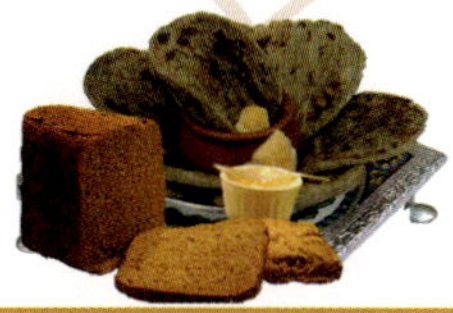

1. Preheat oven to 350°F. Grease and flour a 9 x 5 inch bread baking pan or can even use a greased cookie sheet to make a circular loaf.
2. In a large bowl sift together the flour, baking soda, and salt.
3. In another small bowl add lukewarm water, sugar and yeast, mix well and cover with lid for 10 minutes. When the yeast mixture is bubbly on top, the yeast is activated.
4. Add yeast mixture, cinnamon powder, yogurt/buttermilk, baking soda and softened butter into the flour mixture. Mix well.
5. Now add the nuts and orange zest. Knead the dough very well till all the nuts are mixed well in the dough.
6. Set the dough aside to rise for 2 hours. Knead one more time and place the dough in a loaf pan and bake it on 350°F for 40 minutes.
7. Cool, slice and serve with butter.

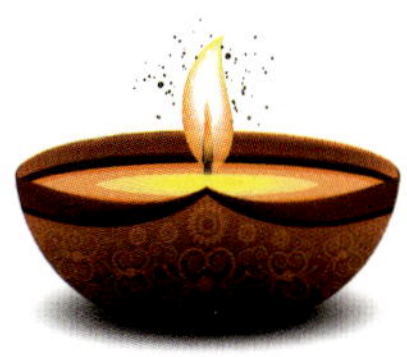

Oatmeal Whole Wheat Bread

Wholesome and slightly sweet – perfect for sandwiches or can enjoy by itself

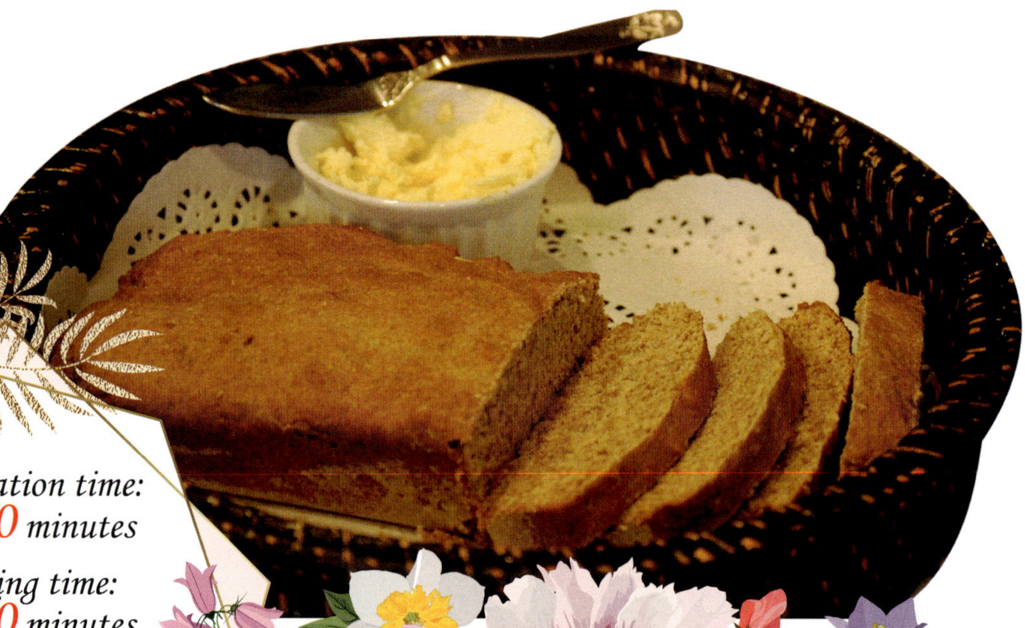

Preparation time: 20 *minutes*

Cooking time: 20 *minutes*

Servings: 16-18 *slices*

Ingredients

- 2 cups rolled oats, ground in blender
- 2 cups whole wheat flour
- 1 ¼ tablespoons baking powder
- ⅓ cup vegetable oil
- 2 cups whole milk
- ½ teaspoon plain yogurt
- 1 tablespoon honey
- 1 teaspoon salt

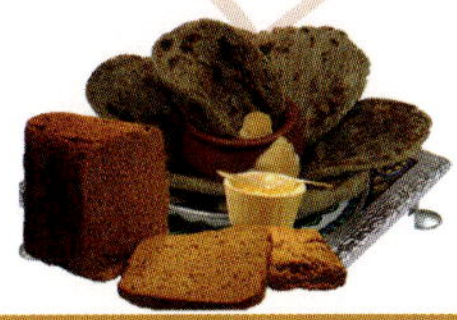

Process

1. Preheat oven to 350°F.
2. In a large bowl, combine oatmeal, flour, baking powder, yogurt and salt.
3. In a separate bowl, dissolve honey in vegetable oil and stir in the milk.
4. Combine both mixtures and knead until a soft dough is formed.
5. Make the dough into a ball and place on a lightly greased baking rectangular pan size 9 x 5 x 3.
6. Bake for approximately 20 minutes. If you tap the bottom of the loaf and it sounds hollow, that means it's baked.
7. Remove from oven and cool for 10 minutes. Turn it over on a cooling rack. Slice and enjoy.

Focaccia Bread

An Italian flat sheet baked bread with strong flavors of rosemary, basil and olive oil

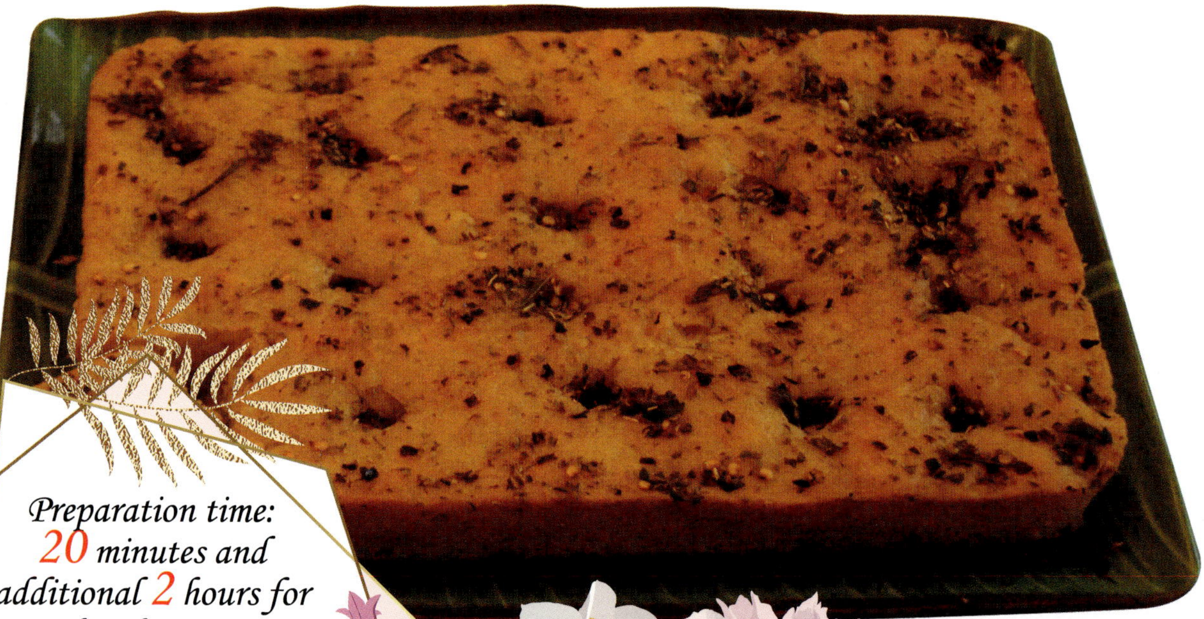

Preparation time:
20 minutes and additional 2 hours for dough to rise

Cooking time:
35-40 minutes

Servings:
24 slices

Ingredients

- 2 cups all-purpose flour
- ¼ cup semolina flour
- 1 ½ teaspoon instant active dry yeast
- 1 ¼ teaspoon Kosher salt
- 1 teaspoon sugar
- 2 tablespoons olive oil
- 1 cup milk (lukewarm)
- 1 teaspoon crushed oregano powder
- 1 teaspoon crushed red pepper

For Garnishing

- 3 tablespoons olive oil
- 2 teaspoons fresh rosemary, chopped (can use dry if not available)
- ¼ cup fresh basil, chopped (can use dry if not available)
- 1 tablespoon crushed red pepper

Process

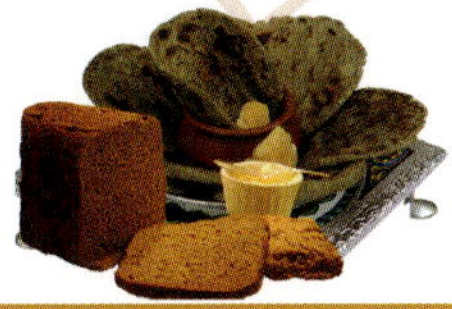

1. In a small pan heat milk till it is lukewarm, dissolve sugar in it and then sprinkle the yeast and allow to rest for ten minutes until the yeast is active. You will observe a layer of bubbles on top of milk.
2. In a large bowl mix together all-purpose flour, semolina flour, crushed pepper, oregano powder and salt. Add the active yeast warm milk from step 1 and olive oil (listed in the dry ingredients) and mix together till it forms a soft dough.
3. Knead the dough well till it becomes smooth and elastic. Coat the dough with some olive oil so that it does not dry out.
4. Keep the dough in big bowl. Cover it with dry or wet clean cloth. Allow the dough to rest in warm place for 2 hours.
5. Dough will double in size. Knead it one more time with a little bit of olive oil.
6. Pre-heat oven to 425°F.

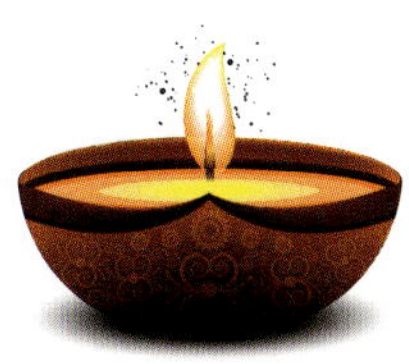

7. Place dough ball in a greased medium size baking pan and press dough into an even shape of the pan. With the finger gently make indentations one inch apart all over the dough.
8. In a small bowl mix together 2 tablespoons of olive oil, crushed red pepper and chopped basil and rosemary. Spread this oil mixture on top of the dough evenly.
9. Bake the bread in an oven for 20 minutes at 425°F temperature.
10. Enjoy this bread either hot or cold with pasta or any dip.

Cooking tips:

a. Onion slices and garlic added to the oil mixture can be spread on the bread before baking.

b. All-purpose flour can be replaced with whole wheat flour for a healthier bread but the texture of that will be firmer.

Carrot Lemon Rice

A mildly spicy rice, containing shredded carrot and a hint of lemon-lime

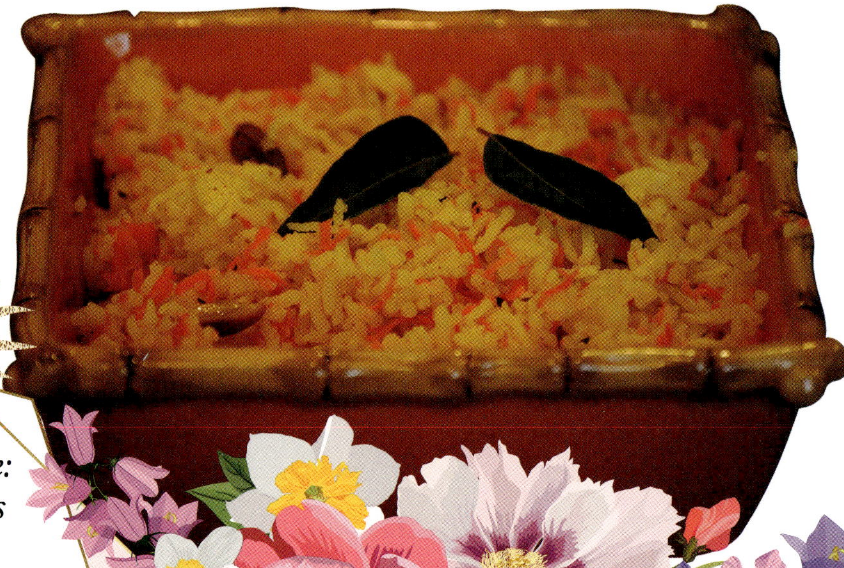

Preparation time: 15 *minutes*

Cooking time: 20 *minutes*

Servings: 5 *(8 oz. servings)*

Ingredients

- 1 cup basmati rice
- 1 teaspoon urad dal
- 1 teaspoon chana dal
- ½ cup roasted peanuts
- 3-4 carrots, peeled and shredded
- 3 red chillies
- 1 teaspoon mustard seeds
- 1 teaspoon cumin seeds
- 1 teaspoon turmeric
- ½ teaspoon asafoetida
- 10 curry leaves
- 3 green chillies, slit
- ¼ cup lemon juice (or a little less as per taste)
- 2 cups water
- 1 tablespoon ghee
- 1 teaspoon salt or to taste

Process

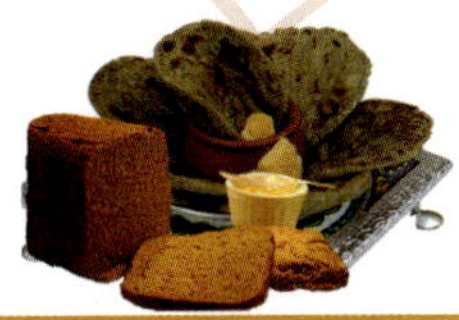

1. Cook rice with double water. Let it cool a little.
2. Heat ghee in a pan. Add mustard seeds and let them splutter. Add cumin seeds, urad dal, chana dal, red chillies, asafoetida, turmeric, green chillies and curry leaves. Sauté till the dals turn golden brown.
3. Then add shredded carrot and cook it for 4-5 minutes.
4. Now, add roasted peanuts and cook another minute and turn off the heat.
5. To the cooled rice, add lemon juice, salt and the sautéed mixture.
6. Mix well and serve with yogurt, buttermilk and pickles.

Healthy option tips: White rice can be substituted with brown rice or quinoa for a healthier entrée. Shredded carrots can also be substituted with spinach purée.

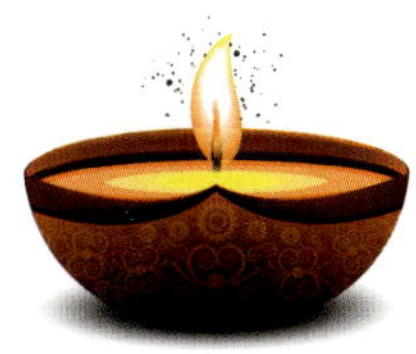

Spinach and Corn Rice

A rice dish that contains spinach, as well as sweet corn, mixed in with spices

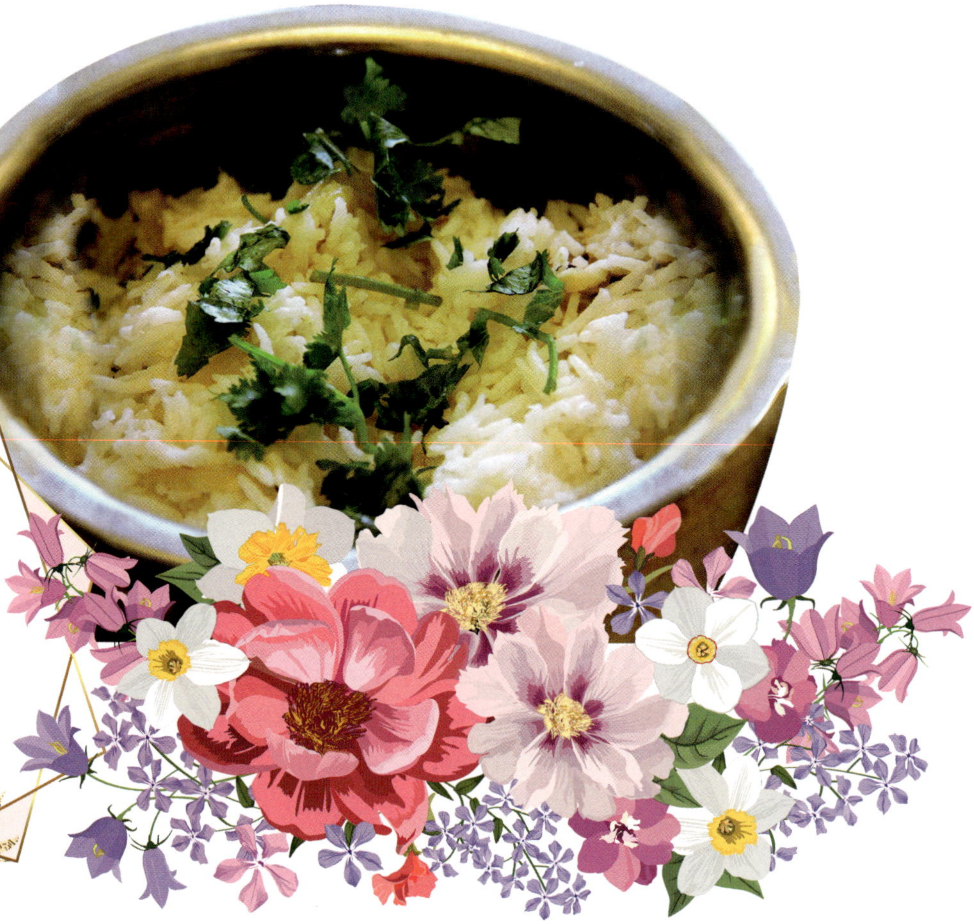

Preparation time: 15 *minutes*

Cooking time: 25 *minutes*

Servings: 6 *cups (8 oz. servings)*

Ingredients

- 1½ cups basmati rice
- 2 cups chopped spinach
- 1 cup frozen corn kernels
- 10 or 12 cashews
- ½ teaspoon cumin seeds
- ¾ teaspoon black pepper powder
- 4 green cardamoms
- 4 cloves (optional)
- 1 bay leaf
- pinch of cinnamon powder
- 3 tablespoons of lemon juice
- ¼ cup cilantro for garnish
- 3 cups water
- salt to taste

Process

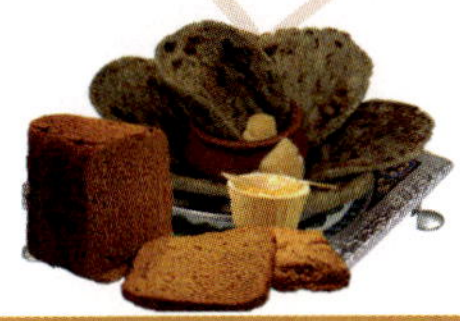

1. Rinse rice with water and keep it aside for 30 minutes.
2. Heat oil in a nonstick pan of rice cooker/or a pan and add cumin seeds, bay leaf, cardamoms, cloves, and cashews.
3. After the ingredients above have turned a little bit brown, add chopped spinach and corn into the mixture.
4. Sauté for a minute and gently mix in the rice.
5. Add 3 cups of water, salt, black pepper, and a pinch of cinnamon and lemon juice.
6. Mix well and cook in a rice cooker/pan.
7. Once cooked, garnish rice with cilantro and serve with buttermilk/lassi or yogurt.

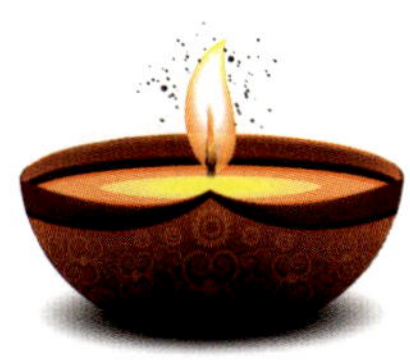

Tamarind Rice

A tangy and sour rice with a strong flavor of tamarind

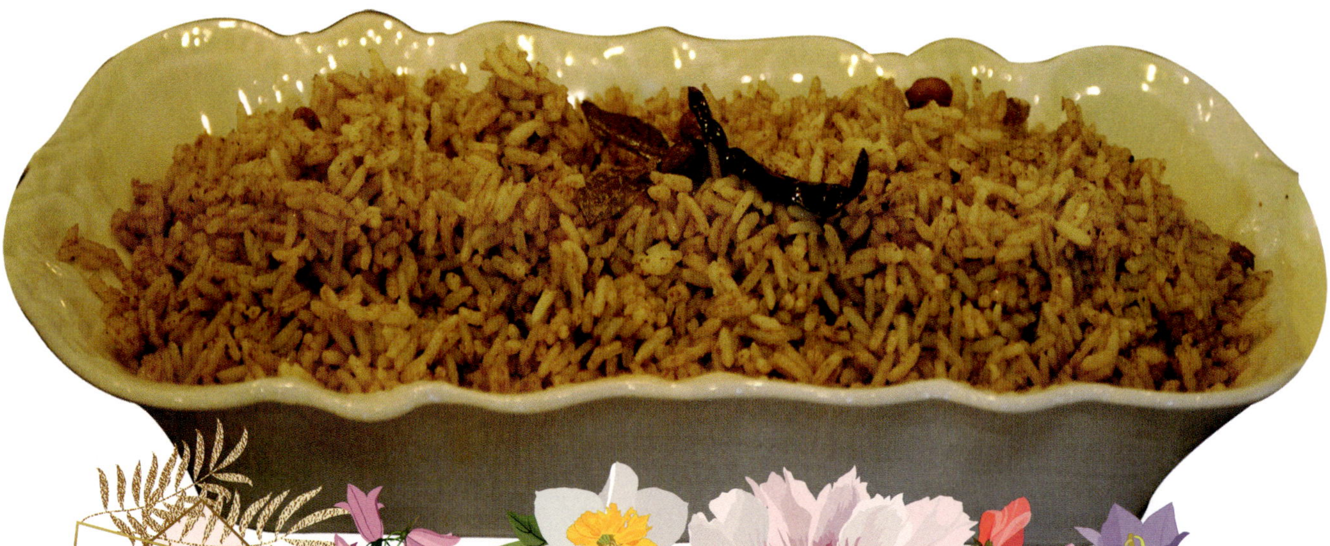

Preparation time: 15 *minutes*

Cooking time: 30 *minutes*

Servings: 3 *(8 oz. servings)*

Ingredients

- 1 cup uncooked rice-equivalent to 3 cups of cooked and cooled rice
- 2 teaspoons or small lemon size tamarind paste, or 1 tablespoon amchur powder instead of tamarind or 1 oz. or 2 tablespoons tamarind
- 1 cup hot water for tamarind water/ amchur water or tamarind pulp
- ¼ teaspoon mustard seeds
- 1 dried red chilli
- 4-5 curry leaves
- ¼ teaspoon asafoetida
- ¼ teaspoon turmeric powder
- 2 tablespoons peanuts
- ¼ cup chopped cilantro for garnish
- 2 cups water
- 2 tablespoons oil
- salt to taste

For spice powder

- ½ teaspoon chana dal (split Bengal gram)
- ½ teaspoon urad dal (split skinless black gram)
- ¼ teaspoon mustard seeds
- ½ teaspoon cumin seeds
- ¼ teaspoon peppercorns
- ½ teaspoon fennel seeds
- 5-6 curry leaves
- 2 dried red chilli
- 1 teaspoon dry coriander seeds

Process

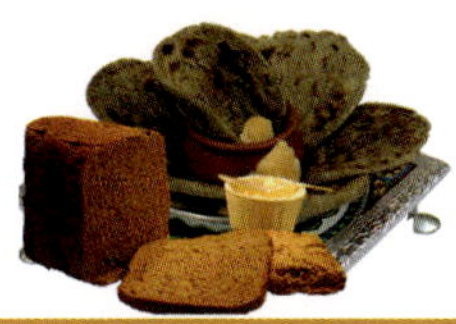

1. Roast all ingredients for spice powder in a nonstick skillet till all the dals turns golden brown, let it cool and make a powder in a dry grinder bowl.
2. While spices are cooling make tamarind water. If using tamarind paste or amchur powder, then dissolve it into 1 cup of hot water. If using tamarind then soak the tamarind in hot water for 15-20 minutes, mash it with hands and strain the pulp and keep it aside.
3. Cook 1 cup of rice with double water to make about 3 cups cooked rice. Cool the rice to room temperature before using it (prefer not to add salt while cooking rice).
4. Heat oil in a pan on medium heat. Once hot, add mustard seeds. Let them pop. Then add dry red chilli and curry leaves. Cook for 30 seconds.

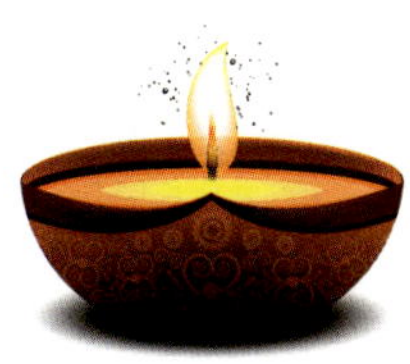

5. Then add peanuts and roast till they turn golden brown. Then add the tamarind water, followed by spice powder, turmeric powder, asafoetida and salt. Mix well and let it cook till it is reaches a thick consistency.
6. Add cooked rice to it. Mix well until the masala spreads evenly on the rice.
7. Garnish with cilantro and serve warm.

Ingredient tip: For better taste, use Sona Masuri rice to prepare Tamarind rice.

Bise Bele Bath

A delicious one pot meal – combination of rice, lentils and vegetables

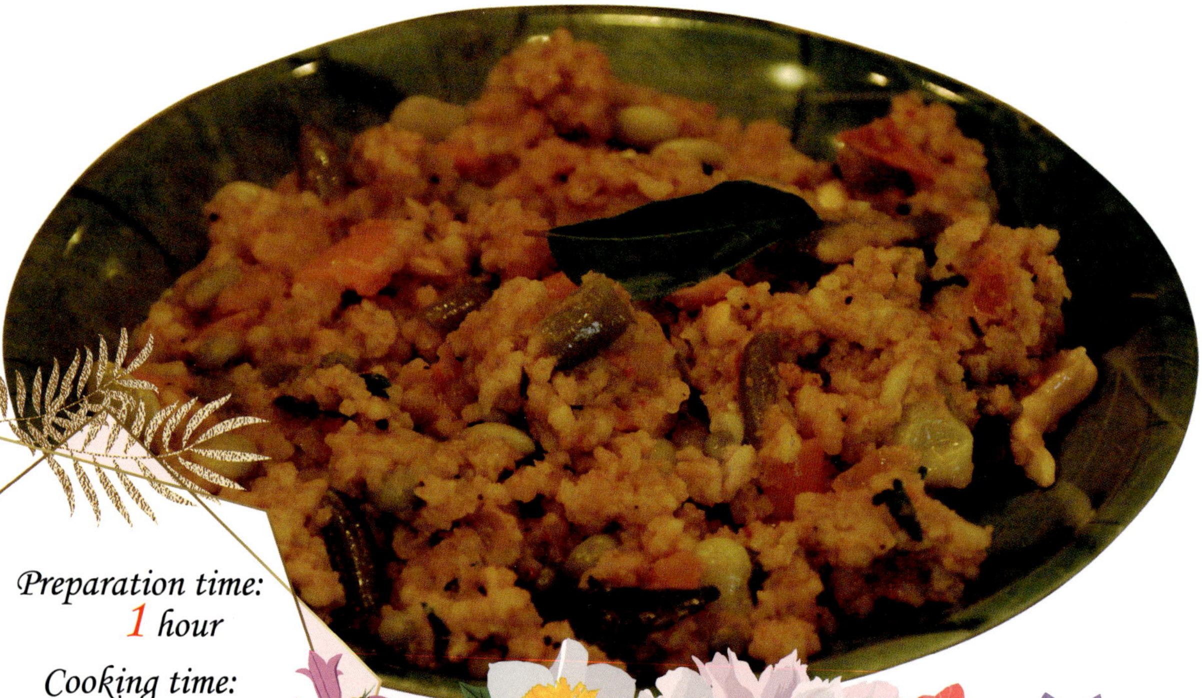

Preparation time: 1 *hour*

Cooking time: 2 *hours*

Servings: 6-8
(4 oz. bowls approx.)

Ingredients

For bise bele bath powder (Step 1)

- 1 ½ teaspoon chana dal
- ½ teaspoon urad dal
- ½ teaspoon rice (uncooked)
- 1 teaspoon coriander seeds
- ½ teaspoon cumin seeds
- 1-inch cinnamon stick
- 3-4 black peppers corns
- 4-5 red chillies
- ½ cup coconut, grated
- 1 stalk curry leaves
- Water (as much as needed for creating a chutney consistency)

For main dish

- 1 cup toor dal
- 1 cup rice
- 2 cups vegetables such as beans, carrots, potatoes, peas, ridge gourd etc., coarsely chopped
- 1 onion, sliced (optional)
- 2 tomatoes, finely chopped
- 1 bell pepper, sliced
- 1 cup raw peanuts (optional)
- 1 tablespoon jaggery
- 1 teaspoon tamarind
- cilantro for garnish
- salt to taste

For tempering (Step 6)

- 2-3 tablespoons of oil
- 1 tablespoon mustard seeds
- 1 tablespoon chana dal
- 1 tablespoon urad dal
- ½ teaspoon cumin seeds
- pinch of asafoetida

Process

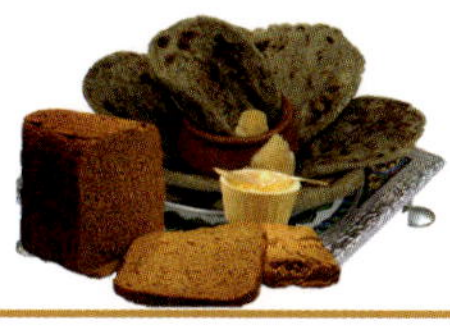

1. For preparing bise bele bath powder roast chana dal, urad dal, coriander seeds, curry leaves, cinnamon, black pepper, cumin seeds, red chillies, rice (½ teaspoon) until it turns brown.
2. Grind the above ingredients with the coconut and some water to a chutney consistency.

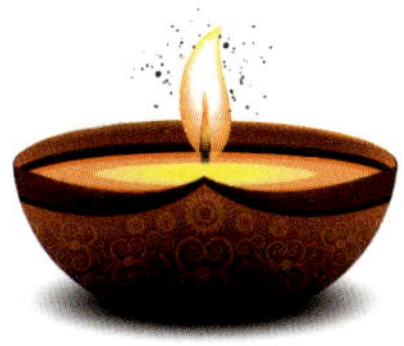

3. Boil 1 cup of toor dal with 4 cups of water in an open vessel until it is half cooked.
4. Add 1 cup of rice to it and all the cut vegetables.
5. Once these vegetables are cooked, reduce the heat and let it slow cook.
6. In a separate pan, heat oil for tempering and add mustard, cumin seeds, chana dal, urad dal and asafoetida.
7. When fragrant add onions (if using), and once brown, add bell pepper.
8. Once bell peppers are partially cooked, add tomatoes and let it cook.
9. Now add the bise bele bath powder, some jaggery, tamarind, and salt to taste.
10. Mix the items (steps 6 to 9) into the main vessel containing cooked dal, rice and vegetables.
11. Simmer for another 10 minutes until all the ingredients are blended.
12. Garnish with cilantro and serve warm with raita made with cucumbers and tomatoes.

Optional tip: Raw peanuts may be added to this dish, either while cooking the dal or later to the tempering if a crispy taste is preferred.

Himachali Pulao

A slightly sweet rice, containing dried and fresh fruits

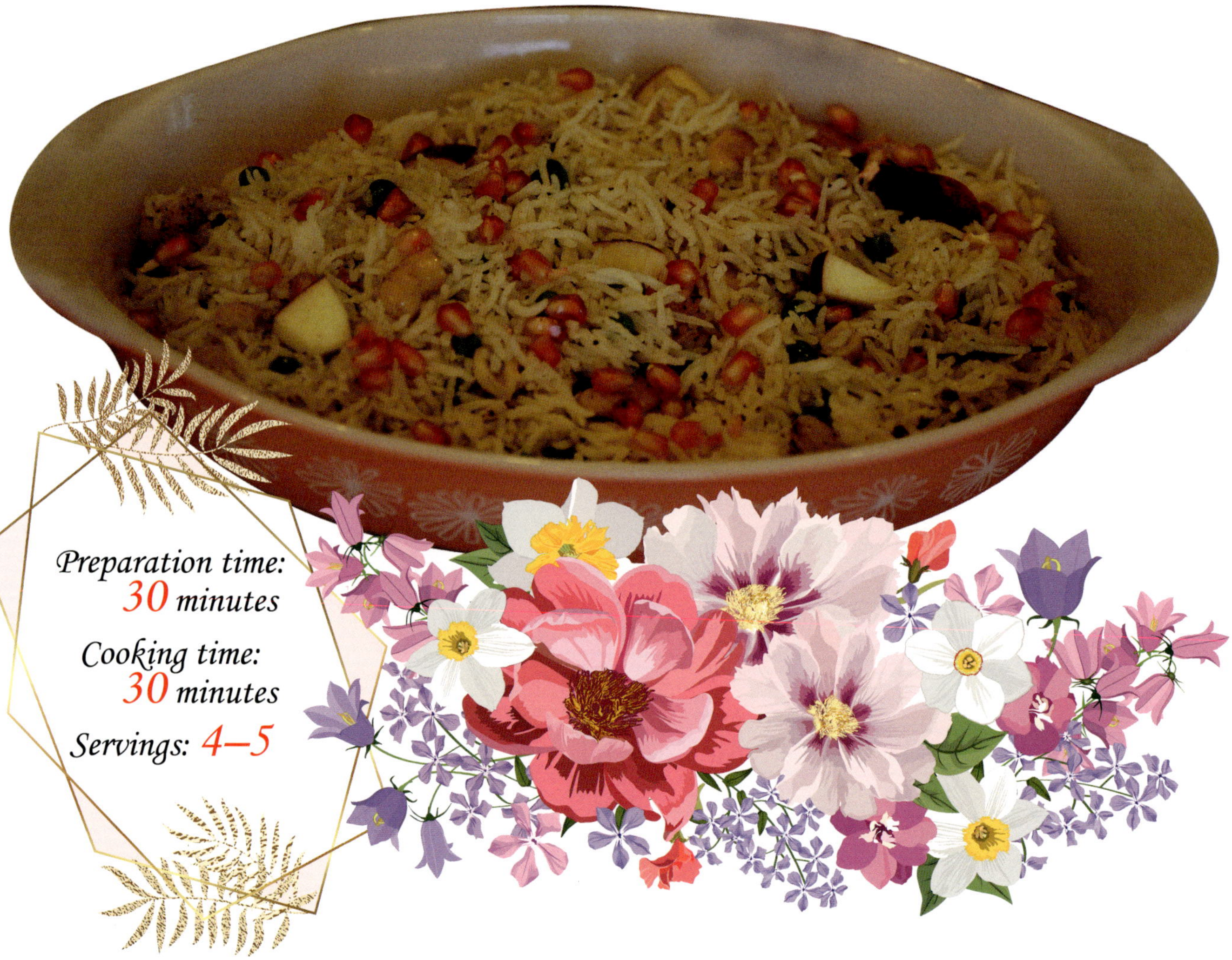

Preparation time: 30 *minutes*

Cooking time: 30 *minutes*

Servings: 4–5

Ingredients

- 1 ½ cups Basmati rice
- 1 apple, chopped in small cubes
- ½ cup fresh pomegranate seeds
- ½ cup fresh green peas
- 10 cashew nuts
- 10 raisins
- 1 teaspoon garam masala powder
- 2 bay leaves
- 2-3 black cardamoms
- 4 green cardamoms
- 3 sticks of cinnamon
- few strings of saffron
- ½ cup of milk
- 2 tablespoons ghee
- 2 teaspoons of sugar
- water 4 cups
- salt to taste

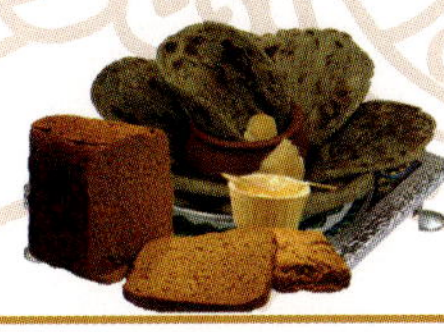

Process

1. Wash basmati rice and soak for half an hour.
2. Boil 4 cups of water in a saucepan. Add the rice. When rice is cooked, drain out the water and keep the rice aside.
3. In a non-stick heavy pan, add 2 tablespoons of ghee and heat on low flame for 2 minutes. To this add bay leaf, black cardamom, green cardamom and cinnamon sticks. Let them cook till fragrant.
4. Add green peas and a pinch of salt. Then add cashew nuts and raisins. Keep stirring the mixture in the pan for 5 minutes on low fire.
5. Now, add the rice. Mix it well with the masala in the pan.
6. In a separate pan, heat milk to lukewarm temperature and add saffron to it. Add this milk-saffron mix to the rice pan.
7. Next, add in the apple cubes and pomegranate seeds.
8. Last, add salt as per taste, sugar and garam masala powder. Mix it all well and let it cook for another 5 minutes on low heat with the lid on the pan.
9. Serve warm with yogurt or raita.

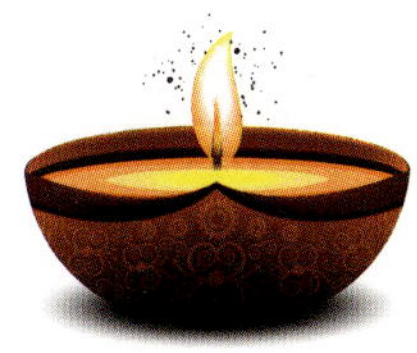

Mithai

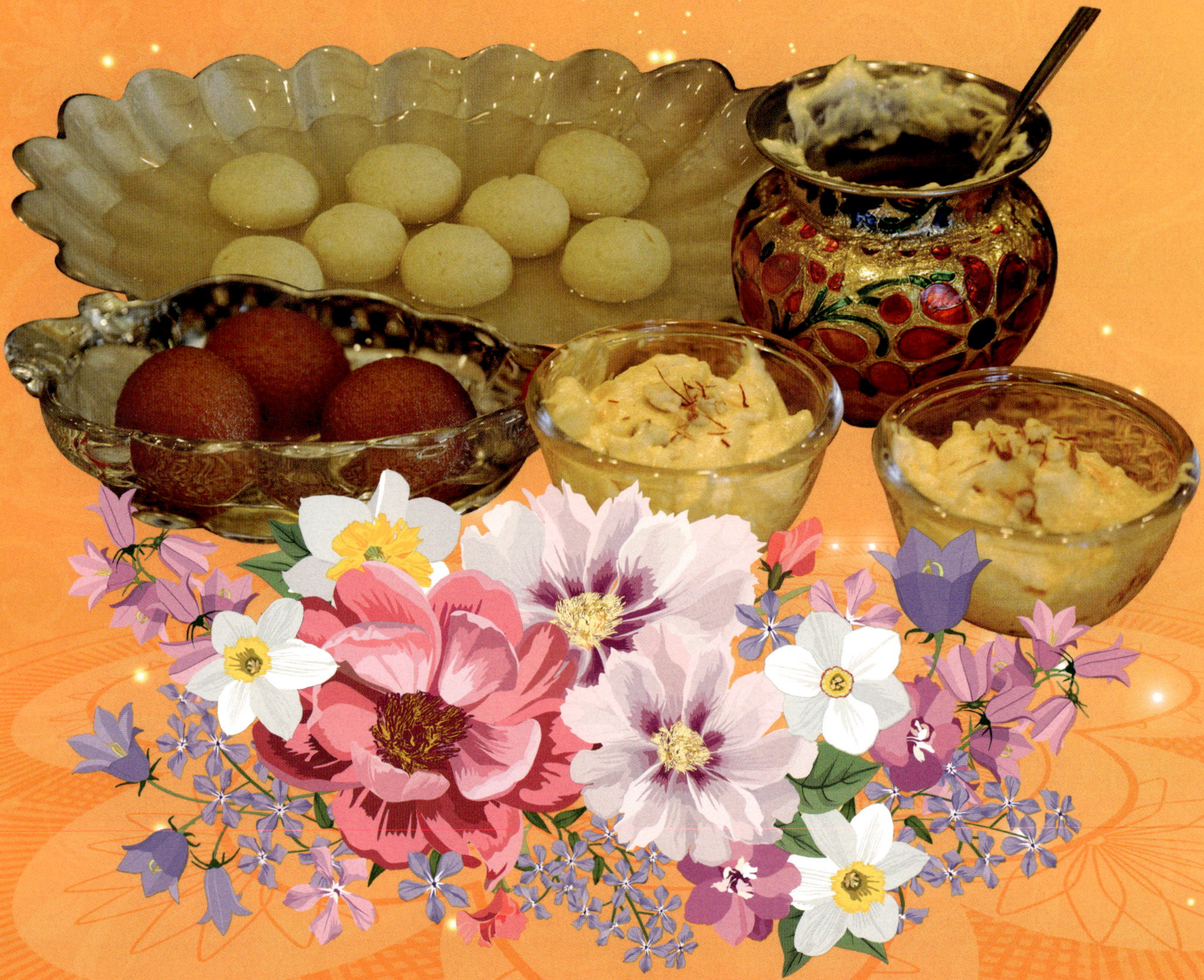

Perfect as bhog offerings this chapter includes sweet blissful delights such as *gulabjamuns, rasagullas, burfis and* more that never fail to please and are ideal for divine occasions. *Double ka meetha, almond and cashew cookies, sesame peanut flax chikki,mango shrikandh* and *kulfi* are other choices to pick from.

To make festive indulgence more nutritious we have selected recipes that are chock full of nuts and dry fruits, seeds such as sesame and flax, and have the goodness of fruits – mangoes, dates and coconut. Sometimes if the recipe permits we have substituted the white sugar with brown or jaggery, replaced all-purpose flour with healthier grains.

Many of these are traditional family recipes and they all complete the festival and special occasion meals, or may simply be enjoyed as after meal desserts!

1. Double ka Meetha
2. Gulab Jamun
3. Besan Burfi
4. Walnut Burfi
5. Peda
6. Kopra Pak
7. Date Nut Roll
8. Gud Papdi
9. Sesame Peanut Flax Chikki
10. Almond and Cashew Cookies
11. Rasagulla
12. Mango Shrikandh
13. Kulfi

Double Ka Meetha

An easy to cook, rich Hyderabad delicacy. Also, known as "Shahi Tukda"

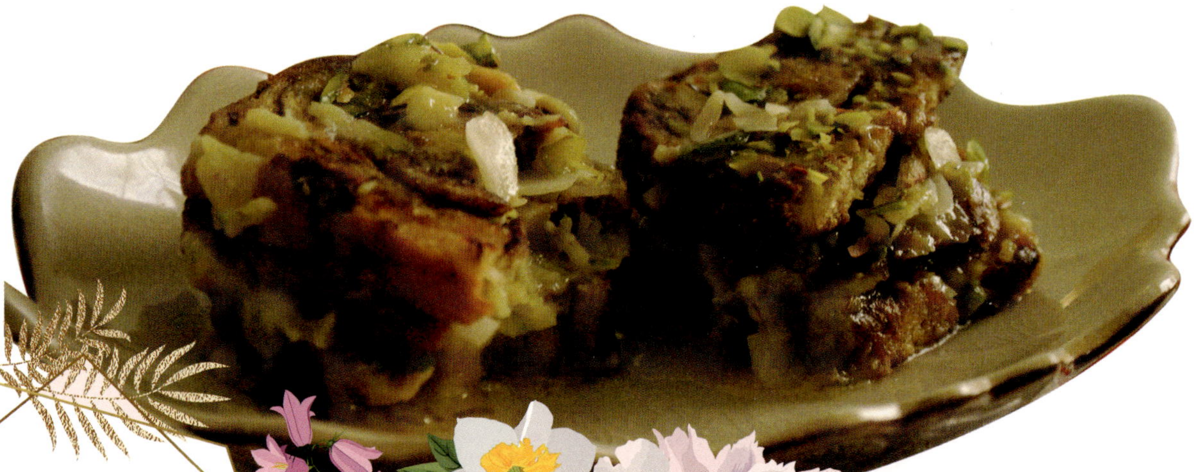

Preparation time: 20 *minutes*

Cooking time: 40 *minutes*

Servings: 4

Ingredients

- 3 slices white bread, sliced into quarters
- ¾ cup brown sugar, or 1 cup shredded jaggery
- dry fruits–almonds, cashew nuts and raisins to taste
- 3 cloves of green cardamom, crushed
- 1 cup milk
- ½ cup ghee

Process

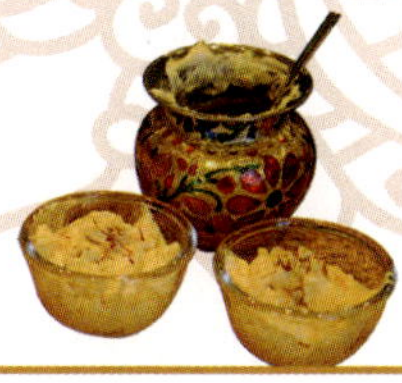

1. In a skillet melt ghee on a low heat setting.
2. Now, add the quartered bread slices. Keep toasting them on both sides till they are brown. Set aside the slices.
3. In a saucepan, add 1 cup of milk and 3 crushed cardamoms. Boil, then keep it on low heat.
4. In a separate vessel, add jaggery and pour 4 tablespoons water. Heat it enough so that the jaggery melts and starts dissolving in water. Continue to boil until it is a viscous syrup.
5. As soon as the jaggery syrup is ready, mix it with the cardamom flavored hot milk.
6. Now add the ghee toasted bread slices.
7. Add crushed dry fruits–almonds, raisins and cashew nuts. You may also roast them in some ghee before mixing for added flavor.
8. Cook for about 5 minutes on low heat until you achieve a creamy or desired consistency taking care that the bread holds its shape and does not become mushy.

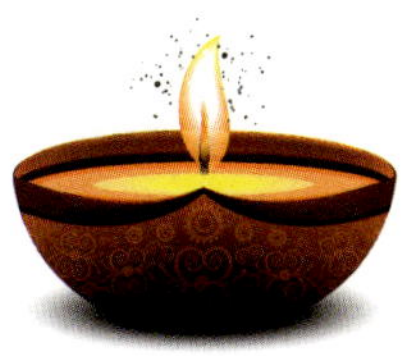

Gulab Jamun

Melt in your mouth, heavenly brown balls soaked in sugar syrup

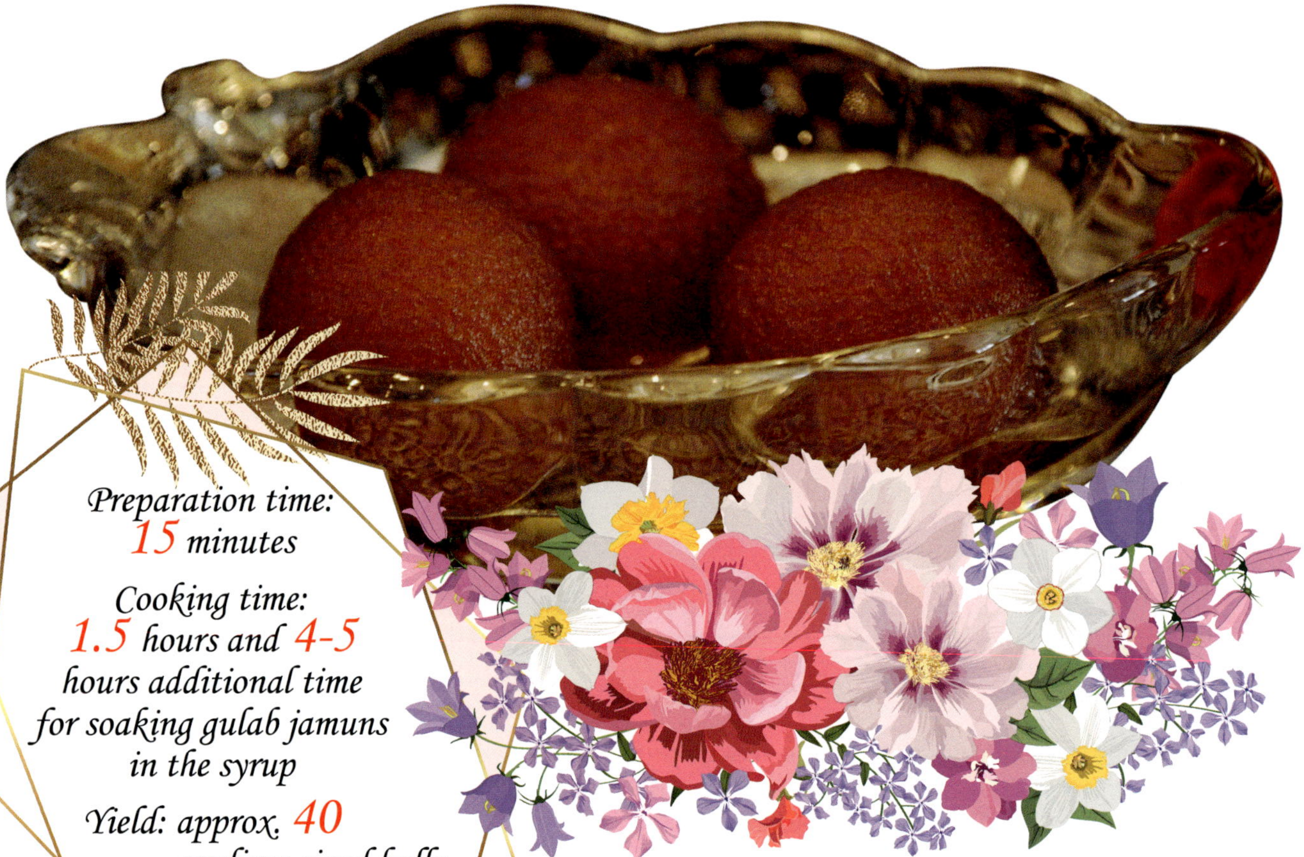

Preparation time:
15 minutes

Cooking time:
1.5 hours and 4-5 hours additional time for soaking gulab jamuns in the syrup

Yield: approx. 40 medium sized balls

Ingredients

For gulab jamuns

- 1 ½ cups milk powder, Carnation
- ¾ cup Bisquick (pancake mix)
- 3 tablespoons melted butter
- 1 cup whole milk approx. or as much needed to make dough
- oil for frying

For the syrup

- 3 cups sugar
- 5 cups water
- 5-7 coarsely ground green cardamoms

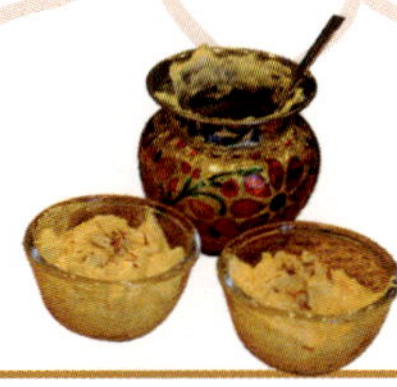

Process

1. Prepare the syrup with sugar, water and cardamoms. After letting the syrup boil for about 5 minutes, keep it warm.
2. In a big bowl mix the two dry ingredients, milk powder and Bisquick. Now add the melted butter and using whole milk prepare a soft dough, which is kind of sticky at first but can be rolled into balls later.
3. Make medium sized balls (¾ inch). After soaking in the sugar syrup, they will double in size. Keep them covered with a moist cloth to prevent drying.
4. Now fry these balls gently in the heated oil on medium heat by stirring or shaking the kadai continuously till they are cooked to a golden-brown color.
5. These can be immediately put in the sugar syrup. Leave them for several hours or overnight for best results. Serve warm or at room temperature.

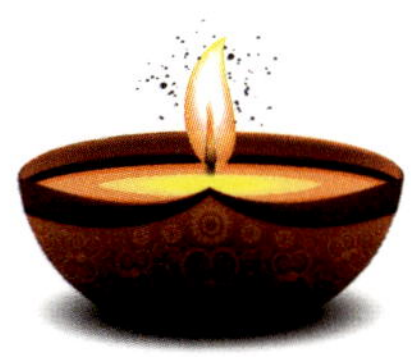

Besan Burfi

An all-time favorite dessert with nuts and flavored with cardamom

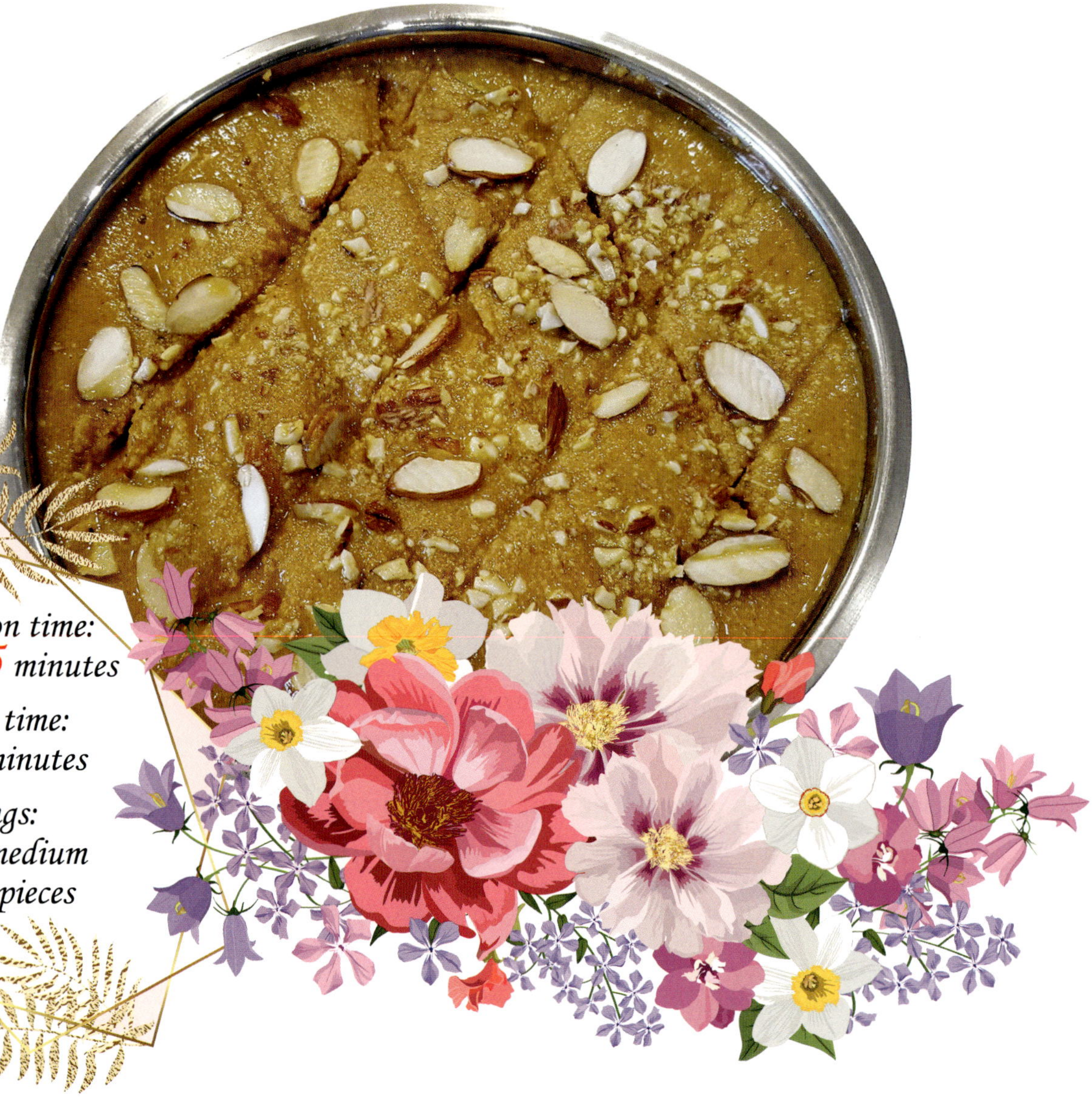

Preparation time:
10-15 *minutes*

Cooking time:
30 *minutes*

Servings:
40 *medium size pieces*

Ingredients

- 2 cups gram flour, preferably fine
- 1 cup powdered sugar
- ½ teaspoon green cardamom powder
- 12 almonds, sliced
- 10-12 pistachios, chopped
- 1 cup pure ghee, or a little less than 1 cup

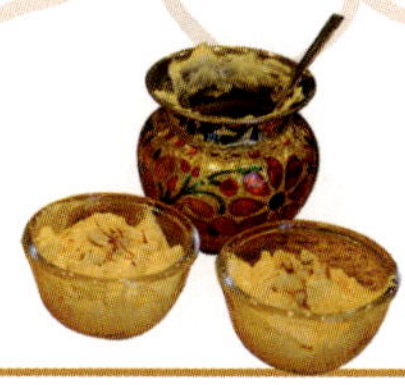

Process

1. Heat the ghee in a non-stick pan. Add the gram flour and roast on low heat, stirring continuously, for 10-15 minutes or until it starts changing color and becomes golden brown and is fragrant.
2. Add the cardamom powder, pistachio and almond slivers (save some for garnish/decoration) and mix. Remove from the heat and set aside to cool.
3. Add the powdered sugar and mix well.
4. Grease a shallow tray with ghee. A 10-inch steel plate works great.
5. Pour the gram flour mixture into the tray and spread it evenly with a greased spatula or using the bottom of a steel bowl (katori).
6. Garnish with remaining almonds and pistachios. Cool and cut into square or diamond shaped pieces and serve.
7. Burfi may be stored in an airtight container for about 2 weeks.

Cooking tip: If the burfi breaks when taking it out, heat the tray/plate for a few seconds. When the ghee melts the pieces will slide off easily.

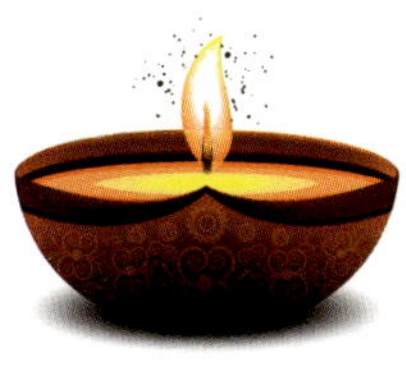

Walnut Burfi

Quick, easy and tasty fudge like dessert

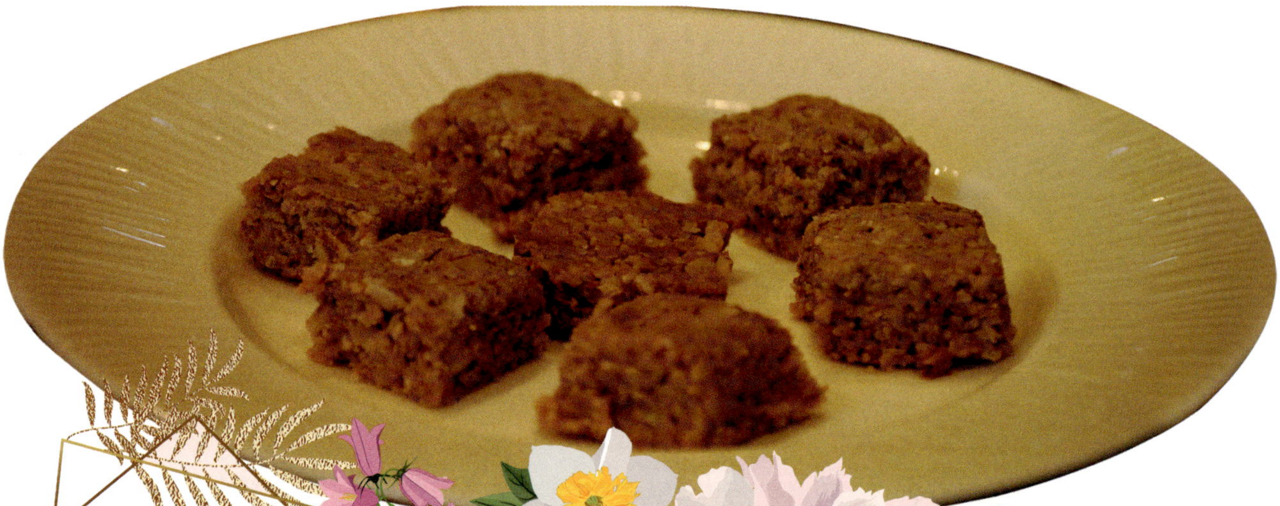

Preparation time: 15 *minutes*

Cooking time: 30 *minutes*

Yield: 30-40 *pieces*

Ingredients

- 3 cups walnuts coarsely ground
- 2 cups sugar
- 1 cup nonfat dry milk
- 2 teaspoons ghee (optional)
- 1 cup water

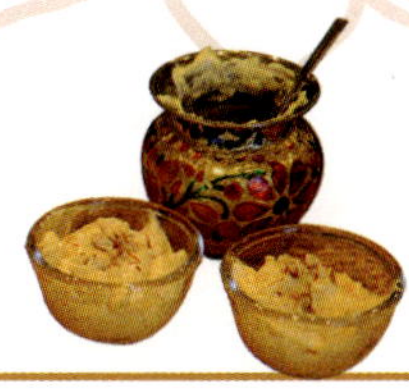

Process

1. In a deep vessel or kadai boil sugar and water to make 1 ½ thread sugar syrup.
2. To this syrup now add the coarsely ground walnuts.
3. Next add the nonfat dry milk and ghee, and keep stirring and mixing for another 5 minutes. Turn off the heat, leaving the vessel on the stove. Let it cool a little.
4. Grease a 10 x 13- inch cookie sheet with ½ inch thickness and spread the mix.
5. Let it cool for half an hour. Cut in desired pieces and serve.

Cooking note: The 1 ½ thread syrup refers to the thickness of the syrup or chasini. When you take a few drops of the syrup between index finger and thumb and then open them, you will observe one or more fine sugar strings/threads. If there is one string, it is one thread syrup/chasini and so on. More the threads, denser and thicker is the syrup.

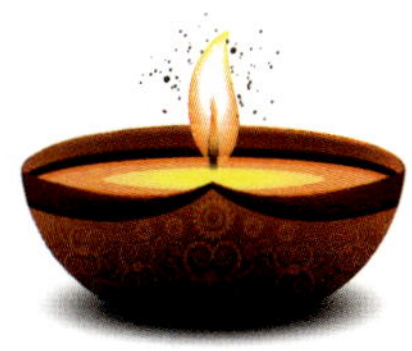

Peda

A rich and fudge-like dessert made from condensed milk and milk powder

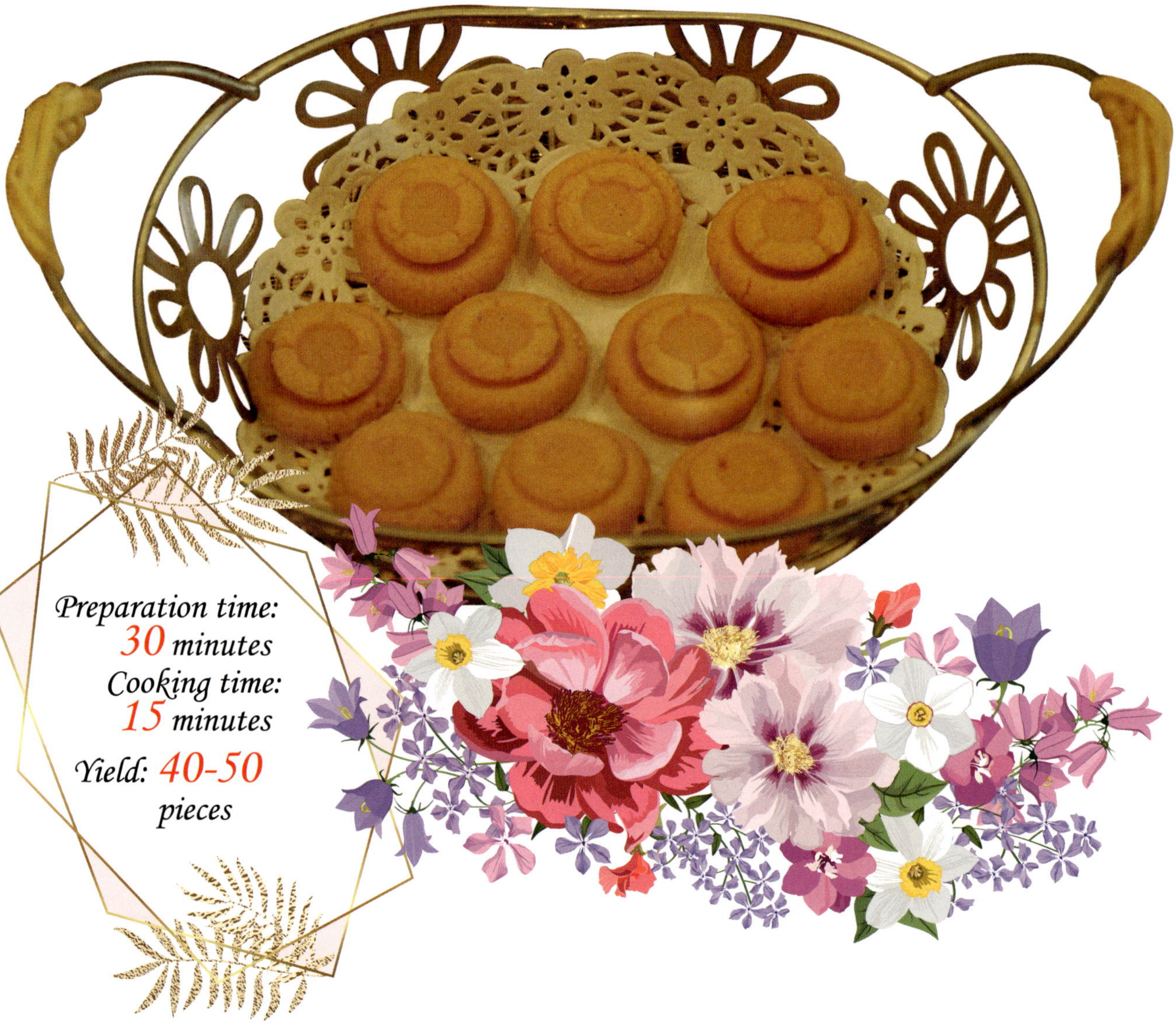

Preparation time: 30 *minutes*
Cooking time: 15 *minutes*
Yield: 40-50 *pieces*

Ingredients

- 2 cups dry milk powder
- 2 cans condensed milk
- 1 stick unsalted butter (8 tablespoons)
- few strands of saffron
- ¼ cup nuts

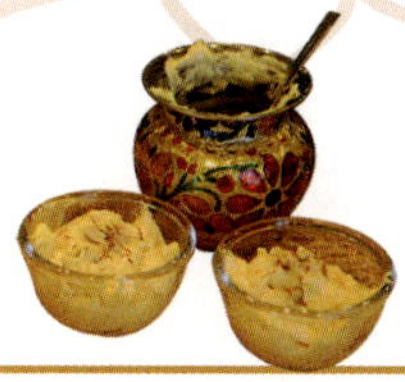

Process

1. In a deep bowl, melt butter and then add the condensed milk. Mix the two well.
2. Now, add the dry milk powder a little at a time. Mix well ensuring that mixture is smooth, with no lumps.
3. Heat in the microwave on medium high stirring at regular intervals (approx. 5 minutes–3 times) and making sure that the mixture does not overflow from the bowl. This step needs to be monitored depending on the heat of the microwave. Can check at shorter intervals.
4. Continue to heat and mix until mixture thickens in consistency.
5. Spread in a 2-inch pie plate (9-10" pie dish), decorate with nuts and refrigerate for 3-4 hours.
6. Cut in pieces or different shapes as desired.

Cooking tip: Use a deep bowl with contents filling just half of it. When heated, the mixture tends to bubble up and can spill over in the microwave if the bowl is small.

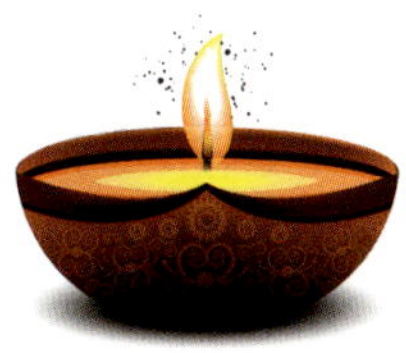

Kopra Pak

A sweet coconut dish with saffron and cardamom flavors

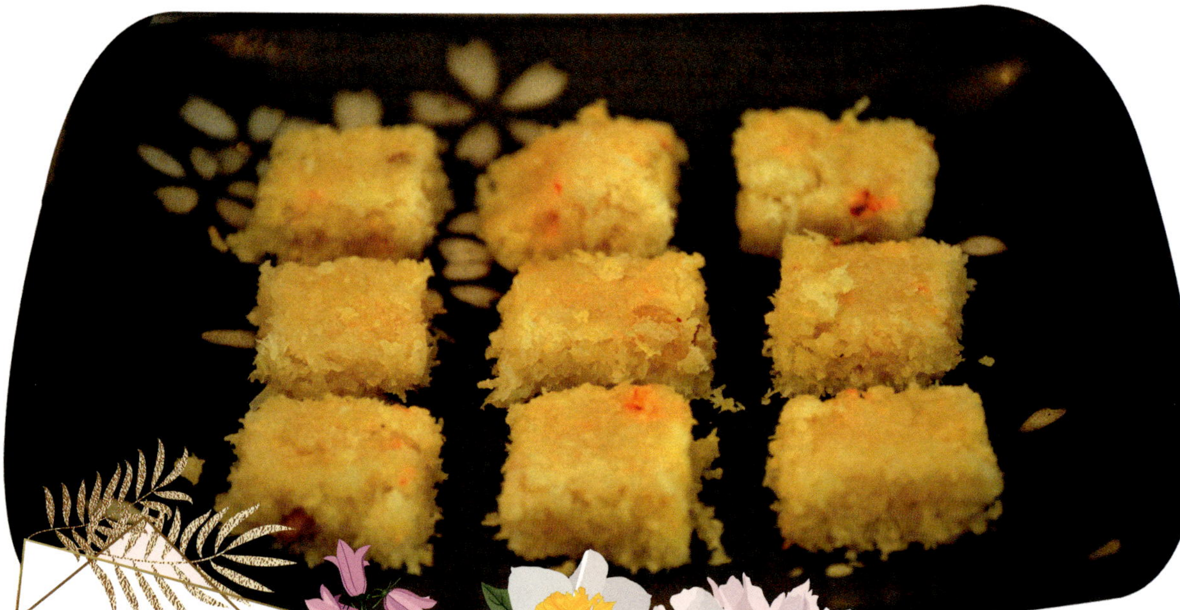

Preparation time: 10 *minutes*

Cooking time: 30 *minutes*

Yield: 25 *pieces*

Ingredients

- 3 cups dry coconut, finely shredded
- 14 oz. can sweetened-condensed milk
- 1 cup ricotta cheese (part-skim)
- 1 teaspoon cardamom, powdered (8-10 green cardamoms)
- 1 teaspoon ghee
- 2 to 5 strands saffron
- ¼ cup warm milk for soaking saffron (soak for 10 minutes)
- powdered pistachio for garnishing (optional)
- wax paper for layering the flat baking tray

Process

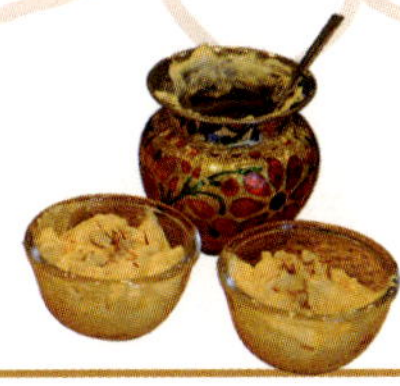

1. In a small bowl, soak saffron strands in milk. Keep aside.
2. In a shallow non-stick pan, roast shredded coconut for 5 minutes on medium heat.
3. Add ghee, sweetened condensed milk, ricotta cheese and cardamom powder. Mix all these ingredients together. Continue to stir and cook for approximately 2-5 minutes, till the ingredients clump together. Remove from heat.
4. Layer wax paper on flat baking sheet and pour the coconut mixture onto the baking sheet. Spread it evenly.
5. Sprinkle powdered pistachio on top (optional). Refrigerate for an hour and then cut into pieces.
6. If stored in the refrigerator, the Kopra Pak remains good for about 10 days.

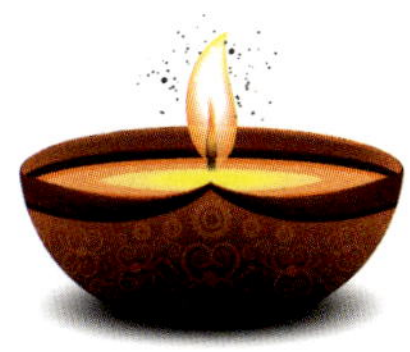

Date Nut Roll

Simply nature's ingredients, dates and nuts used to roll out this healthy and tasty dessert

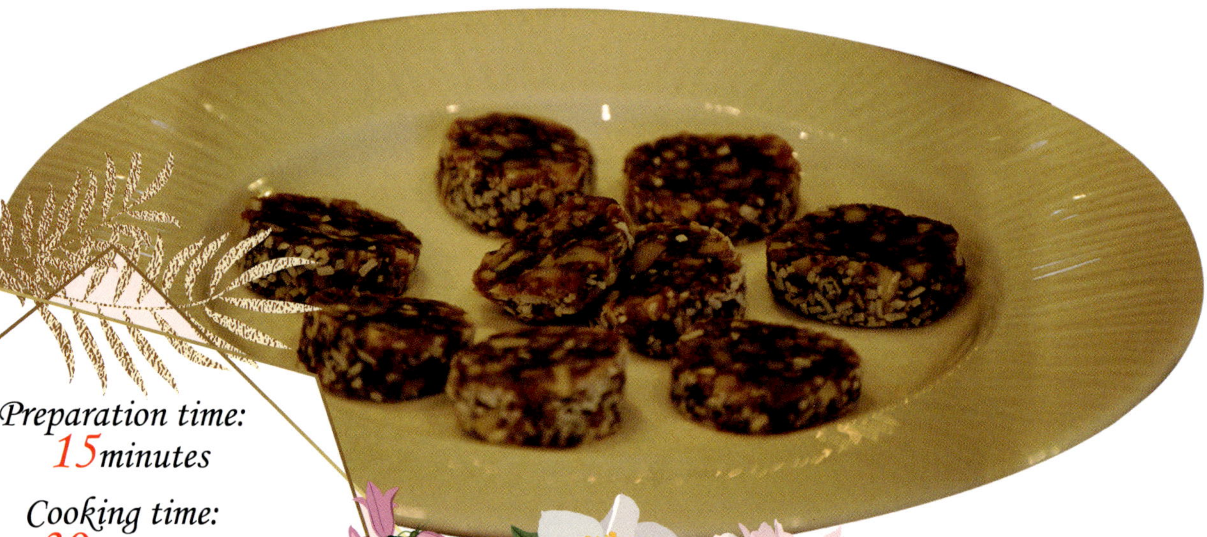

Preparation time: 15 *minutes*

Cooking time: 30 *minutes*

Refrigeration time: 30–40 *minutes*

Servings: 12 *(approx. 3 pieces per serving)*

Ingredients

- 1 cup medjool dates, pitted and chopped
- ¼ cup pistachios, chopped
- ¼ cup walnuts, chopped
- ¼ cup cashews, chopped
- ¼ cup almonds, chopped
- 1 tablespoon ghee

For garnishing

- 3 teaspoons powdered pistachio
- 3-4 teaspoons dried shredded coconut

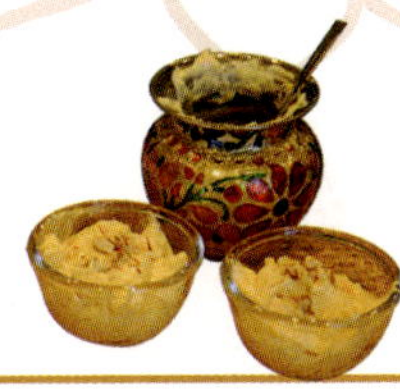

Process

1. In a bowl, mix all the chopped dry fruits–pistachios, walnuts, cashews and almonds and keep aside.
2. In a shallow non-stick pan warm 1 tablespoon ghee, and add chopped dates. Cook while stirring for 3 to 5 minutes or until the dates becomes soft and mushy.
3. Remove from heat and transfer the cooked dates to a platter. Let this mixture cool down.
4. Once it is comfortable to handle, mix the date mixture and chopped nuts in a bowl with your hand to form a dough.
5. Divide this dough like mixture into two parts, and roll them into 2 cylinders. Tightly wrap these cylinders in aluminum foil or plastic wrap.
6. Refrigerate for 3 hours. Remove from foil or plastic wrap. Cut them into ½ inch slices.
7. Garnish with shredded coconut and powdered pistachio by sprinkling on each piece.
8. These can last up to a month in airtight containers.

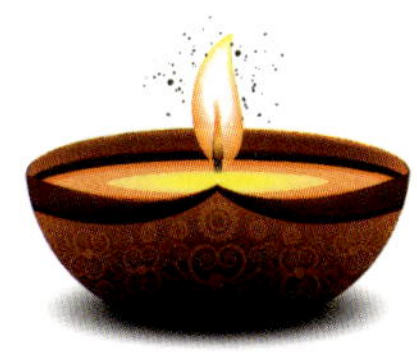

Gud Papdi

A popular dessert made with jaggery and wheat flour to satisfy sugar cravings

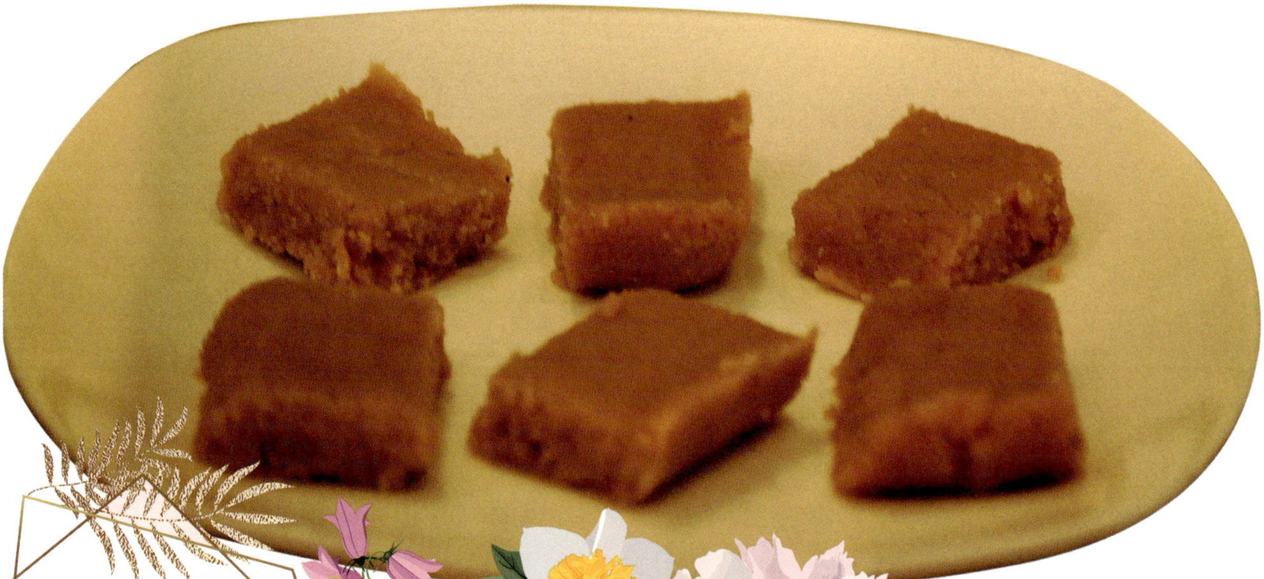

Preparation time: 10 *minutes*

Cooking time: 20 *minutes*

Yield: 24 *pieces*

Ingredients

- 1 cup whole wheat flour
- 1 cup grated jaggery
- ½ cup ghee
- 1 teaspoon cardamom powder
- 2 tablespoons milk
- finely chopped nuts

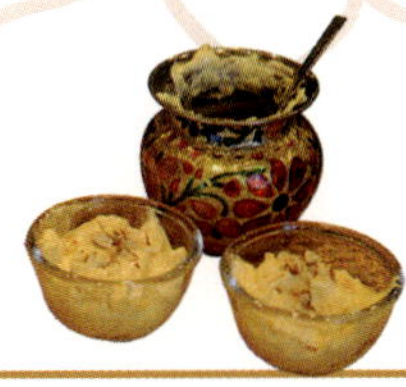

Process

1. In a wide pan heat the ghee.
2. Add the flour slowly and roast until golden brown. The mixture should start coming together and become fluffy.
3. Remove from heat and add the grated jaggery along with the cardamom powder.
4. Now, add milk and keep stirring until it becomes like a lump.
5. Nuts can be added at this time or used as garnish, or both.
6. Spread the mixture in a greased pan (or an 8” pie dish). Let it set for 5 minutes and then cut into diamond or square shaped pieces.
7. Gud papdi stays good for 30 days or even more.

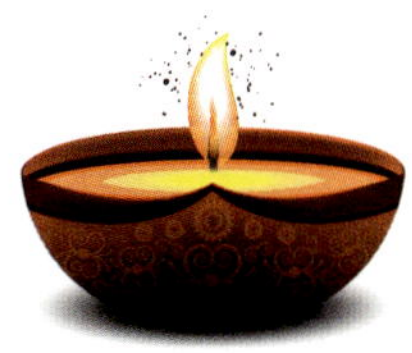

Sesame–Peanut–Flax Chikki

A great winter nourishing sweet treat and a rich source of iron

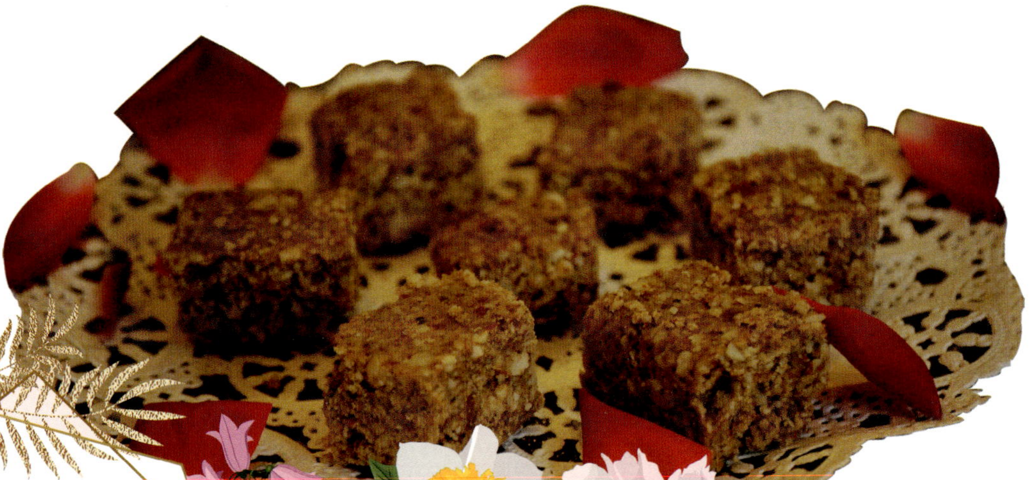

Preparation time: 15 *minutes*

Cooking time: 25 *minutes*

Yield: 50 *pieces*

Ingredients

- 1 cup roasted sesame seed powder
- 1 cup roasted peanut powder
- ½ cup roasted shredded coconut powder
- 3 teaspoons roasted flaxseed powder
- 2 tablespoons ghee
- 1 ½ cup jaggery, chopped
- 2 teaspoons cardamom powder
- 4 teaspoons water

Process

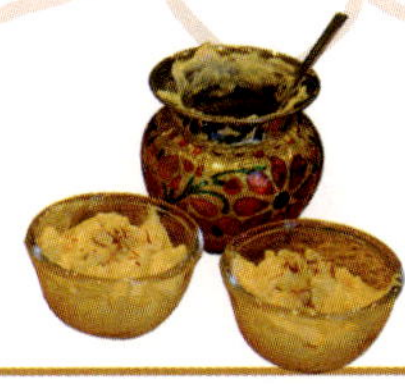

1. In a heated non-stick pan, add ghee and chopped jaggery.
2. Cook on a medium heat for 1 to 2 minutes, stirring continuously.
3. Add water to the jaggery. The jaggery powder should melt and form a liquid like consistency.
4. Turn off the heat. Now, add the roasted sesame seeds powder, peanut powder, flaxseed powder, coconut powder and cardamom powder. Mix very well.
5. Working quickly, spread this mixture thinly on a greased plate and then draw lines on this sheet to mark the desired shape of the Chikki.
6. After it cools down, the pieces break apart easily. These can be stored for about a month in an air tight container.

Cooking tip: This sweet is an excellent nourishing choice during fasts. The mixture can also be shaped as ladoos instead of chikki.

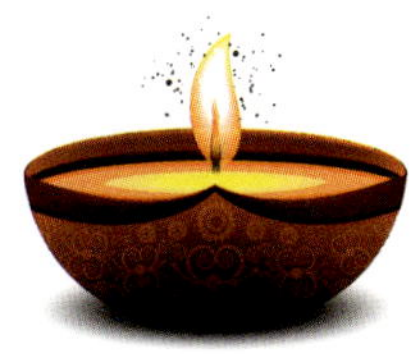

Almond and Cashew Cookies

A vegan and gluten free delight to enjoy with milk or tea

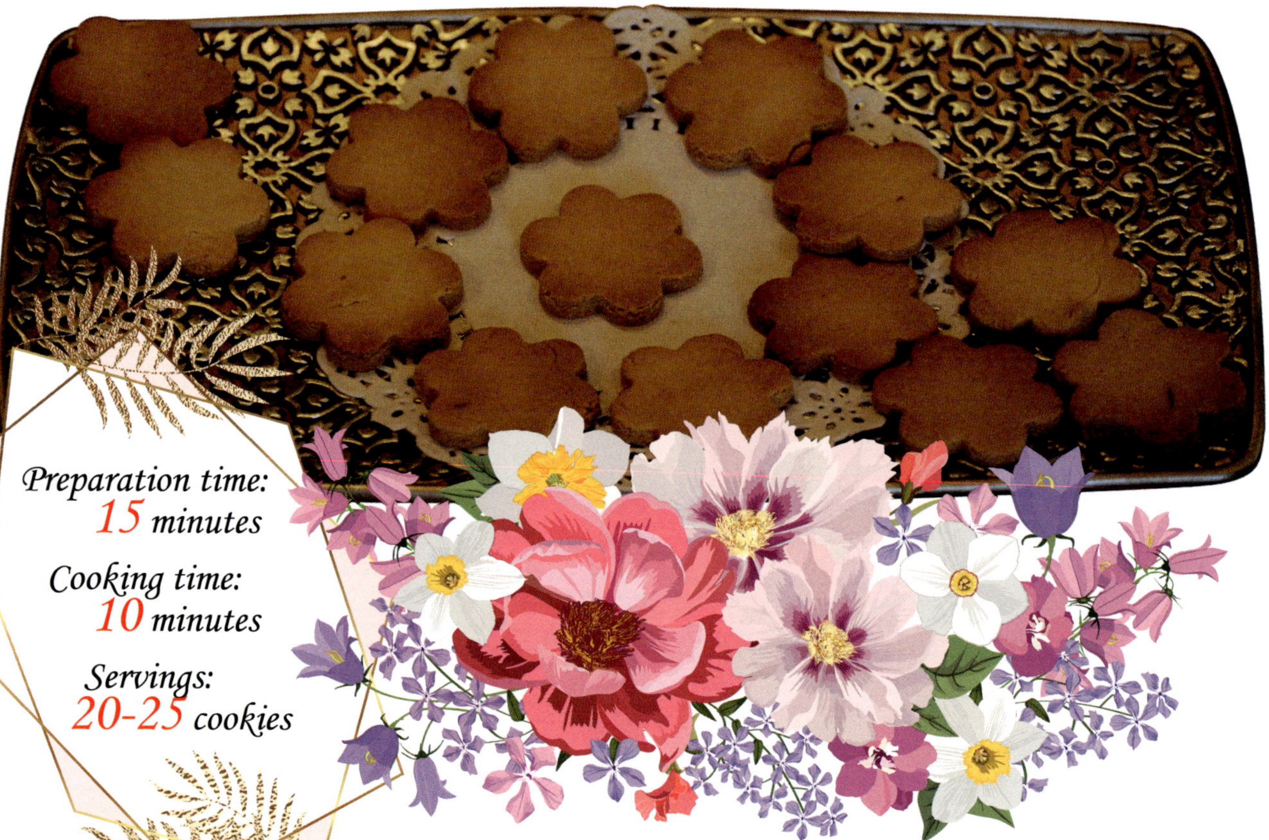

Preparation time: 15 *minutes*

Cooking time: 10 *minutes*

Servings: 20-25 *cookies*

Ingredients

- 1 ½ cups of almond meal
- 1 ½ cups of cashew powder
- 1 teaspoon of cardamom powder
- 1 cup brown sugar
- 5-6 strands of saffron
- ¼ cup almond milk (approx.)

Process

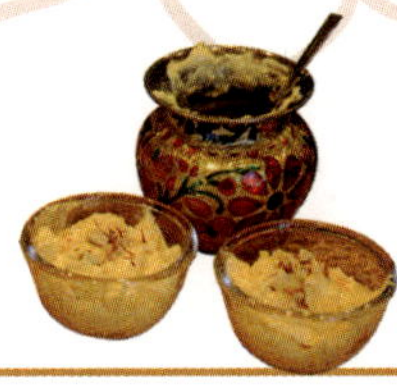

1. Preheat oven to 350°F.
2. In a big bowl, mix all the above ingredients into a tight dough using a hand mixer or stand mixer.
3. Roll out the entire dough to 2-5 mm thickness on a saran wrap, otherwise it will stick to the surface.
4. Cut into various shapes with cookie cutters and bake at 350°F for 10 minutes on a cookie sheet or silpad.
5. Cool for 5 minutes and serve.

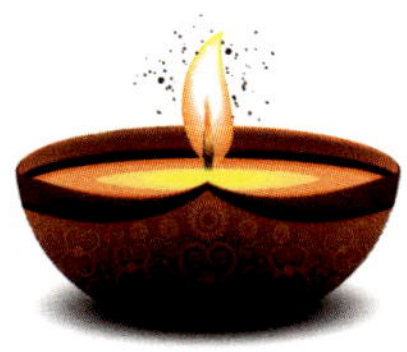

Rasagulla

Mouthwatering spongy cottage cheese balls immersed in light sugar rose syrup

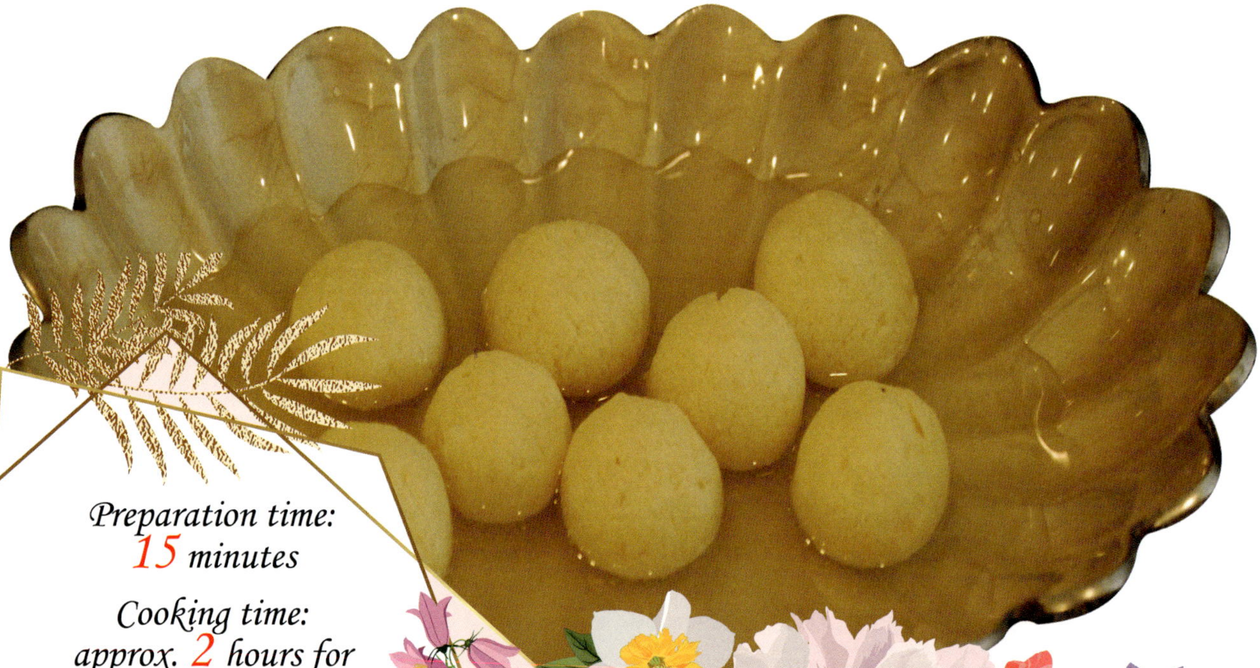

Preparation time:
15 minutes

Cooking time:
approx. 2 hours for rasagullas cooked in 2 batches (refrigeration time is additional 3-4 hours)

Yield: 20-25 medium size rasagullas

Ingredients

For Rasagullas

- ½-gallon 2% milk
- 1/4 cup white vinegar
- few threads of pure saffron (optional)
- 1/4 cup lukewarm water

For Syrup

- 2 cups sugar
- 7 cups water for syrup
- ½ teaspoon rose water (optional)
- ¼ teaspoon green cardamom powder

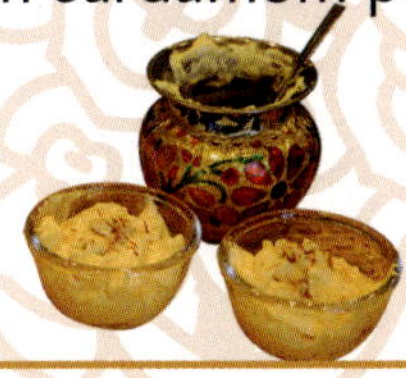

Process

1. ***Making paneer for rasagullas***: Bring milk to boil on medium heat in a pot. Mix lukewarm water and vinegar. Pour it in boiling milk while stirring slowly with a spoon. Let the milk curdle. Turn the heat off and leave for 2 minutes. If milk does not curdle you can add some more vinegar while milk is still hot.
2. Drain curdled milk in a cheese or muslin cloth. Rinse this paneer under cold running water. Tie up the cloth and hang it or put it under heavy weight to drain excess water. Refrigerate for an hour.
3. ***Making syrup***: - Add the sugar and water to a wide pan and bring to boil. Add cardamom and rose water.
4. Meanwhile in a food processor blend paneer to soften. Knead it well to make a smooth dough. Take small portions of this and make ¾-1-inch balls with a soft hand.
5. Add these paneer balls in boiling sugar syrup. Cover the pan with an air tight lid and cook for around 12 minutes on medium heat. Lift and slightly shake the pan sideways few times to separate the paneer balls. Turn the heat off and leave the rasagullas in the pan for 5-10 minutes and then transfer with syrup to a wide shallow casserole.
6. When the syrup cools to lower temperature (still warm) garnish with saffron and refrigerate for 2-3 hours before serving. Serve cold.

Cooking note: Paneer balls must have enough space to float around when immersed and cooked in the sugar syrup. A wide shallow pan is most suitable. If needed they can be cooked in two batches.

Optional tip: By adding rasgullas to thickened, sweet milk flavored with cardamom and saffron, you can make delicious rasmalai.

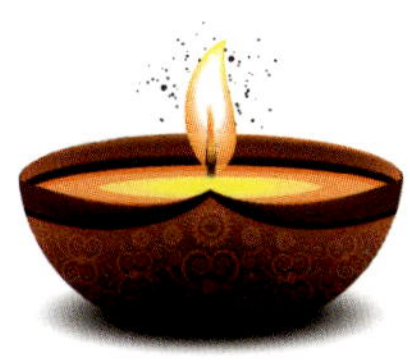

Mango Shrikhand

A Western Indian sweet mango flavored dessert made with strained yogurt

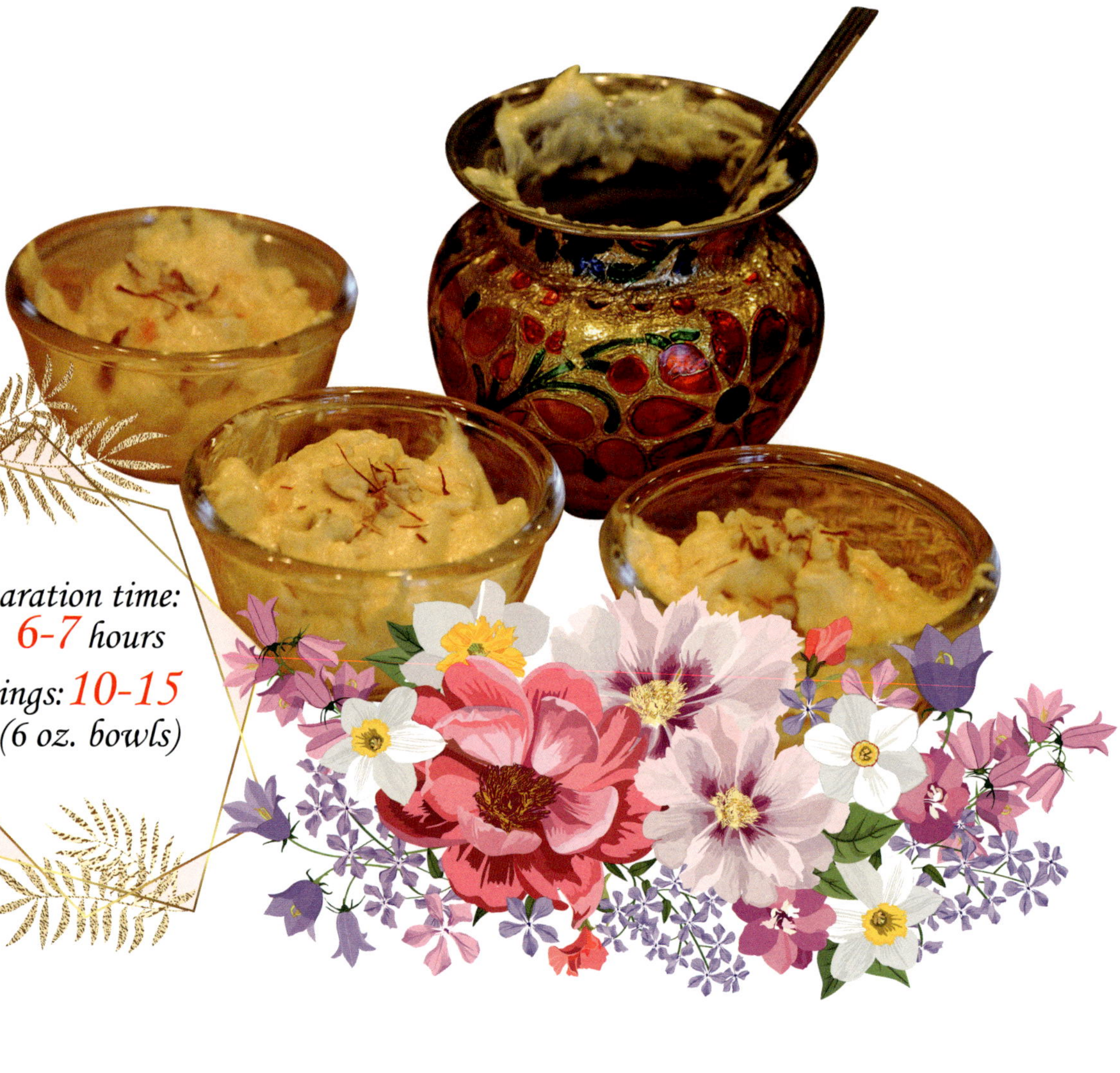

Preparation time: 6-7 *hours*

Servings: 10-15 *(6 oz. bowls)*

Ingredients

- 2 cups Greek plain yogurt
- 1 cup fresh mango purée, ripe and sweet mango
- ½ cup powdered sugar or to taste
- 3 tablespoons pistachio, shelled
- 5-7 almonds
- ½ teaspoon cardamom powder
- saffron few strands, soaked in 2 tablespoons warm milk
- few mango bits, pistachios, and almonds for garnishing

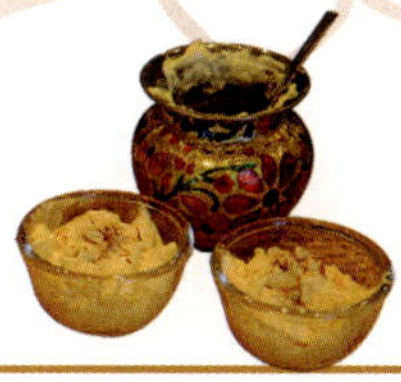

Process

1. Transfer the Greek yogurt to a muslin cloth laid over a bowl. Tie the cloth and hang it overnight to drain out the excess water. This can be done in the refrigerator itself to prevent the yogurt from going sour. Transfer to a mixing bowl after about 6-7 hours.
2. Soak pistachios and almonds in hot water for 10-15 minutes. Remove skin and chop into small pieces.
3. Simultaneously, soak the saffron strands in warm milk for about 10-15 minutes.
4. Add powdered sugar to the yogurt and mix well until the sugar dissolves.
5. Then, add the soaked saffron and milk, chopped nuts, mango purée and cardamom powder. Mix well to obtain a creamy fine texture. Save some nuts, mango pieces for garnishing.
6. Refrigerate for an hour. Then, pour in serving bowls. Garnish and serve chilled.

Alternate tip: Flavored yogurt can be used to make shrikhand of different flavors. Dry fruit shrikhand can be made with other chopped nuts, dates and figs.

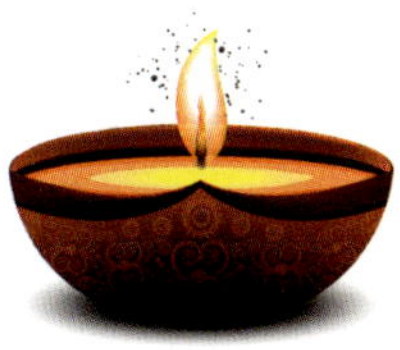

Kulfi

An easy to prepare creamy frozen summer delight made with milk and nuts

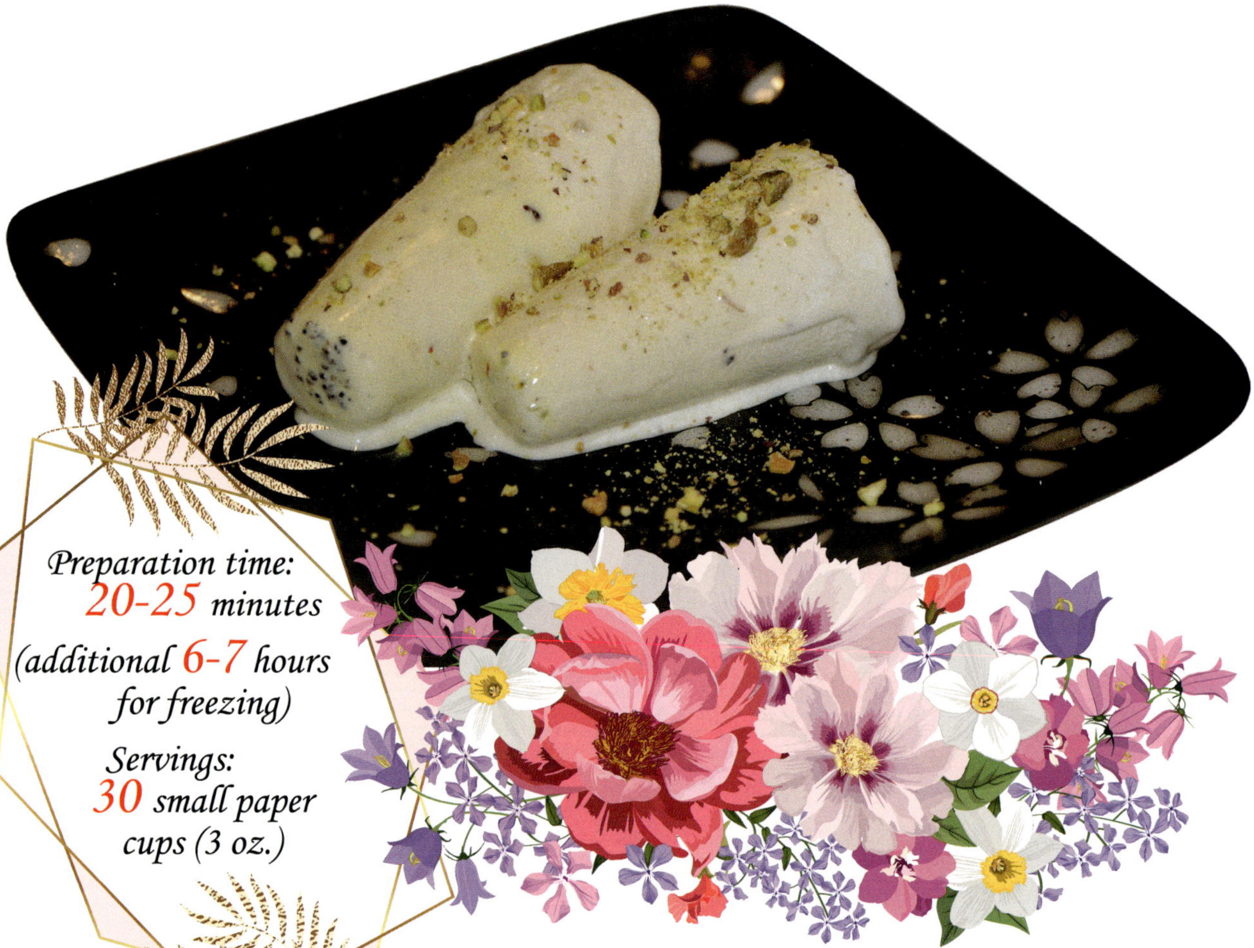

Preparation time:
20-25 *minutes*
(additional 6-7 *hours for freezing)*

Servings:
30 *small paper cups (3 oz.)*

Ingredients

- 14 oz. can of condensed milk
- 14 oz. can of evaporated milk
- ½ cup of full fat or 2% milk
- 16 oz. container of frozen whipped topping (such as Cool Whip), thawed
- 4-5 slices of white bread with crust
- ½ teaspoon cardamom, ground
- 8-10 threads of saffron
- ½ cup of pistachios, coarsely chopped

Special utensils:

- Kulfi molds, or small flat containers with lids. Aluminum kulfi molds are preferable. Small disposable paper cups covered with aluminum foil or just popsicle molds may be used.

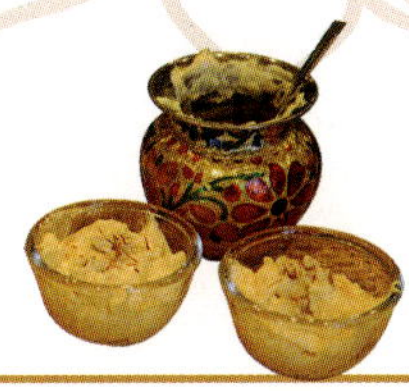

Process

1. In a small bowl, mix the saffron strands with 1 tablespoon of milk. Warm this in the microwave for 30 seconds. Keep aside.
2. Combine evaporated milk, condensed milk and whipped cream in a large bowl. Mix all these well with a spoon or hand-held mixer on low speed.
3. Cut the bread into small pieces along with the crust. In a blender, add bread and the remaining milk and blend well. Pour this into the whipped cream mixture from above.
4. Now, add the saffron mix, ground cardamom, and pistachios to the mixture, keeping aside 1 tablespoon of pistachios for garnishing. Mix well.
5. Pour into kulfi molds or other containers. Freeze for at least 6-7 hours.
6. Before serving, thaw the kulfi molds for 5 minutes and remove from molds.
7. Garnish with pistachios and serve immediately.

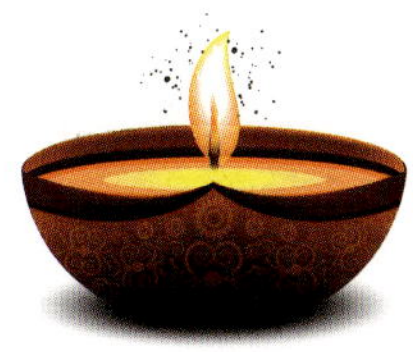

Alternate tip: Kulfi may be flavored with other fruits and nuts. Mango kulfi is one of the more popular flavors.

Cakes and Puddings

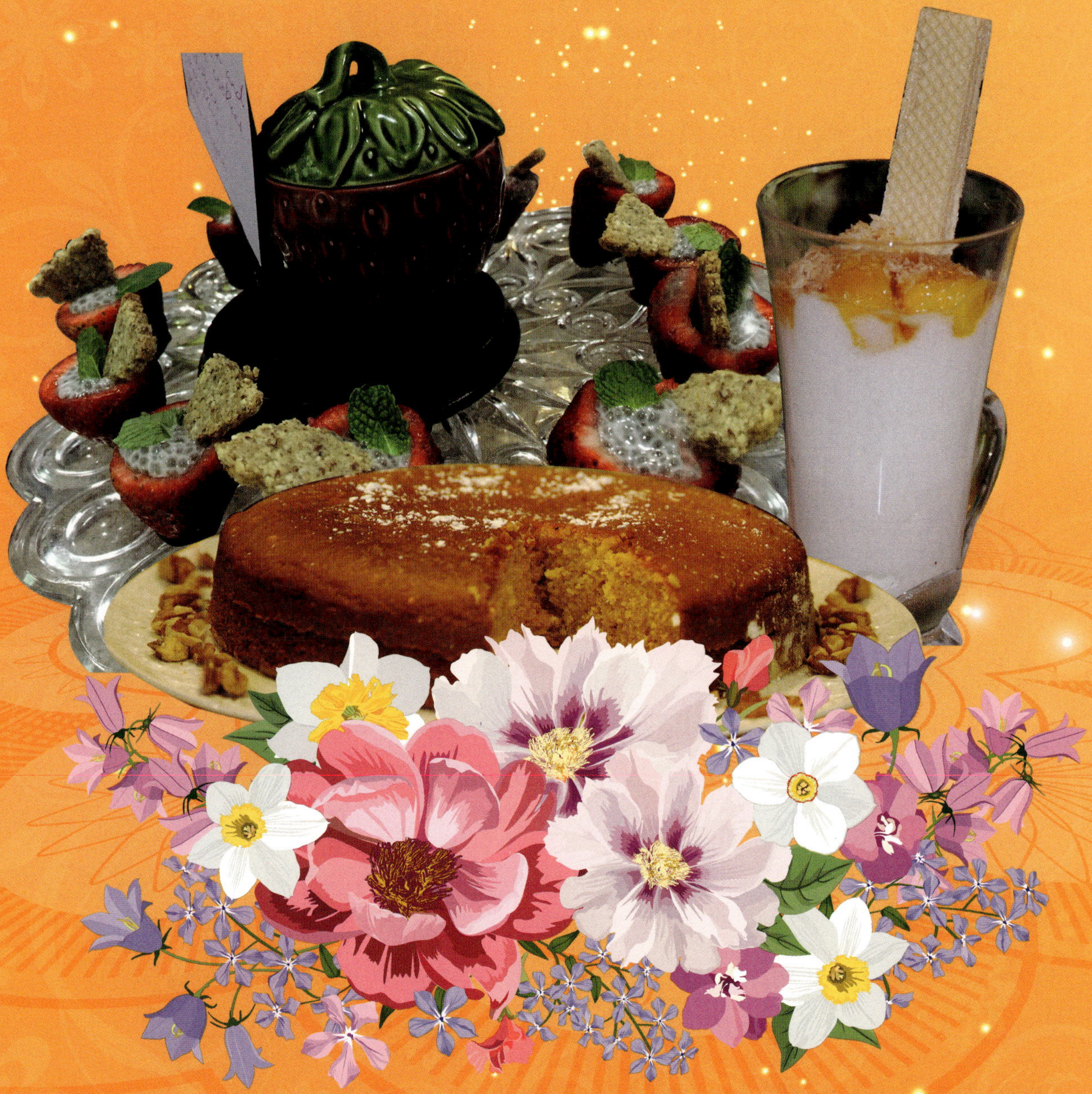

The several types of cake recipes in this section are the perfect bhog choices for birthday celebrations for God and Guru. We have attempted to include recipes having some healthier twist – those with fruits – dates, mangoes, strawberries, bananas; whole grains; nuts and seeds; or, some using brown sugar, jaggery, honey or raisins as sweeteners.

Other selections include the kheer, a traditional bhog recipe cooked in a crockpot. The quick and easy to make *chia berry bowl* and the yummy parfait – a *mango coconut delight* are fun recipes that younger kids can help put together.

1. Banana Nut Cake
2. Date Nut Cake
3. Chia Orange Cake
4. Whole Wheat Mango Cake
5. Sooji Cake
6. Chia Berry Bowl
7. Mango Coconut Delight
8. Kheer

Banana Nut Cake

A moist and delicious wholesome cake

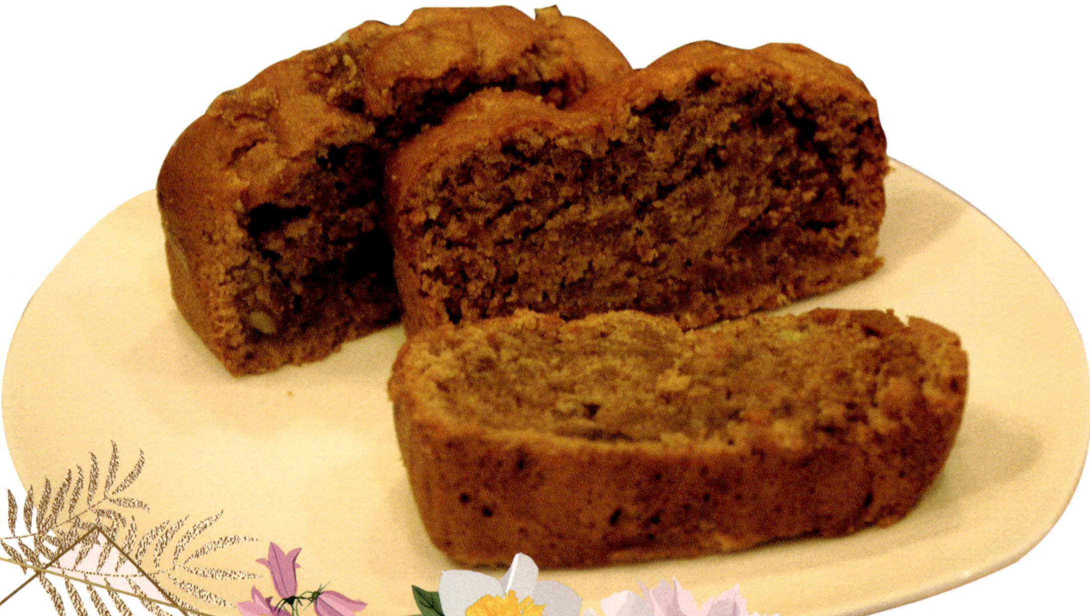

Preparation time: 10 *minutes*

Baking time: 30-35 *minutes*

Servings: 10

Ingredients

- 1 big ripe banana, mashed
- ½ cup walnuts
- 1 cup whole wheat flour
- ½ cup all-purpose flour
- 1 cup (little less than) sugar
- ½ teaspoon baking soda
- ½ teaspoon baking powder
- ½ cup oil
- 1 cup milk or water

Process

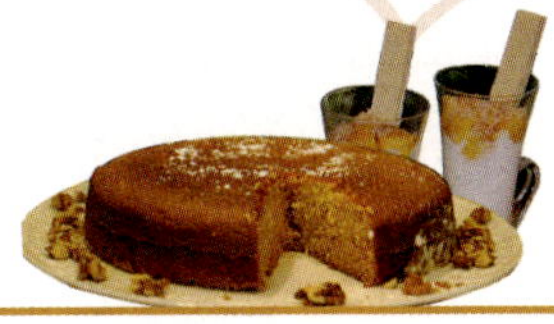

1. Preheat oven to 350°F.
2. Sift together whole wheat flour, all-purpose flour with baking soda and baking powder.
3. In a mixing bowl add sugar and mashed banana gradually to the sifted flour. Add all the other ingredients (walnuts, oil, water) and mix gently with a wooden spoon.
4. Grease and dust a 5 x 7 baking pan with all-purpose flour. Pour batter into the pan and bake for 30 to 35 minutes or until a toothpick comes out clean.
5. Remove from the oven and let it cool for 10 minutes. Slice into pieces and serve.

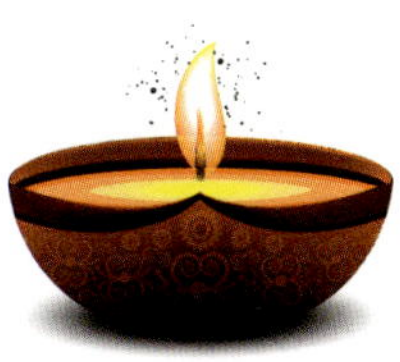

Date Nut Cake

A dense cake with a nutty flavor and health benefits of dates

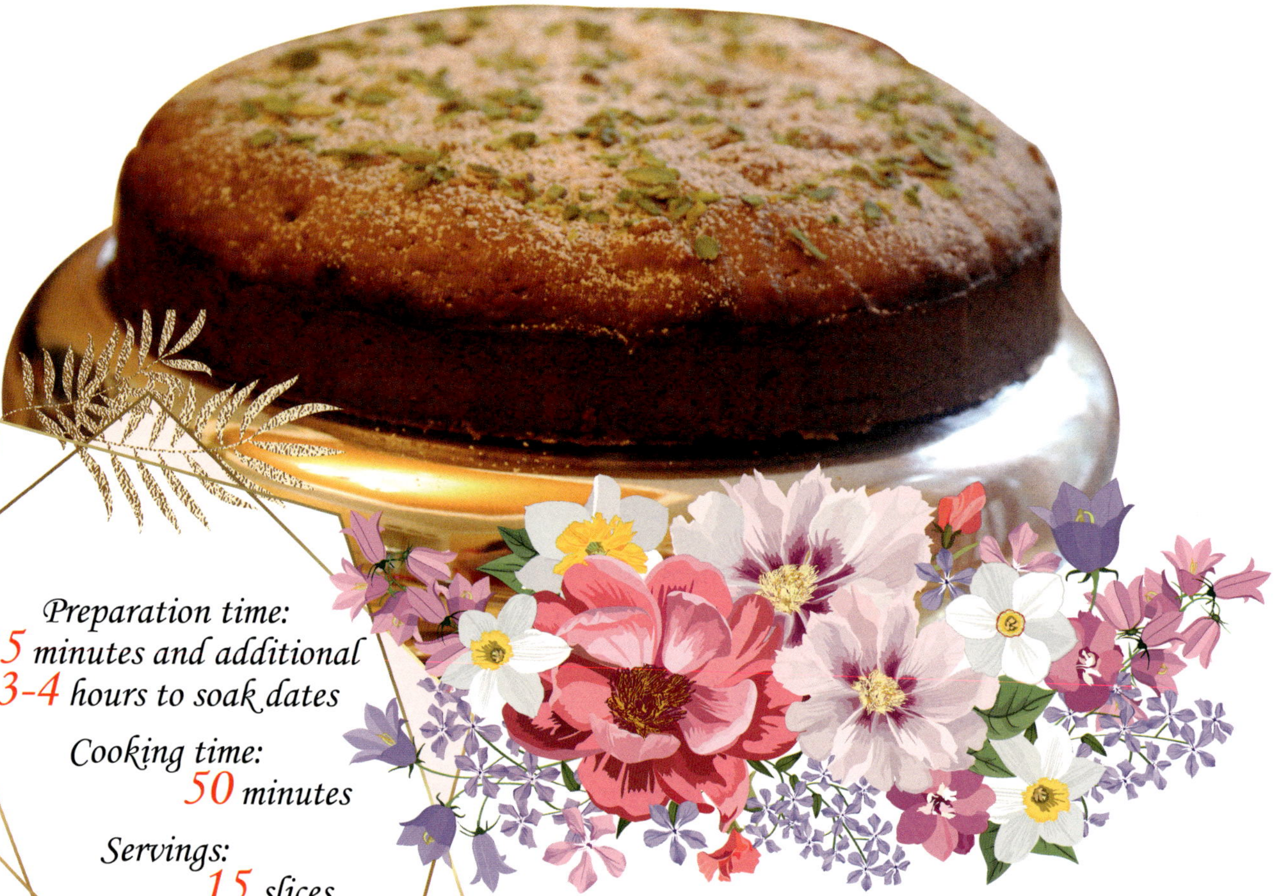

Preparation time:
15 *minutes and additional*
3-4 *hours to soak dates*

Cooking time:
50 *minutes*

Servings:
15 *slices*

Ingredients

- 16-18 dates, pitted and chopped, soaked in milk for 3-4 hours
- ¼-½ cup walnuts, chopped
- 1 cup all-purpose flour, or use whole wheat flour
- 2-3 teaspoons brown sugar
- ½ teaspoon baking soda
- ½ cup oil
- ¾ cup milk (whole, for soaking dates)

Process

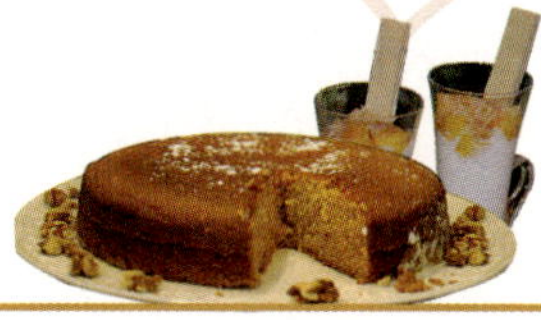

1. Pre-soak the dates in milk for 3-4 hours until soft.
2. Preheat oven to 350°F.
3. Grind the pre-soaked dates into a fine paste in a blender.
4. In a mixing bowl, add oil, baking soda, brown sugar and the flour and mix these well. To these add the blended dates.
5. Now add the walnuts to the batter and mix in gently with a spatula.
6. Grease a 9-inch round baking pan with oil and dust with all-purpose flour.
7. Pour in the batter and bake for 40-50 minutes or until the toothpick comes out clean.
8. Remove from the oven and let it cool for 10 minutes. Slice into pieces and serve immediately. Cake tastes best when warm.

Optional note: Walnuts may be replaced by other nuts such as pecan nuts.

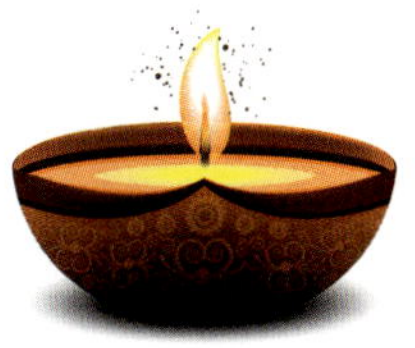

Chia Orange Cake

A moist dense cake made with nutritionally rich Chia seeds and citrusy flavors

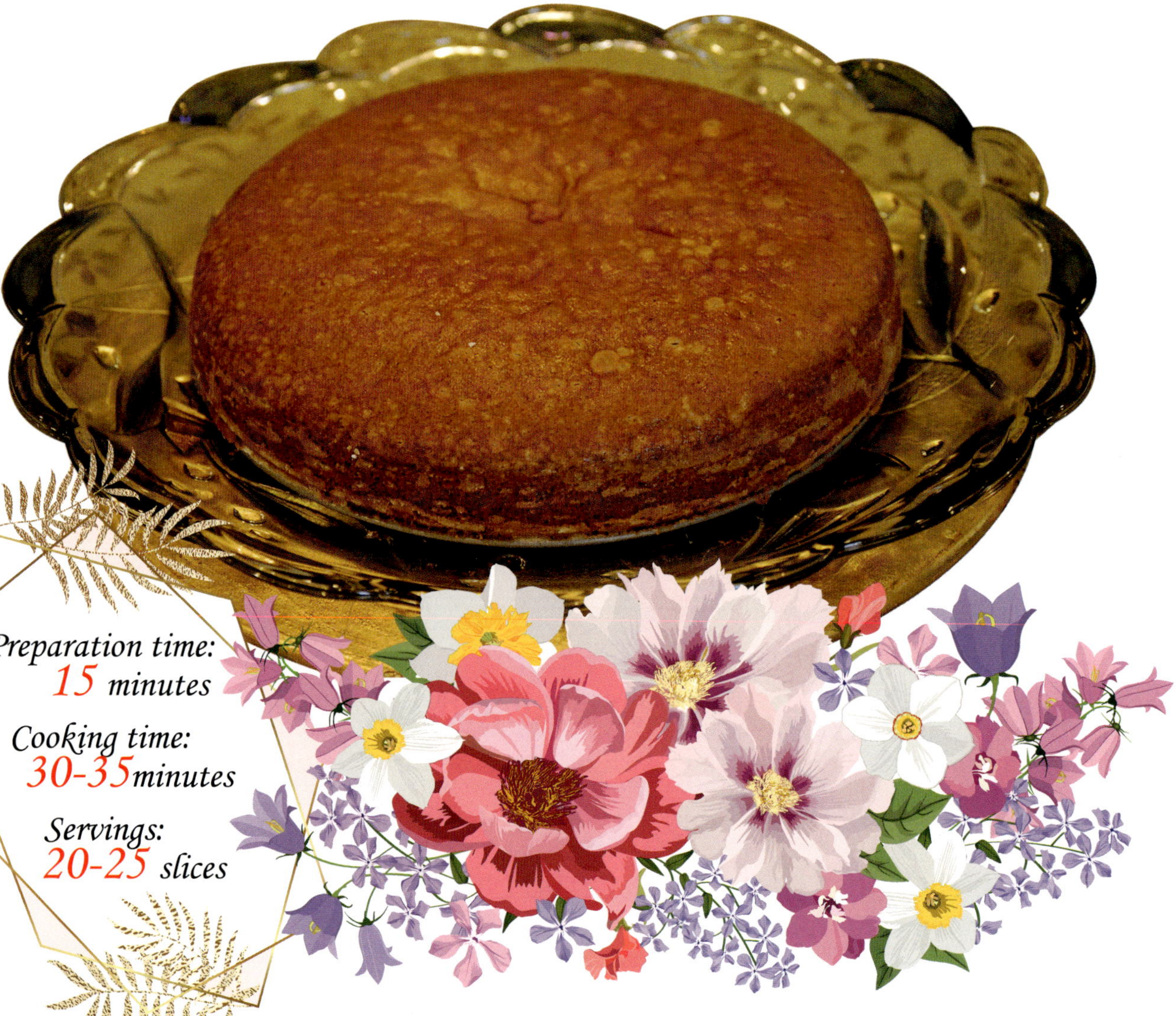

Preparation time: 15 *minutes*

Cooking time: 30-35*minutes*

Servings: 20-25 *slices*

Ingredients

- 3 cups unbleached all-purpose flour
- 2 cups sugar
- 1 teaspoon baking soda
- 1 teaspoon baking powder
- ½ teaspoon salt
- 2 tablespoons chia seeds
- ½ cup orange juice
- 2 teaspoons lemon juice
- 1 tablespoon orange rind
- 1 cup oil
- 1 ½ cup milk (whole)
- 4 tablespoons water for soaking chia seeds
- 8 oz. Cool Whip

Process

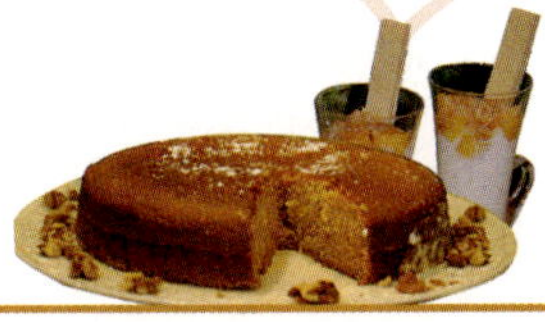

1. Soak chia seeds in 4 tablespoons water for 15 minutes.
2. Preheat oven to 350°F.
3. Sift flour, baking soda, baking powder and salt together into a bowl. Then add sugar and stir well. Now add oil, chia seed mixture and milk to flour mixture and mix well.
4. Mix in orange juice, lemon juice and orange rind.
5. Pour the batter into 8 x 8 x 2 baking pan (or 9-inch round pan) which has been sprayed with oil and dusted with all-purpose flour and bake for 30-35 minutes in the preheated oven or until a toothpick comes out clean.
6. Let the cake cool in the pan. Once cool, flip the pan upside down to remove the cake. Decorate with Cool Whip and serve.

Decoration Note: Icing made with whipping cream and sugar may be used instead of Cool Whip if desired.

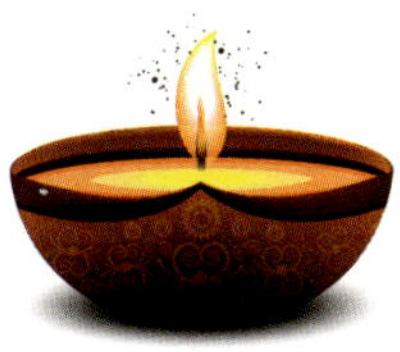

Whole Wheat Mango Cake

A healthier version of the rich, tropical mango cake

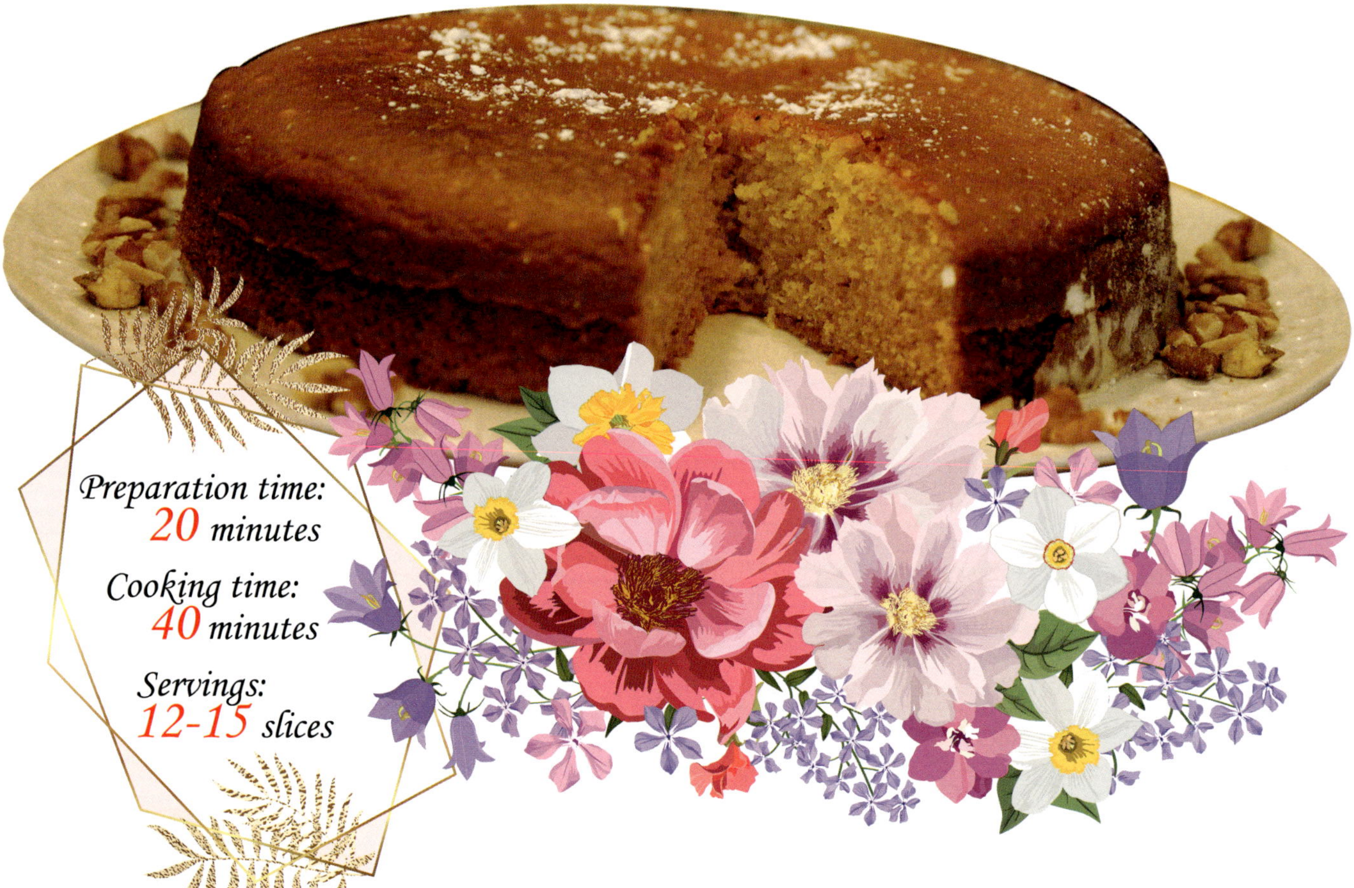

Preparation time: 20 *minutes*

Cooking time: 40 *minutes*

Servings: 12-15 *slices*

Ingredients

- 2 mangoes, cut into small pieces (any variety of sweet ripe mangoes. Add 1 more if using for decoration.)
- 2 cups whole wheat flour
- 1 cup unbleached all-purpose flour
- 1 ½ cups sugar
- 2 teaspoons baking soda
- ½ cup walnuts (optional for decoration)
- 2 tablespoons powdered sugar (optional for decoration)
- 1 cup oil
- 1 cup milk
- ½ cup water

Process

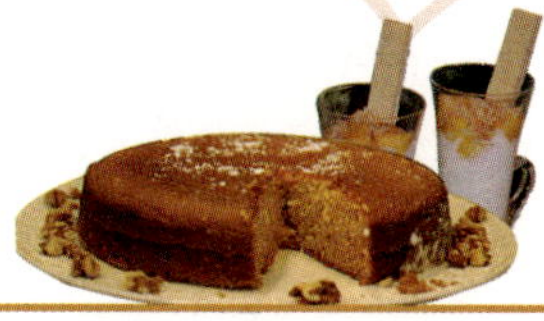

1. Preheat oven to 350°F.
2. Grease a 9 x 13 rectangular pan (or 9-inch round pan) with butter or cooking spray and dust with all-purpose flour.
3. Sift flour and baking soda in a bowl. Add sugar, cut pieces of mango and oil. Add water and milk to the mixture. Mix well and pour into the baking pan.
4. Bake for 40 minutes or until toothpick comes out clean.
5. Once cake is cooled, decorate with mango slices or walnuts and powdered sugar.
6. Slice and serve at room temperature.

Alternate option: In case mangoes are not available, a 16 oz. can of mango pulp may be used instead.

Sooji Cake

A healthy cake with drier grainier texture and nutty taste to enjoy with tea

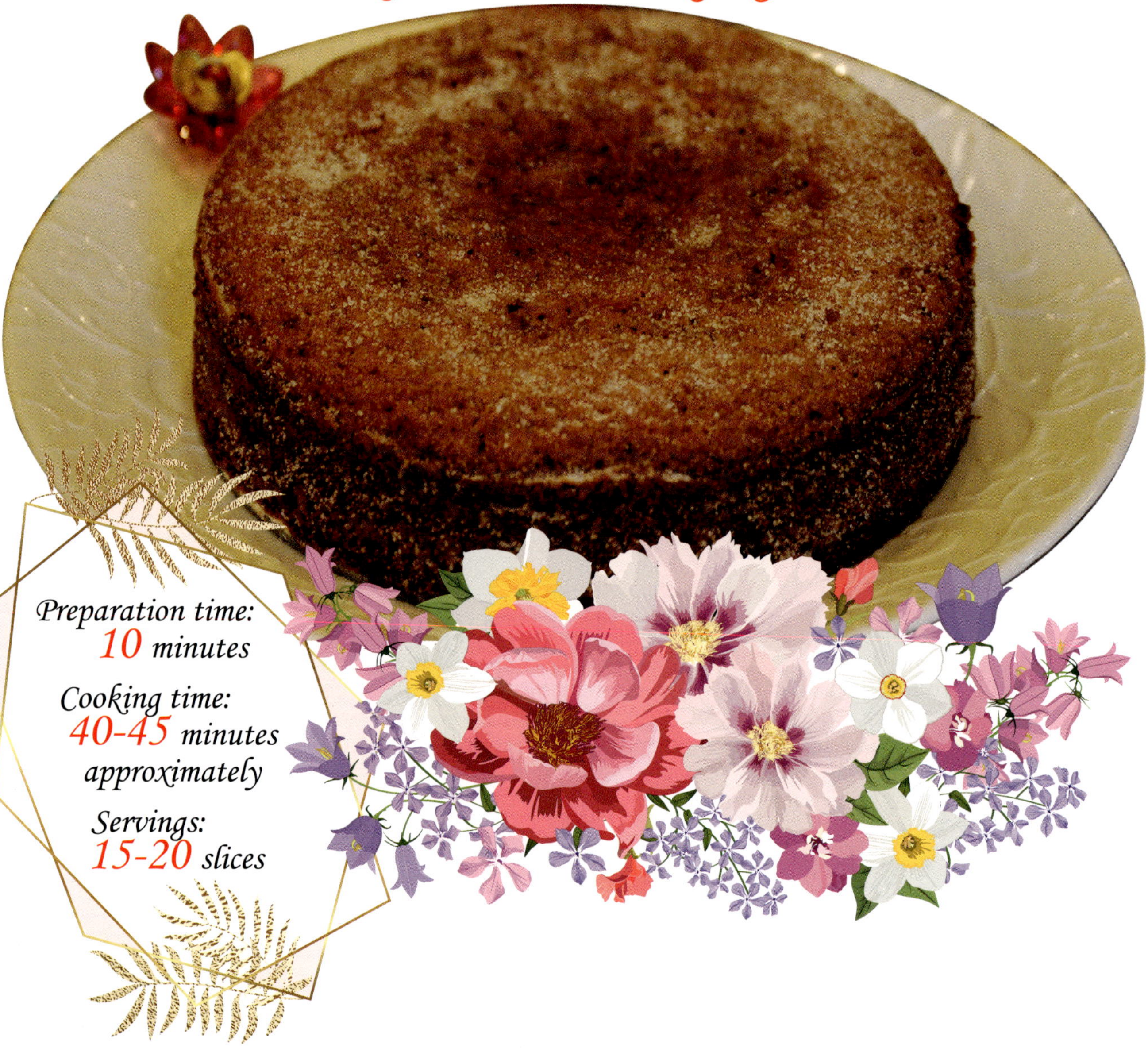

Preparation time: 10 *minutes*

Cooking time: 40-45 *minutes approximately*

Servings: 15-20 *slices*

Ingredients

- 1 cup fine sooji (semolina)
- ½ cup sugar
- ½ teaspoon leveled baking soda
- ¼ teaspoon crushed cardamom
- ½ cups walnuts, finely chopped
- 6 teaspoons oil
- 1 cup yogurt
- 20 raisins
- powdered sugar for decoration

Process

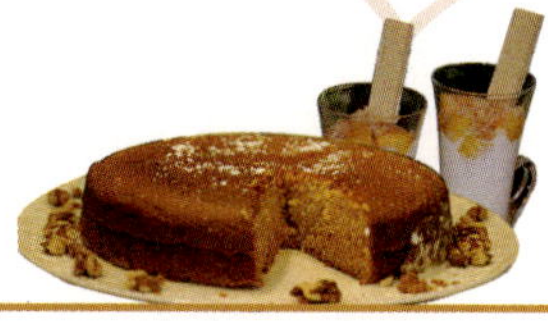

1. Preheat oven to 300°F. Grease and dust an 8 x 8 x 2 square pan (or, 6-8-inch round pan).
2. Combine sooji, sugar, baking soda, cardamom, raisins and walnuts. Mix well. Now add oil and curd and beat for 2-3 minutes.
3. On the lower rack, bake for approximately 40-45 minutes or until toothpick comes out clean.
4. Once cake is cooled, decorate with powdered sugar.
5. Slice and serve at room temperature.

Optional tip: For people with sweet tooth an extra quarter cup of sugar may be added. Also, pineapple, orange or mango fresh fruit pieces may be added for enhanced flavors.

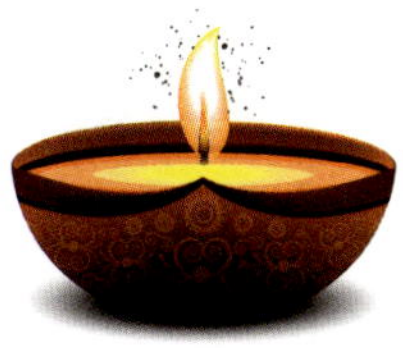

Chia Berry Bowl

Super easy, delicious, and nutrient dense dessert. Kids love it!

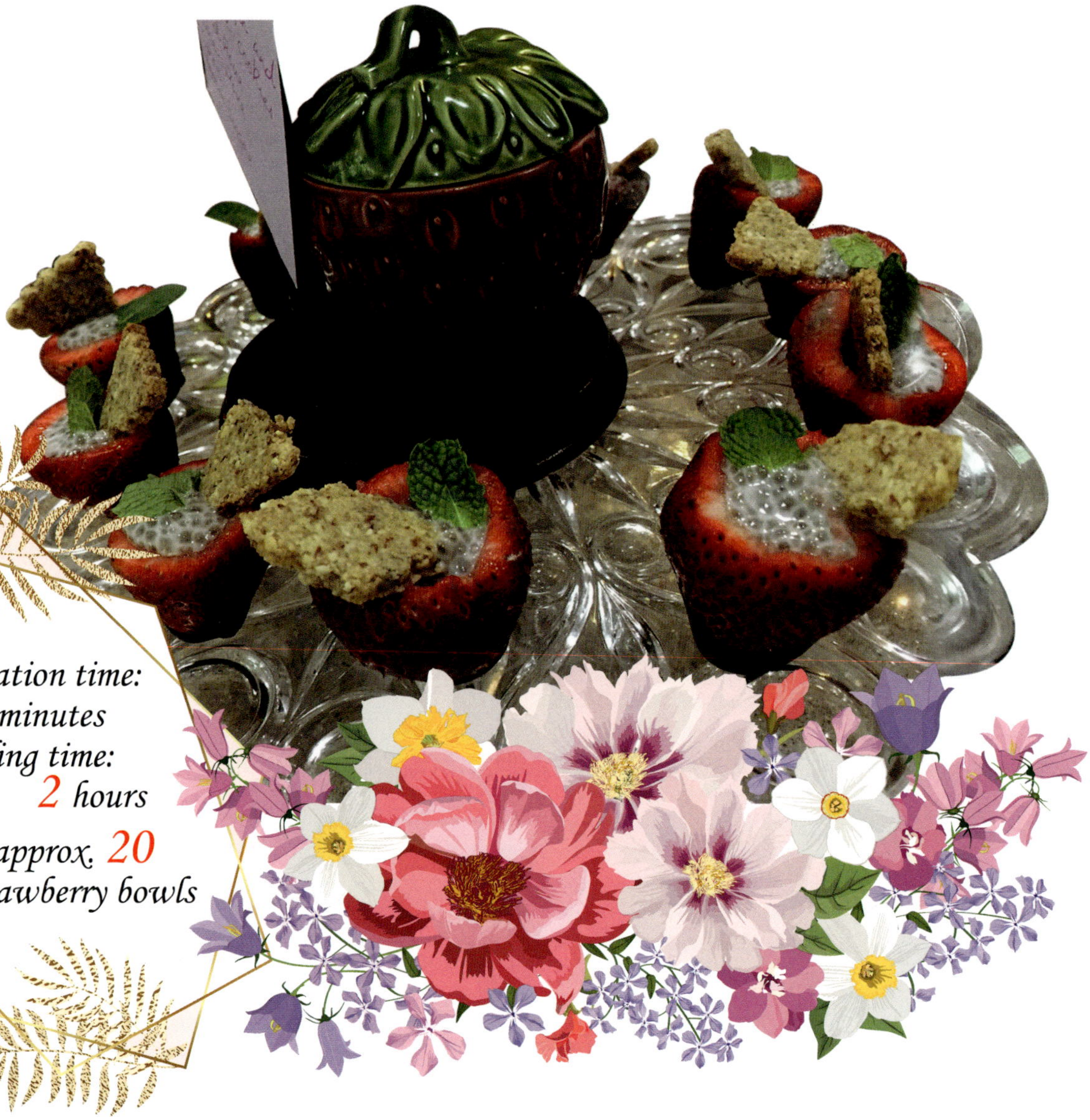

Preparation time: 30 *minutes*
Chilling time: 2 *hours*
Makes approx. 20 *strawberry bowls*

Ingredients

- ½ cup chia seeds
- fresh strawberries (approx. 20)
- 2 cups unsweetened almond, hazelnut or regular milk
- 2 tablespoons raw honey
- 1 teaspoon vanilla extract (optional)
- ½ teaspoon cinnamon
- topping: mint leaves, blueberries and cookies
- dark chocolate for dipping base of strawberries (optional)

Process

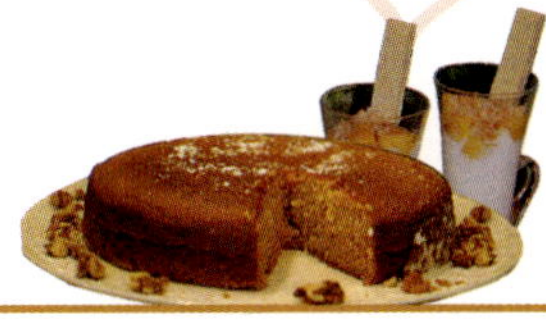

1. Combine chia seeds, milk, honey, vanilla extract and cinnamon in a jar. Cover and shake vigorously.
2. Chill the mix in the jar for at least 2 hours to let the chia seeds expand and form a gel-like substance to make the pudding.
3. Slice the base of the strawberries so that they can stand without support. Scoop strawberries just enough to fill the pudding. If desired dip the strawberries from the base in dark chocolate.
4. Top with mint, blueberries and a cookie.

Mango Coconut Delight

A quick and easy summer dessert

Preparation time: **10** *minutes*

Servings: **4-5**

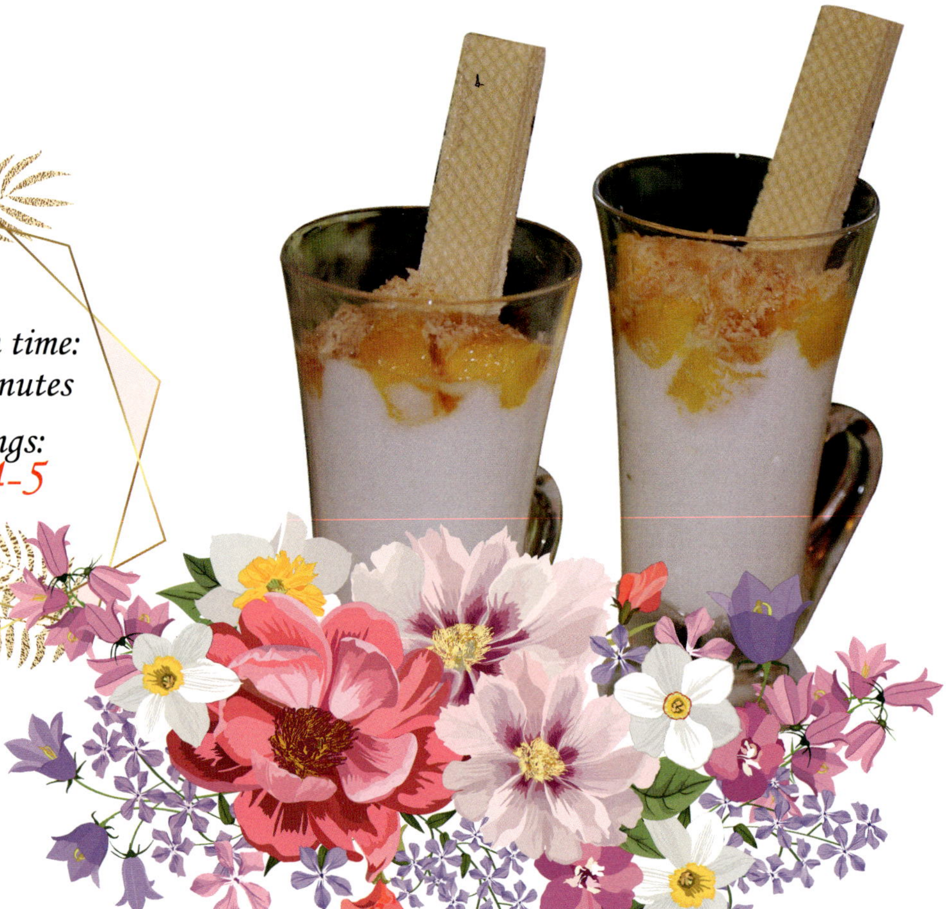

Ingredients

- 2 cups plain yogurt or ice cream (low-fat or nonfat)
- 2 tablespoons honey or maple syrup
- 1 ripe mango, medium size (peeled, pitted, and cut into ½ inch cubes)
- 1 cup coconut flakes (lightly toasted)
- 5 butter cookies for decoration (such as Belevita, thin wafers)

Process

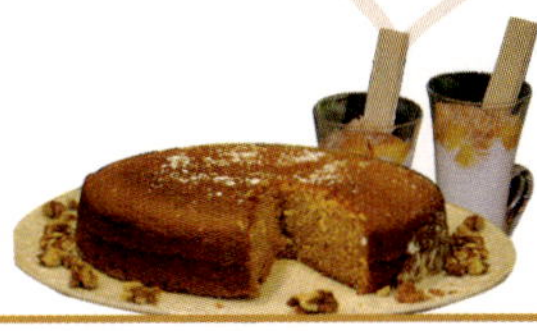

1. Scoop yogurt or ice cream in a parfait cup.
2. Top with mango pieces and coconut flakes. Drizzle honey or maple syrup.
3. Serve with a cookie.

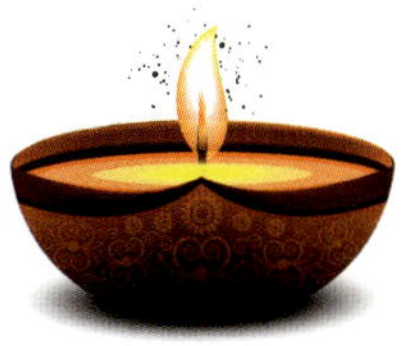

Kheer

Creamy mix of milk, rice and nuts—easy to prepare traditional delight

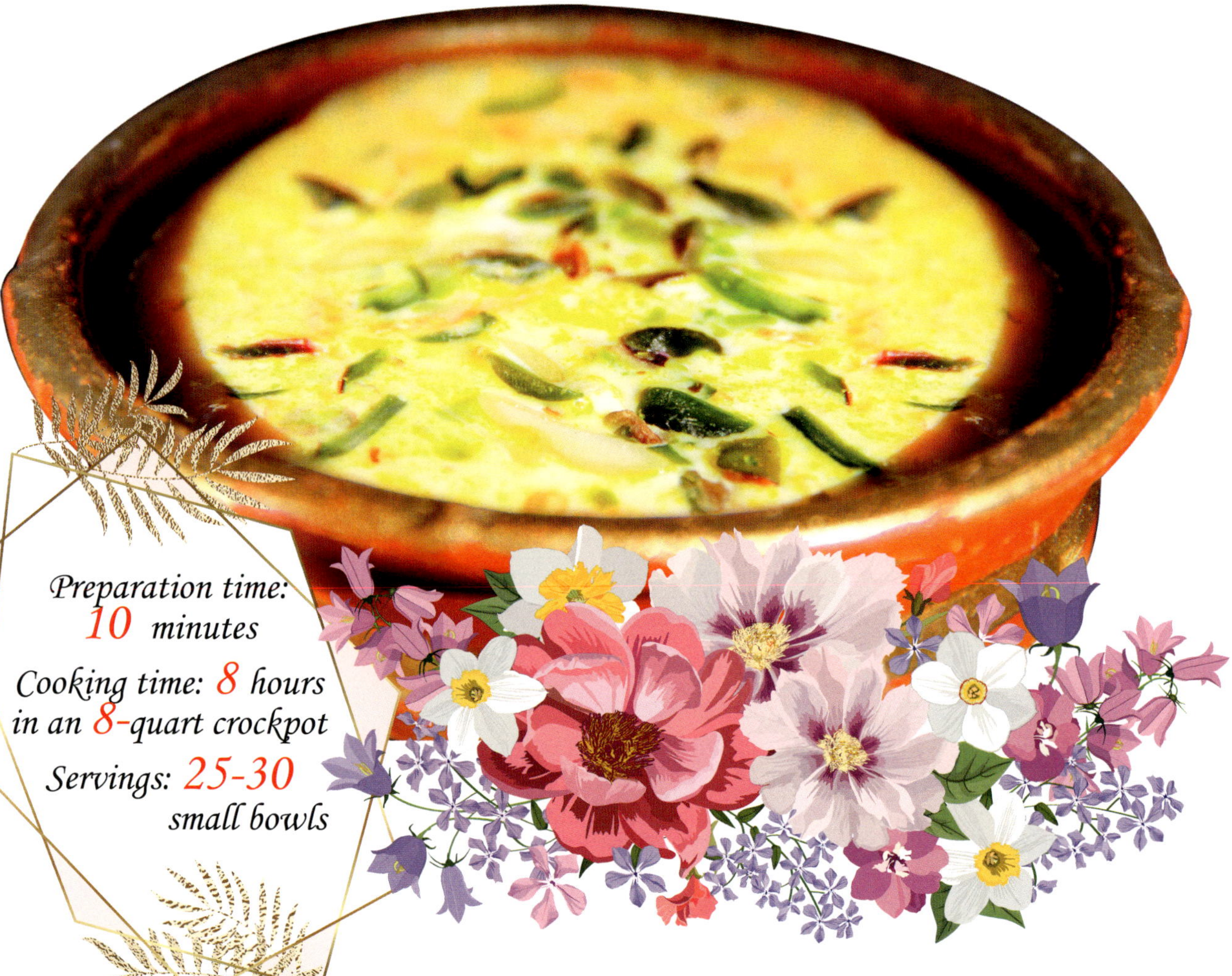

Preparation time: 10 *minutes*

Cooking time: 8 *hours in an* 8*-quart crockpot*

Servings: 25-30 *small bowls*

Ingredients

- 1 gallon milk (whole)
- 1 cup rice
- 1 ¼ cup sugar or jaggery
- 4-6 strands of saffron
- ½ cup mix of nuts-pistachios, almonds or others, chopped
- 1 teaspoon ghee

Process

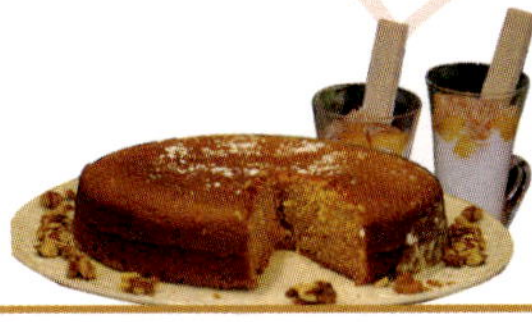

1. Wash and soak rice for about 10 minutes.
2. Grease an 8-quart crockpot with ghee.
3. In the greased crockpot pour in whole milk. Then add the drained rice and a few strands of saffron.
4. Cook on low for about 8 hours stirring every few hours.
5. Add sugar or jaggery and your favorite nuts. Mix well and simmer for about 30 minutes.
6. Kheer may be served hot or cold.

GLOSSARY

(The commonly used Indian culinary terms are in italics.)

A

All-purpose flour – *maida*, a versatile finely milled flour used for making breads like *naan* and savory snacks like *samosas*, and, also baking cakes and pastries.

Almond meal - almond flour made from ground almonds.

Amchur - tangy mango powder, used as a souring agent, made from drying green unripe mangoes.

Apple butter - more concentrated than applesauce. Apples are cooked till the sugar in the apples crystallizes to a deep brown color and a dense buttery texture. A quick substitute for tamarind chutney.

Asafoetida - ***hing***, a pungent powder used in Indian cooking as it aids digestion.

Atta - **whole wheat flour**, widely used for making unleavened flat breads (*rotis, paranthas, puris*). Also known as a *chapati* flour.

B

Baingan - **eggplant**, also known as brinjal.

Barley flour - ***jau* flour**, made from barley grains.

Basil, or sweet basil - a widely used herb in different cuisines of the world. Used dry and as fresh leaves.

***Basmati* rice** - literally means 'full of flavor.' It is the finest aromatic long-grain rice known as the 'prince of rice' from the Indian subcontinent.

Bay leaf - ***tej patta***, aromatic leaves used in cooking, also called Malabar leaf.

Besan - **gram flour** made from Bengal gram. A versatile flour having a nutty flavor used to make *paranthas/rotis, pakoras* and crêpes with its batter, sweets, or used for thickening curries.

Bharta - vegetables mashed and cooked in aromatic spices, *baingan bharta* being the most popular, where the *baingan* is roasted and then cooked with onions, tomatoes and spices.

***Bhindi* - okra** or 'ladies' finger, a vegetable.

Boondi – deep fried droplets made with *besan* batter.

Buckwheat flour - *kuttu ka atta*, an energizing fasting food that is used to make *rotis, puris* and *paranthas.*

Burfi - milk-based sweet, like fudge, made with nuts, flours and different flavors.

C

Canola oil - a vegetable oil.

Cardamom - *elaichi*, pods with seeds, are of two kinds - small green ones and big black ones. They are used as pods or as a powder for their strong and distinct flavor.

Carom seeds - *ajwain*, used to flavor rotis/paranthas, in roasted potatoes, and in some curries. Have additional health benefits too.

Chaat - Indian street food, savory layered snack, made with a blend of tangy, sour and sweet tastes and ingredients.

***Chana dal* - Bengal gram**, a yellow colored skinned split lentil with a sweet and nutty flavor used in variety of vegetable dishes. It can be cooked as a dal, or used as a spice for tempering, as in southern India.

Chapati - a flat bread made with whole wheat flour and water on a '*tawa*', a circular griddle. *Chapatis* are often smeared with oil or *ghee* on top before serving. The term roti is in this book is used synonymously with a *chapati.*

Chasani - sugar syrup of different consistencies referred to as one-thread/tar or two-thread used for various Indian sweets such as *gulab jamuns.*

Chia - a seed of Mexican origin, a superfood rich in omega-3s and other nutrients, like basil or *sabja seeds.*

Chick peas - garbanzo beans, a legume very similar to gram, *kabuli chana*. Rich in protein and fiber.

Chilla - savory pancake made with flour, lentils and spices.

Chivda - roasted munching snack usually made from grains (*poha* or flattened rice, puffed rice), roasted lentils, spices, and nuts.

Cilantro - *dhania*/coriander, a pungent herb used to garnish Indian dishes.

Cinnamon - ***dalchini***, the brown, quill like bark of the cinnamon tree, used in its dried tubular form or as a ground powder.

Clove - ***laung***, flower buds that aid digestion, a pungent aromatic spice that may be used ground or whole.

Coconut - ***nariyal***. The edible white meat of the fruit (also a nut/seed) with a fibrous husk and hard shell, grows on palm trees and is used in many sweet and savory dishes and widely prevalent in coastal cuisines of India.

Coconut oil - ***nariyal ka tel***. Very heat stable, so it makes an excellent choice as a cooking and frying oil.

Coriander - see cilantro.

Coriander powder – see ***dhania*** powder.

Cumin - ***jeera***, an abundantly used aromatic spice in many kinds of dishes used both as whole seeds or ground as powder.

Curry - 'stew-like' dish made with onions-tomatoes masala, spices and seasonings having gravy or a sauce.

Curry leaves - ***curry patta***, used for flavoring in many dishes. Have health benefits too.

Cutlet - flat crispy shallow fried patty made with mashed potatoes, vegetables and binding materials.

D

Dalia - dry roasted *chana dal*.

Dals **(pulses)** - A primary source of protein in a vegetarian diet, these are dried seeds of plants such as beans, lentils and peas. Egs. chickpeas (*kabuli chana*), split black chick peas (Bengal gram or *chana*), black gram (*urad dal*), red lentils (*arhar*) and yellow lentils (*moong*).

Dhania powder - **coriander powder**, grounded from coriander seeds, extensively used in Indian cooking.

Dhokla - steamed spongy cakes made from a fermented batter of chickpeas and rice. A Gujarati staple.

Dosa **or** ***dosha*** - a rice lentil crêpe made with fermented batter. It may be filled with a spicy mixture. A South Indian staple.

Drumstick – ***sajjan-ki-phalli***. Used in *sambar*.

E

Egg substitute - 1 tablespoon flax seed powder plus 3 tablespoons warm water, mix well, turns gooey after 7 to 8 minutes of letting it sit.

ENO salts – sodium bicarbonate and citric acid, are an antacid drug, also used in cooking. Available in Indian grocery stores.

F

Fennel powder - ***saunf***, are ground fennel seeds have an anise-like flavor and a sweet aroma.

Fenugreek - ***methi***, an herb, both seeds and leaves are used in cooking. Fresh leaves are also cooked as a vegetable and stuffed in flat breads.

Flax seed - ***alsi***, a superfood seed that has many antioxidants. Used ground or whole in vegetables, yogurt, oatmeal, cereals. Also used as an egg substitute in baking.

G

Garam masala - a blend of ground spices used in many Indian dishes.

Garlic - ***lahsun.***

Gatte - cooked gram flour dumplings added to curries or to rice dishes.

Ghee - **clarified butter**, made by melting butter and separating the fat from the solids. Has a very high smoking point and is also used in traditional religious rituals.

Ginger - ***adrak***, fresh root ginger. Commonly used minced, as a paste, chopped or slivered, it has many medicinal benefits.

Gobi - **cauliflower.**

Gram Flour - see ***besan***.

H

Haldi - **turmeric**, a root that belongs to the ginger family, is an ancient spice and is used extensively in Indian cooking in its ground form giving cooked dishes the distinct yellow color. An anti-inflammatory, it also has other medicinal properties.

Holy basil - ***tulsi*** or ***tulasi***, the most sacred plant, is used in religious offerings and in cooking. Also has great medicinal properties and is used in herbal teas to reduce stress and anxieties.

I

Idli - steamed rice cakes made with fermented rice and lentil batter.

J

Jaggery - ***gud***, completely unrefined sugar, having minerals and nutrients is eaten raw or used to sweeten curries, dals and used to prepare many traditional deserts and sweet snacks. Healthier alternative for white sugar.

Jowar - **sorghum or white millet**. It is gluten free and has incredible health benefits. Can be used whole in soups, curries or ground as a flour in making rotis and parathas.

K

Kadai - **the Indian wok**, popularly used in Indian cooking.

Kadhi - Punjabi dish made with yogurt and *besan*.

Kala namak - **black salt**, rock salt.

Kamut puffs – puffed whole grain wheat, also known as Khorasan wheat originating from Iran.

Karela - **bitter gourd**, vegetable.

Katori - small bowl made of steel.

Kheer - sweet rice pudding made with whole milk.

Kokum or ***cocum***, a very sour edible fruit. When dry, used as a souring agent.

Kopra - dried meat of the coconut.

Kulfi – is the Indian equivalent of ice-cream. Made from milk, cream and sugar it is flavored with pistachios, saffron etc. Comes in different flavors, mango being very popular.

Kuttu ka aata – see buckwheat flour.

L

Lauki – doodhi, is bottle gourd, a light vegetable as it contains a lot of water and other nutrients.

Lemongrass - has citrus flavor, and is used as herb and flavoring in curries, soups and curry pastes or even tea. Used predominantly in Thai and Vietnamese cuisines.

M

Maida - see all-purpose flour.

Makhana - **fox nuts**, lotus seed.

Makhani - rich, creamy gravy made with butter.

Makki ki roti - A Punjabi staple, made from corn flour and traditionally served with *'sarson da saag.'*

Mango – ***aam***, sweet and tangy tropical fruit.

Masalas – refers to dry spices, also to the base made for curries and dishes made with onions, tomatoes etc.

Masoor dal - skinned split red lentils that are of orange color.

Methi - see fenugreek.

Mint – ***pudina***, a widely used herb known for its digestive properties. It is used to make *chutneys*, and *raitas* and drinks such as tea and *aam panna*, it adds freshness and flavor.

Moong dal - skinned split *mung* beans.

Moong **sprouts** – Sprouted whole *moong* dal, is considered even more nutrient rich.

Muli **or** ***Mooli*** **– white long radish** also known as daikon (Japanese). Has a slightly peppery taste and crunchy texture having a high water content. They are used in salads, stuffing for paranthas or cooked as a vegetable.

Mustard seeds – ***Rai*** **or** ***Sarson***. The kind used in Indian cooking are tiny and black or brown in color. They are profusely used in some regional cuisines for tempering and pickles such as South Indian.

Muslin cloth – ***mulmul ka kapda***. Plain weave cotton cloth, similar to cheese cloth, used for straining *paneer* (cottage cheese) or *shrikhand*, etc.

N

Naan - a popular North Indian leavened bread, made from *maida* or all-purpose flour. Originally made in clay ovens or tandoors.

O

Orange zest – the ingredient derived from scraping the outer skin of oranges to flavor foods such as cakes.

P

Pakoras - deep friend fritters made with potatoes and vegetables made by dipping in *besan* batter. A popular snack food.

Palak - spinach.

Paneer - **cottage cheese** made by curdling milk with vinegar or lemon/lime juice.

Parantha - a bread; richer version of chapati, crispy, sometimes stuffed with vegetables or paneer and cooked with ghee/oil on a griddle.

Peda - small, round sweets made from condensed milk.

Peppercorns – ***kali mirch ke dane***. Mostly black but they can be other colors too. They are used whole, or ground as black pepper.

Pistachios - ***pista***, green nuts used in many desert recipes and commonly used for garnishing such as in *kulfi*.

Puri - unleavened deep-fried bread served on special occasions served with vegetables, chanas, *halwa* etc.

R

Rai - see mustard seeds.

Raita - spiced whisked yogurt with grated or chopped vegetables or *boondi* etc. A cooling side dish.

Rajmah - **kidney beans**. Rajmah served with rice is a popular Indian meal.

Rava - see sooji.

Raw mango - unripe sour mango used in making pickles, *aam panna.*

Red chilli - ***lal mirch***, used as whole, as flakes or as a powder, adds heat and color to the dishes.

Ridge gourd - ***turai***, a commonly used vegetable in India, like zucchini in taste.

Rind - outer skin of a fruit or vegetable, used to flavor or decorate.

Rock salt - see ***kala namak.***

Rose water - flavoring agent in Indian deserts such as rasagullas.

Roti - related to the French word "rôtie," meaning toasted bread. These are made from whole wheat (*aata*), millet (*bajra*) or sorghum (*jowar*) or other grains. Term loosely used to refer to *chapatis* too.

S

Sabja seeds - also commonly known as *tukmaria* seeds or *falooda*, are the seeds of sweet basil. They look like chia seeds.

Sabudana - tapioca root, can be used in dishes like *kheer* or *vada*. A popular fasting food.

Sabzi - general term for any Indian vegetable dish.

Saffron – ***kesar***, used for its exquisite flavor and orange coloring used as a finishing touches in Indian desserts and rice dishes.

Sagu - coconut-based curry flavored with spices.

Sambar **powder** - a southern Indian spice mix for vegetable curries.

Sambar **vegetables** - some vegetables that give sambar a more authentic feel include chayote (kind of squash), *dosa kai* (yellow cucumber) and *sufed Kaddu* (white pumpkin or white winter melon), *hara kela* (plantain).

Sesame seeds - ***til.***

Shrikhand - sweet dessert made from strained yogurt.

Silpad - nonstick mat.

Sooji - **semolina flour**, also known as *rawa* or cream of wheat.

Sorghum flour - see *jowar*.

Soya flour - grinded soya beans flour.

Split pigeon peas – see *toor dal.*

T

Tahini – A condiment used in Mediterranean cooking. Paste made from toasted ground sesame seeds and oil.

Tamarind - ***Imli***. A pod like fruit used to prepare tamarind chutneys and a popular souring agent in Southern India. Also available as paste or concentrate.

Tava - a cast iron griddle used for making chapatis/rotis/paranthas.

Thali - big stainless-steel plate with lips.

Thepla - A Gujarati staple, flat bread made with whole wheat, *besan* and fenugreek leaves.

Til - sesame seeds, black, brown and white with their nutty crunch and sweet flavor are a healthy food used in sweets, regular dishes or tempering on dhoklas etc.

Toor dal* or *Tuvar, Toovar - split pigeon peas, dark yellow in color, look like chana dal, are an extensively used dal in Indian cooking.

***Tulsi* leaves** - see holy basil.

U

Urad dal – cooked whole as in *dal makhani,* or split and skinned is used to make as a tempering spice in South India, or for preparing batters for idli, dosa batters and is cooked as dal too.

V

Vada – a deep fried, savory ball (often donut shaped) made with ground lentils and spices.

W

Whole wheat flour – see *aata.*

Whole *moong* beans – unsplit green dal.

OTHER PUBLICATIONS

1. Science of Healthy Diet
2. Art of Mind Management
3. Bhagavad Gita, The Song of God
4. Essence of Hinduism
5. Spiritual Dialectics
6. Yoga for Mind, Body, and Soul

BOOKS FOR CHILDREN

1. My Best Friend Krishna

2. Mahabharat - The Story of Virtue and Dharma

2. Healthy Body Healthy Mind – Yoga for Children

3. Bal-Mukund Wisdom Book

4. Festivals of India

5. Saints of India

6. Inspiring Stories for Children – set of 4 books

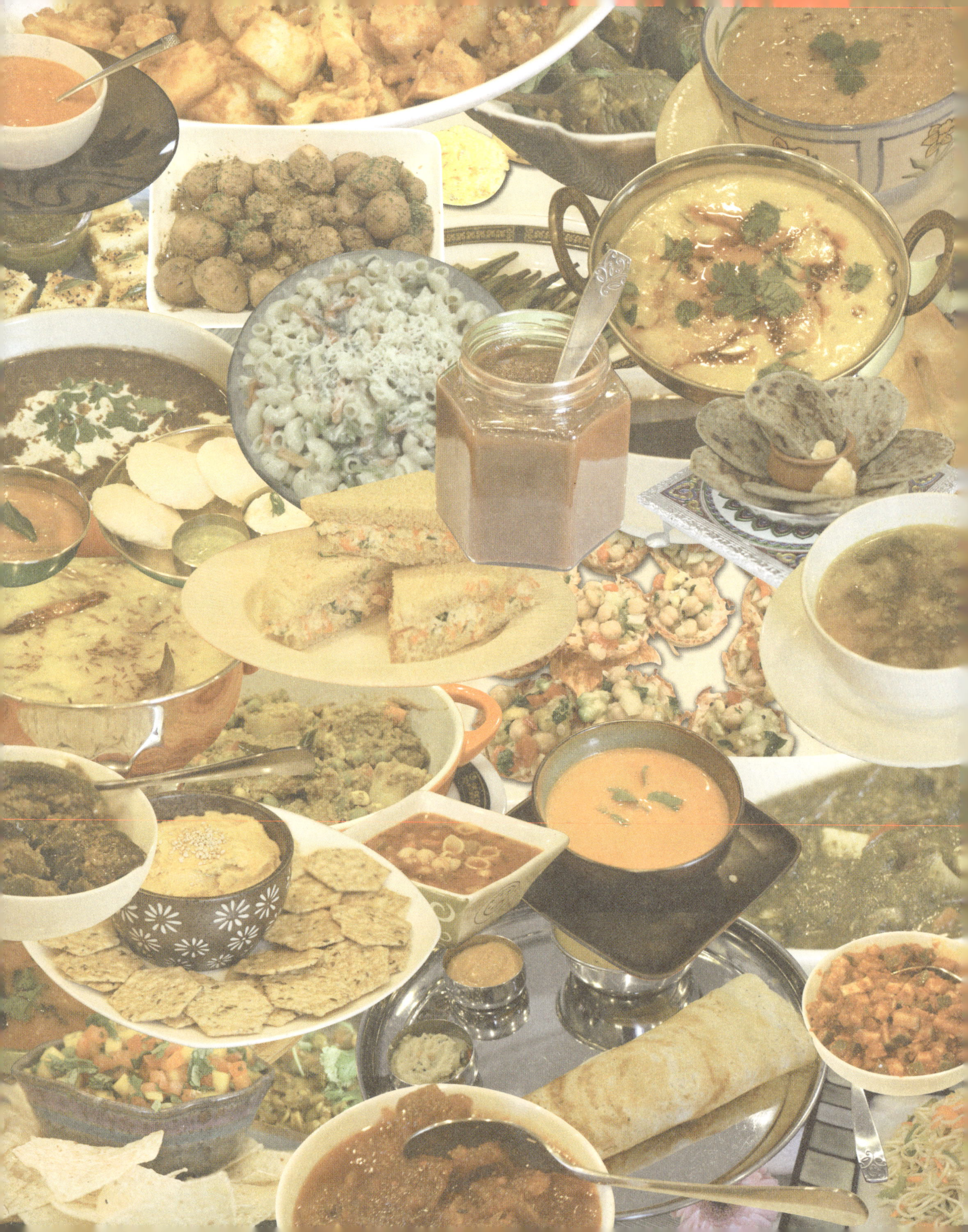